Statistical Methods
in Genetic Epidemiology

Statistical Methods
in Genetic Epidemiology

DUNCAN C. THOMAS

OXFORD
UNIVERSITY PRESS

2004

OXFORD
UNIVERSITY PRESS

Oxford New York
Auckland Bangkok Buenos Aires Cape Town Chennai
Dar es Salaam Delhi Hong Kong Istanbul Karachi Kolkata
Kuala Lumpur Madrid Melbourne Mexico City Mumbai Nairobi
São Paulo Shanghai Taipei Tokyo Toronto

Copyright © 2004 by Oxford University Press, Inc.

Published by Oxford University Press, Inc.
198 Madison Avenue, New York, New York, 10016
http://www.oup.com

Oxford is a registered trademark of Oxford University Press

Library of Congress Cataloging-in-Publication Data
Thomas, Duncan C.
Statistical methods in genetic epidemiology / Duncan C. Thomas.
p. cm. Includes bibliographical references and index.
ISBN 0-19-515939-X
1. Genetic epidemiology–Statistical methods. I. Title.
RB155.T468 2004 616′.042–dc21   2003053096

9 8 7 6 5 4 3 2 1

Printed in the United States of America
on acid-free paper

To Nina

Preface

The field of genetic epidemiology is still quite young. Although its parent disciplines of epidemiology and genetics have been flourishing for over a century, the first use of the two terms in combination appears to have been in 1954 in a chapter entitled "Genetics and Epidemiology" in a classic textbook on human genetics (Neel and Schull, 1954). It wasn't until the 1980s that the term *genetic epidemiology* came into widespread use with the establishment of the journal *Genetic Epidemiology* in 1984 and the International Genetic Epidemiology Society in 1992. The first edited book on the subject was published in 1978 (Morton and Chung, 1978), followed soon thereafter by two textbooks (Morton, 1982; Morton et al., 1983). For many years, the best text on the subject has been Khoury, Beaty, and Cohen's *Fundamentals of Genetic Epidemiology* (1993), which I have used as a reference in my own classes since I started teaching this subject, supplemented with the more detailed book on linkage analysis by Jurg Ott (1999), now in its third edition. As of this writing, however, there is no book on the market that adequately covers the entire field, particularly the explosive development in recent years of methods for association studies.

This text is a broad overview written at a level that should be accessible to graduate students in epidemiology, biostatistics, and human genetics. Its primary aim is to bridge these fields, particularly those of genetic epidemiology and statistical genetics, so that investigators from the two disciplines can communicate and collaborate more effectively. The book's main focus is on the design and statistical analysis of family-based studies, but genetic applications of traditional population-based epidemiologic (cohort and case-control) studies are also discussed.

In an effort to make the book self-contained, I asked my molecular epidemiology colleague, Dr. Sue Ingles, to contribute a chapter on basic principles of molecular biology. In the space available, it is possible to provide only a cursory introduction to these principles and rapidly evolving laboratory techniques, so the reader interested in more detail is encouraged to use one of the many outstanding textbooks on the subject, such as *Human Molecular Genetics 2* (Strachan and Read, 1999). I have also included brief reviews of basic principles of Mendelian inheritance (Chapter 3), epidemiology and statistics (Chapter 4), and of population genetics (Chapter 8), but there are likewise many excellent books on these subjects (see, for example, the two-volume series by Breslow and Day [1980, 1987], the standard epidemiology text by Rothman and Greenland [1998], and the population genetics texts by Hartl [2000] and Balding et al. [2001]).

Genetic epidemiology is closely related to many other fields: *population genetics* with its focus on the evolutionary processes that have led to the distributions of genes we see today, related to normal variation in common traits as well as disease; *clinical genetics* with its focus on individual patients or high-risk families rather than whole populations; *molecular genetics* with its focus on molecular mechanisms rather than statistical associations; and *human genetics* with its focus on the determination of disease or normal traits by genes rather than the environment. Genetic epidemiology is particularly closely related to *molecular epidemiology,* which focuses on the use of biochemical methods in traditional epidemiologic studies, including such aspects as exposure biomarkers and early markers of disease that are beyond the scope of this book, but tends not to rely as heavily on the use of family studies as genetic epidemiology does (Khoury and Dorman, 1998). The statistical methods used in the service of genetic epidemiology are also commonly known as *statistical genetics,* a well-developed field of its own (see, for example, Balding et al., 2001), but presented here with emphasis on its applications to genetic epidemiology. Finally, the area of *genomics,* focusing on the DNA sequence of the entire genome and its variation across populations, and the *bioinformatics* tools used to organize all this information, are also relevant but touched upon only briefly in this book.

Chapter 1 provides a nontechnical overview of the process of genetic epidemiology, illustrated with examples drawn mainly from the literature on breast cancer genetics. These examples are described in greater detail in the chapters that follow. In telling this story, I assume some familiarity with the basic terminology of genetics, but the reader should feel free to skip ahead as needed to the next couple of chapters, where these concepts are defined in greater detail. The next three chapters provide some basic concepts that will be necessary for the rest of the book but might be skipped by readers with the appropriate background—biological for Chapter 2, genetic for Chapter 3, and statistical for Chapter 4.

Beginning in Chapter 5, the process of genetic epidemiology is developed in greater detail, starting with familial aggregation and then continuing in

Chapter 6 with segregation analysis. The statistical techniques of linkage analysis are described in Chapter 7.

The next four chapters are broadly concerned with association studies, which can be used in a number of distinct ways. Chapter 8 provides the basic population genetics principles on which studies of association and linkage disequilibrium rely. Chapter 9 describes the general approaches to testing associations with a single genetic locus at a time; these loci could be either candidate genes or markers in a candidate region that might help localize the causal gene being sought. If the purpose is fine mapping, then these methods might be applied simultaneously to a dense panel of markers in the candidate region using techniques reviewed in Chapter 10. Once the causal gene has been identified and cloned, the methods of Chapter 11 are used to study its epidemiologic characteristics. The concluding chapter (12) illustrates this entire process using the example of colorectal cancer.

Throughout the book, new terminology is indicated in italics where first introduced and the major recurring terminology is defined in the Glossary at the end.

Los Angeles, California   D. C. T.

Acknowledgments

This work has benefitted greatly from the input of many friends and colleagues. I am grateful to my colleagues at the University of Southern California, who have collaborated with me over the years on numerous genetic epidemiology projects and methodologic research in statistical genetics, particularly Jim Gauderman, Kim Siegmund, Dan Stram, Peter Kraft, Robert Haile, Paul Marjoram, Bryan Langholz, Sue Ingles, and Simon Tavaré. Many of them have graciously read numerous drafts of various chapters, offered their suggestions, and even lectured on this material in my graduate courses. I have learned a great deal from their expertise.

I also want to thank my graduate students who diligently waded through early drafts of this book and pointed out numerous mistakes and areas that needed clarification. In particular, I wish to single out several of my teaching assistants over the past few years, who helped me assemble visual aids, research literature, review drafts of the chapters, and helped explain it all to the other students: Peter Kraft, Dajun Qian, Corina Shtir, and Wei Wang. Sheena Lin, Mulugeta Gebregziabher, and Terri Kang offered particularly helpful comments on the penultimate draft in the fall of 2002.

Over the years, I have been encouraged in my pursuit of this field by many distinguished experts from around the world. Quite a few of them served as reviewers of the proposal draft and offered many critical, helpful, and encouraging suggestions. I am particularly grateful to D.C. Rao, John Hopper, Muin Khoury, and Chris Amos, as well as to several other anonymous reviewers.

I am deeply grateful to Corina Shtir, who was my editorial assistant for the last year and a half. In addition to her regular duties as my teaching assistant, she took incredibly detailed notes during my lectures and undertook to rewrite many passages based on our discussions in class. She assisted me with countless organizational details, from library research to organizing copyright permissions to proofreading, but most of all, I discovered that she had remarkable artistic skills. She drew all of the original illustrations in this volume, as well as organized electronic versions of all the previously published figures. I could never have completed this task without her tireless help.

My friend Elizabeth Braunheim also encouraged me throughout the process, and in particular applied her outstanding editorial skills to the first chapter at a time when I was nearing paralysis. My administrative assistant, Jeanette Villanueva, provided all kinds of logistical support. My patient editor at Oxford University Press, Jeff House, was tireless in helping me conceptualize the reorganization of material and leading me through the mysterious process of publishing one's first textbook.

Acknowledgments also go to the National Institutes of Health, which have supported my research and that of my colleagues on which much of the experience described in the book is based.

Finally, to my family and especially to my loving wife, Nina, who survived the inevitable mood swings and the unpredictable hours and never let me lose heart. In loving gratitude, I dedicate the book to her.

Contents

SUMMARY OF COMMONLY USED NOTATION, xix

1. OVERVIEW OF GENETIC EPIDEMIOLOGY, 3
   The Process of Genetic Epidemiology, 4
       Descriptive Epidemiology and Hypothesis Generation, 6
       Familial Aggregation, 11
       Segregation Analysis, 14
       Linkage Analysis, 15
       Fine Mapping and Cloning, 18
       Candidate Gene Association Studies, 19
       Characterizing the Effects of Cloned Genes, 20
   Conclusions, 22

2. BASIC CONCEPTS OF MOLECULAR GENETICS
   (by Sue Ingles), 25
   Chromosomes, 25
   Cell Division, 27
       Cell Cycle, 27
       Mitosis, 28
       Meiosis, 30
   Genetic Recombination, 31
       Meiotic Recombination, 31
       Mitotic Recombination, 32
   DNA, 33
   Gene Expression, 35
       Transcription, 37
       RNA Processing, 38
       Translation, 39
       Post-Translational Modification, 41
   DNA Polymorphism, 42
   Conclusions, 43

3. PRINCIPLES OF MENDELIAN INHERITANCE, 45

Basic Concepts, 45

Mendelian Inheritance at a Single Locus, 50

Classical Autosomal Dominant Inheritance, 53
Classical Autosomal Recessive Inheritance, 54
Classical X-Linked Inheritance, 55
Multiallelic Loci, 57

Mendelian Inheritance at Two Loci, 58

Conclusions, 59

4. BASIC EPIDEMIOLOGIC AND STATISTICAL PRINCIPLES, 61

Basic Probability Theory, 61

Basic Epidemiologic Principles, 64

Study Designs, 65
Measures of Disease Frequency and Association, 67
Interpretation of Epidemiologic Associations, 76

Maximum Likelihood, 77

Generalized Estimating Equations, 86

Markov Chain Monte Carlo Methods, 87

Randomization Procedures, 92

Conclusions, 93

5. FAMILIAL AGGREGATION, 95

Genetic Relationships and Gene Identity, 95

Formal Derivation of φ and Δ, 97

Familial Correlations of Continuous Phenotypes, 99

Familial Risk of Disease, 104

The Concept of Familial Risk, 104
Design Principles, 111
Analytical Approaches, 113

Other Designs, 120

Randomization Tests of Familial Clustering, 120
Twin Studies, 122
Adoption Studies, 126

Approaches to Dependent Data, 129

Genetic Models, 130
Regressive Models, 130
Frailty Models, 131
Generalized Estimating Equations, 134

Conclusions, 135

6. SEGREGATION ANALYSIS, 137

Design Issues, 137

Ascertainment of Families, 137
Sequential Sampling, 139

Classical Methods for Sibships, 141
    Ascertainment Correction, 143
Likelihood Methods for Pedigree Analysis, 146
    General Model, 146
    Polygenic and Mixed Models, 148
    Penetrance Models, 150
    The Elston-Stewart Peeling Algorithm, 153
    Hypothesis Testing, 157
Alternative Methods, 160
    Gibbs Sampling, 160
    Generalized Estimating Equations, 162
Applications to Breast Cancer, 162
Conclusions, 164

7. LINKAGE ANALYSIS, 167
Recombination and Map Functions, 168
Direct Counting Methods, 172
Relative Pair Methods, 176
    Identity by State and by Descent, 177
    Affected Sib Pair Methods, 182
    Affected Relative Pair Methods, 187
    Sib Pair Methods for Quantitative Traits, 188
    Generalized Estimating Equation Methods, 190
Lod Score Methods, 191
    Two-Point Linkage, 191
    Joint Segregation and Linkage Analysis and the
      Mod Score, 196
    Multipoint Linkage and Ordering Loci, 200
    Genome-Wide Scans, 207
    Genetic Heterogeneity, 211
    Gibbs Sampling Methods, 214
Design Issues, 216
    Power and Sample Size, 216
    Selection Bias and Misspecification, 220
Fine Mapping and Cloning of *BRCA1*, 221
Conclusions, 226

8. PRINCIPLES OF POPULATION GENETICS, 227
Distribution of Genes at a Single Locus, 228
    Hardy-Weinberg Equilibrium in Large Populations, 228
    Genetic Drift in Finite Populations, 230
    Effects of Mutation and Selection, 232
Distribution of Genes at Two Loci, 235
    Origins of Linkage Disequilibrium, 238
    Decay of Linkage Disequilibrium, 240
    Estimation of Linkage Disequilibrium, 242

Evolution of Haplotypes, 246

Ancestral Inference, 247

    Coalescent Trees, 247
    Ancestral Recombination Graphs, 250

Conclusions, 251

9. TESTING CANDIDATE GENE ASSOCIATIONS, 253

Distributions of Genes in Affected and Unaffected
    Individuals, 254

    Homogeneous Populations, 254
    Ethnically Stratified Populations, 259
    Families, 261

Design Options for Association Studies, 264

    Cohort Study Designs, 264
    Case-Control Designs, 265
    Parental Controls and the Transmission/Disequilibrium Test, 274
    Family-Based Association Tests, 279

Quantitative Traits, 280

Conclusions, 281

10. LINKAGE DISEQUILIBRIUM MAPPING, 283

Recently Admixed Populations, 283

Isolated Populations, 286

Empiric Methods for Estimating the Location of a Disease
    Gene or Mutation, 288

Haplotype Sharing Methods, 290

Parametric Methods Based on the Coalescent, 291

How Much Linkage Disequilibrium Is There in the Human
    Genome? 294

    Haplotype Block Structure, 295

Conclusions, 302

11. GENE CHARACTERIZATION, 303

Estimation of Genetic Risks, 303

    Cohort and Case-Control Designs Using Unrelated Subjects, 304
    Familial Cohort Study Designs, 305
    Multistage Sampling and Countermatching, 315
    Relative Efficiency of the Alternative Designs, 318

Gene–Environment and Gene–Gene Interactions, 320

    Case-Control Designs, 321
    Case-Only Studies, 323
    Case-Parent Trios, 324
    Gene–Environment Interactions for Breast Cancer, 326
    Relative Efficiency of Alternative Designs for Interaction Effects, 329

Estimation of Gene Frequencies and Carrier Probabilities, 331
Searching for Additional Genes, 335
Conclusions, 338

12. TYING IT ALL TOGETHER: THE GENETIC EPIDEMIOLOGY
OF COLORECTAL CANCER, 339
History, Descriptive Epidemiology, and Familiality, 339
Mechanistic Hypotheses, 343
Models of Carcinogenesis, 343
Cancer Genes, 344
Genomic Instability, 345
Familial Cancer Syndromes, 346
Familial Adenomatous Polyposis, 346
Hereditary Nonpolyposis Colorectal Cancer, 348
Sporadic Cancers, 352
Genetic Alterations in Colorectal Cancer, 352
Pathways: Suppressor and Mutator, 353
Metabolic Pathways, 354
The Relationship Between Polyps and Colorectal Cancer, 356
Discovery of Novel Colorectal Cancer Genes, 356
Implications for Clinical Management, 358
The Future, 358
Genome-Wide Scans for Association and Interactions, 358
Gene Expression Assays, 360
DNA Methylation and Loss of Imprinting, 363
Conclusions, 366

GLOSSARY, 367
REFERENCES, 387
INDEX, 429

Summary of Commonly Used Notation

Variables

N	Sample size (individuals, families, meioses, and so on, depending on the context)
Y	Phenotype
E	Expected value of Y under H_0
G	Trait genotype (with alleles d, D)
M	Marker genotype (with alleles m, M)
H	Multilocus haplotype at loci $\ell = 1, \ldots, L$
X	Random family effect (e.g., frailty)
$\mathbf{S} = (S_m, S_f)$	Parental source indicators
$\mathbf{Z}$	Vector of covariates *or* polygenes *or* Number of alleles shared *IBD Z*
(r, s)	Number of affected and unaffected sibs *or* Number of recombinants and nonrecombinants

Parameters

$\mathbf{f} = (f_0, f_1, f_2)$	Vector of penetrance parameters for genotypes (dd, dD, DD)
$\lambda(t, G, \mathbf{Z})$	Age-specific penetrance (hazard rate) at age t
q	Disease susceptibility allele frequency
$\mathbf{Q} = (Q_0, Q_1, Q_2)$	Vector of genotype probabilities (a function of q) *or* vector of haplotype frequencies

$\mathbf{p}$	Vector of marker allele frequencies *or* segregation ratio p
θ	Recombination fraction
x	Map distance (crossover probability)
α	Proportion of families linked *or* parameter(s) in a covariance model
$\boldsymbol{\tau} = (\tau_0, \tau_1, \tau_2)$	Vector of transmission probabilities
$\mathbf{T} = (T_{g_o, g_m, g_f})$	Array of transition probabilities (functions of θ and/or τ) where subscripts o, m, and f refer to offspring, mother, and father, respectively
$\boldsymbol{\omega} = (\mathbf{f}, q)$	Vector of segregation parameters
δ	Linkage disequilibrium parameter
$\boldsymbol{\mu}$	Vector of expected values E_j of phenotypes within a family *or* mutation rate μ
σ^2	Component of variance (e.g., σ_A^2, additive genetic variance)
$\boldsymbol{\lambda} = (\lambda_s, \lambda_o, \lambda_m)$	Familial relative risks for siblings, offspring, and MZ twins, relative to the general population
h^2, c^2	Heritability and shared environmentality
$\mathbf{C}$	Matrix of phenotypic (residual) covariances within a family
$\mathbf{I}$	The identity matrix
$\mathbf{1}$	A vector of 1s
φ	Kinship coefficients
Φ	Matrix of kinship coefficients
$\boldsymbol{\pi} = (\pi_0, \pi_1, \pi_2)$	Probabilities of sharing alleles identical by descent (IBD) *or* conditional genotype probability given a relative's genotype *or* ascertainment probability π
Π	Matrix of $\bar{\pi} = \pi_1/2 + \pi_2$ proportions of alleles shared IBD
Δ	Matrix of π_2 probabilities *or* disequilibrium parameter for multiallelic loci
$\psi = OR$	Odds ratio
$\boldsymbol{\beta}$	Vector of log OR parameters in loglinear model for covariates and/or genotypes
Θ	Generic vector of model parameters

Functions and derived quantities

$\mathcal{L}(\mathbf{\Theta})$	Likelihood function with parameter(s) $\mathbf{\Theta}$
$\ell(\mathbf{\Theta}) = \ln \mathcal{L}(\mathbf{\Theta})$	Loglikelihood function
$G^2 = 2[\ell(\hat{\mathbf{\Theta}}) - \ell(\mathbf{\Theta}_0)]$	Likelihood ratio test chi square
$\mathrm{lod} = G^2 / 2 \ln(10)$	lod score
χ^2	Chi-square distribution
$\mathcal{N}(\mu, \sigma^2)$	Normal density function (subscript $\mathcal{J}$ denotes dimension of multivariate normal density function)

Note: When bolded, these symbols denote a vector of the corresponding variables, e.g., $\mathbf{Y} = (Y_1, \ldots, Y_n)$ for a family's phenotypes or $\mathbf{M} = (M_1, \ldots, M_L)$ for multilocus marker genotypes. Lower case symbols denote specific values for the corresponding random variables.

Statistical Methods
in Genetic Epidemiology

1

Overview of Genetic Epidemiology

Genetic epidemiology is the study of the joint action of genes and environmental factors in causing disease in human populations and their patterns of inheritance in families (Last, 1993; Morton, 1982; Neel, 1984; Rao, 1985; Thomas, 2000a). Many other disciplines also address aspects of this same overall objective—human genetics, population genetics, clinical genetics, molecular genetics, molecular epidemiology, statistical genetics, genomics, bioinformatics—each from its own perspective. Many other basic and clinical sciences—biochemistry, pathology, and physiology, for example—also contribute. A complete understanding of the etiology of disease requires an interdisciplinary approach drawing on all these fields.

The completion of the draft sequence of the entire human genome (Lander et al., 2001) has opened up many new resources for the study of genetic determinants of disease, but this is only the beginning, not the end, of the process. What remains now is to identify the genes involved in specific conditions, their variation across the population, and how they interact with other factors. With the new tools provided by the Human Genome Project at our disposal, the specific techniques—design, laboratory, statistical—are rapidly changing, but the basic epidemiologic principles remain useful. These are the concepts addressed in this book.

Family studies are the basic approach used by genetic epidemiologists. Of course, the basic designs of conventional risk factor epidemiology—cohort and case-control studies—are also useful for some of our purposes and will be compared with family-based designs where both could be used. The addition of molecular tools to traditional epidemiologic approaches has given birth to a new subdiscipline commonly known as *molecular epidemiology*. This field is in some ways broader (e.g., it encompasses biomarkers of environmental exposure and preclinical disease processes) and in some ways narrower (e.g., it typically does not involve the use of family-based designs) than genetic epidemiology. Although some view the two fields as synonymous and some as fundamentally different (Khoury and Dorman, 1998), no such distinction is made here. The book's emphasis is on the epidemiologic study designs—both population-based and family-based—and the statistical methods of analysis that are needed to investigate the patterns of disease in populations, in relation to both genetic and epidemiologic determinants.

The literature on breast cancer provides an example of this way of looking at disease causation. While we can still explain only a minority of breast cancers by established risk factors, a great deal is already known about both its genetic and its environmental determinants and their interactions. There are few other diseases that so well illustrate this entire research process.

The Process of Genetic Epidemiology

The process of defining the genetic basis of a disease usually follows a progression such as that summarized in Table 1.1:

1. *Descriptive epidemiology.* The pattern of international variation in disease risks and changes in risk among migrants, as well as racial/ethnic, social class, temporal, age, and gender variation, can provide clues to whether genetic or environmental factors are involved.
2. *Familial aggregation.* The first step in pursuing a possible genetic etiology is usually to demonstrate that the disease tends to run in families more than would be expected by chance and to examine how that familial tendency is modified by the degree or type of relationship, age, or environmental factors. This is often based on case-control comparisons of family history or on twin or adoption studies.

Table 1.1 The Process of Genetic Epidemiology

Stage	Description	Chapter
Descriptive epidemiology	Use of routine data to generate hypotheses	1
Familial aggregation	Looking for evidence of clustering in families	5
Segregation analysis	Testing hypotheses about genetic models	6
Linkage analysis	Finding the location of a major gene	7
Fine mapping	Localizing a gene using haplotypes and linkage disequilibrium	10
Association	Testing possible candidate genes	9
Cloning	Determining the molecular sequence of the gene	7
Characterization	Describing the effect of the gene	11

3. *Segregation analysis.* The next step is to determine whether the pattern of disease among relatives is compatible with one or more major genes, polygenes, or shared environmental factors. If major genes seem to be involved, then the parameters of the corresponding genetic model are estimated. Studies of the families of a population-based series of cases are generally used for this purpose.

4. *Linkage analysis.* Blood samples are obtained from potentially informative members of multiple case families and typed for genetic markers at known locations. Markers that are transmitted through families in a manner that parallels the transmission of the disease (*cosegregation*) provide evidence for the general chromosomal location of the gene. Extended families with many cases are particularly informative for this purpose and do not need to be population-based, although large series of pairs of affected siblings can also be used. This search may begin before one has any idea of even which chromosome to examine, let alone where on that chromosome. Beginning with a widely spaced array of markers scattered over the entire genome, one narrows down the search as leads develop, a process known as a *genome scan.*

5. *Fine mapping.* As the search region narrows, other techniques are used to narrow it further. Unrelated cases and controls can be compared on a dense panel of markers over the candidate region to look for associations that could reflect *linkage disequilibrium* with the causal gene (i.e., population associations between the alleles at two loci). Within linked families, *haplotypes* can be constructed from a series of closely spaced, highly *polymorphic* markers (genes that vary between individuals) in the hope of identifying *flanking markers* that represent "convincing" recombinants in single individuals.

6. *Association with candidate genes.* The linked region may include a number of genes with known functions that could be relevant to the etiology of the disease. By comparing the *genotypes* at these candidate loci between cases and controls (population- or family-based), one can test hypotheses about whether they are actually associated with the disease. Of course, such an association could also be noncausal, reflecting linkage disequilibrium with the truly causal gene, as in fine mapping.

7. *Cloning the gene and identifying mutations.* When the candidate region is sufficiently narrow and no candidate gene has been found in that region, DNA from that region can be exhaustively searched for polymorphisms. With various molecular techniques, or more recently the established sequence databases from the Human Genome Project, coding sequences are identified and each can then be screened for polymorphisms. Polymorphisms in cases that are rare in controls are considered to be possibly causal *mutations.* A causal mutation could also occur in a noncoding region (such as a regulatory region); in this case, sequencing of the candidate region—a very labor-intensive process—may be necessary.

8. *Characterizing the gene.* Once the gene has been identified, its structure, the function of each exon, regulatory elements, and other features are studied with molecular methods. The genetic epidemiologist then estimates the frequency of the various mutations and the effect of each on disease risk, including any interactions with age, host, or environmental factors.

Drawing on the genetic epidemiology of breast cancer, I now describe each of these steps in nonmathematical terms, deferring the technical details to later chapters. The general process described here, however, does not always follow this sequence exactly and is perhaps most appropriate for studying major susceptibility genes. For example, an epidemiologist with a biologically based hypothesis about a particular pathway might begin with association studies without going through the steps of segregation and linkage analysis, particularly if the genes of interest are common polymorphisms with low *penetrance* (the probability of the phenotype given the genotype) or if specific gene–environment interactions are of interest.

Descriptive epidemiology and hypothesis generation

Clues about the relative importance of genetic and environmental factors might derive from a number of epidemiologic characteristics.

International variation. Many diseases have 10- or 100-fold variation in age-adjusted incidence or mortality between countries. For example, Figure 1.1 shows a roughly 10-fold variation in age-adjusted female breast cancer rates across 95% of the registries included in *Cancer Incidence in Five Continents* (Parkin et al., 1997), with generally high rates in Western countries (the highest being for Europeans in Zimbabwe, 127/100,000) and generally low rates in Asian countries (the lowest being in Korea, 7.1/100,000). While some of this apparent variation could be artifactual (case definition, incomplete ascertainment, differential access to care and diagnosis, etc.), many of these differences are doubtless real. By themselves, however, they do not indicate whether the explanation is genetic, environmental, or both, but most genetic disorders would be expected to show some international variation corresponding to variation in *allele frequencies* (the population distribution of variants in a gene) and/or in modifying factors. Genetic variation might arise from drift, selection, inbreeding, founder effects, or other population genetics factors discussed further in Chapter 8. Thus, one of the objectives of genetic epidemiology is to determine what proportion of such variation in disease rates might be attributable to variation in the frequencies of susceptible genotypes between populations. Ecologic correlation studies of environmental factors have implicated dietary fat as a risk factor for breast cancer, but the results of analytical epidemiologic studies have been mixed (Prentice and Sheppard, 1990). Ecologic comparisons of hormone levels (Henderson et al., 1996) suggest that these factors might account for some of the much lower rate of breast cancer in Chinese than in Caucasians, suggesting that similar comparisons of the prevalence of polymorphisms in genes on the hormone metabolism pathways might be rewarding. An example of

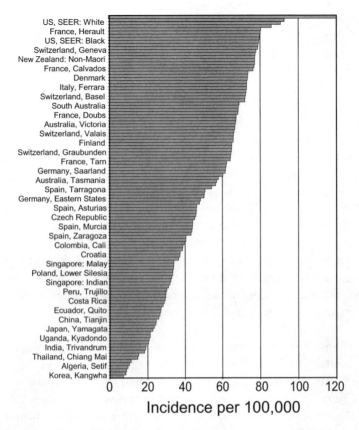

Figure 1.1 International variation in female breast cancer incidence, 1988–1992. (Based on data from Parkin et al., 1997)

such an analysis is the ecologic correlation between the incidence of insulin-dependent diabetes mellitus (IDDM) and the population frequency of the HLA-DR3 and -DR4 alleles (LaPorte et al., 1985; Trucco and Dorman, 1989) or the Asp-57 allele at the HLA-DQβ locus (Bao et al., 1989).

Migrant studies. A bit more insight into whether this international variation is due to genetic or environmental factors comes from studies of migrants (Thomas and Karagas, 1996). If the incidence rates in migrants tend to be more similar to those in their country of origin than to those in their adopted country, this might suggest a primarily genetic origin, whereas if migrants tend to adopt the rates in their country of destination, it might suggest a primarily environmental origin. Frequently, however, we see an intermediate pattern, varying as a function of age at or time since migration, or by the number of generations after migration, suggesting a gradual acculturation process. For example, breast cancer rates for nonwhite migrants to the United States tend to be considerably higher than those in their countries of origin but still lower than those of whites. Rates for white migrants, however, approach those for native-born whites within the first generation (Lilienfeld et al., 1972). Among migrants to Australia from England and Wales, rates approached those of native born persons within 6–16 years, whereas after 17+ years, rates in migrants from Italy and Yugoslavia were still lower than those of native-born Australians (Armstrong and McMichael, 1984; Armstrong et al., 1983). In contrast, the stomach cancer rate among first-generation Japanese male migrants to the United States falls to 72% of those in Japan, while the second-generation rate is only 38% of those in Japan; this rate is still high, however, compared with a relative rate of only 17% among U.S. whites. Such findings suggest that environmental factors (e.g., diet, exercise, and reproductive factors) may play an important role in breast cancer, perhaps through their influence on hormone levels. Such comparisons need to be considered very cautiously, however, since migrants are a highly selected subpopulation and numerous methodological differences in the way rates are computed could confound comparisons.

Racial, ethnic, and socioeconomic variation. Comparisons by race and ethnicity within countries can also shed light on possible etiologic factors and are less subject to methodological artifacts than are international comparisons. Figure 1.2 illustrates the comparison of breast cancer rates *within* the United States for different ethnic groups included in the Surveillance, Epidemiology, and End Results (SEER) registries. For all registries combined, rates for whites are about 14% higher than for African-Americans, and for other races the patterns tend to mirror those seen internationally, being generally low for Asians, Native Americans, and Latinas. These comparisons, like the international comparisons, could reflect either genetic or environmental factors, including socioeconomic factors. For example, breast cancer rates are strongly related to social class, being almost 50% higher in the highest quintile than in the lowest, which could easily confound comparisons of race. Nevertheless, some of this difference may be explainable on the basis of established reproductive risk factors, such as delayed first full-term pregnancy (Pike et al., 1983).

There is an important divergence of opinion in both the scientific and lay press about whether the concept of *race* has any scientific meaning. In part, this debate is supported by evidence from the Human Genome Project that there is greater diversity in genotypes between individuals within races than there are systematic differences between races (Yu et al., 2002). An editorial in the *New England Journal of Medicine* (Schwartz, 2001), for example, argued that "Race is a social construct, not a scientific classification" and

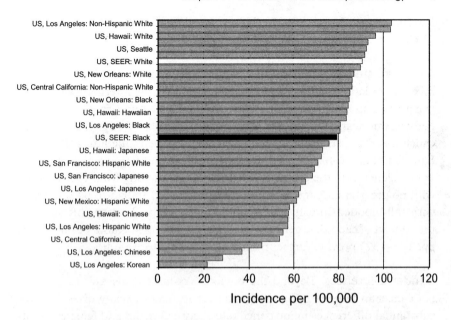

Figure 1.2 Racial variation in female breast cancer incidence in the United States, 1988–1992. (Based on data from Parkin et al., 1997)

further that "attributing differences in a biologic end point to race is not only imprecise but also of no proven value in treating an individual patient." A companion editorial (Wood, 2001) argued instead for "the identification of the genetic determinants of the reported racial differences, rather than attention to the external phenotypic manifestations of race." As we shall see in Chapters 8–11, however, it is often important in genetic research to control for ethnic or racial origins in testing hypotheses about specific genes since different races clearly have different disease rates (as illustrated in Fig. 1.2) and different frequencies of many genotypes (Cavalli-Sforza et al., 1994). There are also numerous examples of differential responses to environmental agents or drugs by different racial groups (Wilson et al., 2001; Wood, 2001). Another article (Wilson et al., 2001) and the accompanying editorial (Anonymous, 2001) argued in favor of using a genetically defined categorization of race (with techniques that are described in Chapter 9) rather than self-reported race in studying variability in drug response. Risch et al. (2002) and Burchard et al. (2003) discuss this issue in detail and argue forcefully for the importance of considering race and ethnicity in genetic epidemiology, while favoring the use of self-identified ethnicity rather than a purely genetic definition that would not encompass cultural factors that may also be relevant. For further discussion of this sensitive issue see Cooper (2003), Cooper et al. (2003), Karter (2003),

Kaufman and Cooper (2001), Kittles and Weiss (2003), Lin and Kelsey (2000), and Phimister (2003).

Admixture studies. One way to examine the effect of race is to study admixed populations—those that have resulted from the intermarriage of two genetically dissimilar populations such as African-Americans, Latinos, or Native Americans. We are not aware of any studies of this type for breast cancer. In the case of non-insulin-dependent diabetes mellitus (NIDDM), Knowler et al. (1988) studied the Pima Indians and found a clear gradient in prevalence with the extent of Indian heritage, ranging from 15% in those with no great-grandparents who were full-blooded Indian to 60% in those with full-blooded Indian great-grandparents. We will revisit this study in the context of candidate gene associations in Chapter 9. Khoury et al. (1993, pp. 133–137) provide further discussion of admixture studies.

Gender differences. Beyond the obvious sex-limited diseases (e.g., ovarian cancer in females and prostate cancer in males), many diseases show substantial differences in incidence rates between males and females or differences in other epidemiologic characteristics associated with the disease. Indeed, colorectal cancer (reviewed in Chapter 12) is one of the few cancers with nearly equal incidence rates in the two genders. On the other hand, the occurrence of a disease normally limited to one sex or the other can yield interesting clues; for example, breast cancer in males is a common feature in the familial syndrome associated with *BRCA1* but not *BRCA2*. The reasons for such differences are manifold, including genetic factors (X and Y chromosomes and mitochondrial DNA), hormonal differences (which are partially under genetic control), and developmental or environmental differences (e.g., occupational exposures, smoking habits). Thus, except for simple recessive *X-linked* diseases (diseases caused by genes on the X chromosome), it is difficult to interpret gender effects specifically in light of genetic and environmental factors.

Age effects. For many diseases that occur in both familial and sporadic forms, a common observation is that the familial form tends to occur at younger ages. This pattern is seen in both breast and colorectal cancer, as reviewed in Chapters 5 and 12, respectively. A classic example is retinoblastoma, a rare childhood tumor of the eye that can occur in one or both eyes. Knudson (1971) noted that the bilateral form is predominantly familial and the unilateral form is predominately sporadic. Furthermore, familial cases occurred usually in the first year or two of life, while nonfamilial cases were distributed more uniformly throughout early childhood. These observations led to the *two-hit* hypothesis of carcinogenesis (discussed further in

Chapter 12) that two mutations in a tumor-suppressor gene are required to produce a tumor. One of these mutations could be inherited (in familial cases) and thus exist in every cell of the body, thereby requiring only a single additional mutation to be acquired *somatically* (i.e., in a tissue cell rather than a germ cell). In nonfamilial cases, on the other hand, the two mutations would both have to be acquired somatically. Hence, they would be unlikely to occur in both eyes and would tend to require longer to develop. Childs and Scriver (1986) reviewed the age distributions of many diseases and found a general tendency for genetic diseases to have an earlier age distribution than nongenetic diseases.

Time trends. Generally, one would not expect a genetic disease to show much variation in incidence over time, although it is theoretically possible that changes in selective forces could produce very gradual changes in allele frequencies from one generation to the next. One would not expect natural selection to have a major influence on genes for diseases like breast cancer that occur primarily after reproductive age. However, improvements in medical treatments for IDDM could have led to higher proportions of diabetic children surviving to reproductive age, thereby increasing the population prevalence of deleterious human leukocyte antigen (HLA) genotypes. It is unlikely, however, that such gradual changes could account for the rapid rise in incidence that was seen over the course of the twentieth century. A more likely explanation would be changes in the prevalence of environmental factors that either have a main effect on disease risks or interact with genetic susceptibility factors.

For an extensive discussion of approaches to hypothesis generation in genetic epidemiology, the reader is referred to Chapter 5 of Khoury et al. (1993) and Chapter 15 of Gordis (1996).

Familial aggregation

The first step in the study of a potentially genetic trait is to see if it tends to aggregate in families, without at this stage having any specific genetic model in mind. The approach to this question depends on the nature of the *phenotype* (the observable outcome, in contrast with the unobserved genes, or *genotype*). In most places, there is no natural sampling frame for families, so *individuals* are selected in some way and then their family members are identified. We call the individual who caused a family to be identified a *proband*. Depending on the endpoint and the sampling scheme, probands are not necessarily diseased individuals even if a binary disease trait is being studied; for example, both affected and unaffected individuals could be probands in a case-control family study design.

For a continuous trait, one might enroll a random series of probands from the general population, together with their families, and look at the pattern of correlations in the phenotype between different types of relatives (sib–sib, parent–offspring, etc.). The resulting correlation matrix is analyzed by *variance components* or *path analysis* techniques to estimate the proportion of variance due to shared environmental and genetic influences. One might also identify families through probands with elevated values of the phenotype or some correlate thereof (e.g., benign breast disease for breast cancer, polyps for colorectal cancer, melanoma for a study of nevi, or heart disease for a study of lipid levels or hypertension). In this case, the analysis needs to allow for the way the families were ascertained, the simplest being to omit the proband from the analysis.

For a rare dichotomous disease trait, one would generally begin with the identification of probands, preferably in some population-based fashion, together with a comparable control series from the same population. For each subject, a structured family history is then obtained, preferably enumerating not just the familial cases but also the family members at risk, together with their ages and times at risk. Independent confirmation of reported familial cases would also be desirable. Two approaches can be taken to the analysis. One method compares cases and controls as independent individuals (or as matched pairs, depending on how they were selected) in terms of *family history* as an exposure variable, using standard case-control methods. The alternative method treats the family members of cases and of controls as two cohorts and uses standard person-years methods to compare their incidence of disease. Chapter 5 discusses the treatment of residual dependencies within the families using this approach.

It has been known for decades that breast cancer tends to run in families, but the familial relative risk is generally fairly small—about 2- to 3-fold. In a relatively early report, Anderson (1974) identified early-onset bilateral breast cancer as conferring a particularly strong familial risk. The alternative approaches to the analysis of familial risk are illustrated by two classic papers, both using the Cancer and Steroid Hormone (CASH) study data. The CASH study (Wingo et al., 1988) was a multi-center, population-based case-control study of breast cancer coordinated by the Centers for Disease Control, using 4730 cases aged 20–54 identified from eight SEER registries and 4688 controls, frequency matched on center and age, identified by random digit dialing. Information on the family history in all first-degree relatives and aunts was obtained by in-person interview, together with extensive information on other risk factors. In the first analysis to be reported, Sattin et al. (1985) compared cases and controls on various classifications of their family histories using standard case-control methods. They reported a 2.3-fold relative risk for any first-degree family history, rising to 14 if both a mother and a sister were affected. The relative risk was also somewhat higher if the affected relative was under age 45 than if she was older (2.8 vs. 1.9). In the second analysis, Claus et al. (1990) treated the family members as a cohort of individuals who had been at risk since birth and analyzed their risk of breast cancer in relation to their *exposure* to a case or a control. They reported age-specific incidence rates and showed that the rate ratio depended on the age of the case and the number of other affected family members.

Randomization tests. Randomization tests can be used with either case-control data or large population-based series of families. The basic idea is to compare some index of familiality for the observed families with a distribution of hypothetical families of the same structure, obtained by repeatedly randomizing the assignment of individuals to families. For example, applying this approach, Schwartz et al. (1991) found that families of young-onset breast cancer patients had greater heterogeneity in risk than expected (an excess of both high and low risk), whereas the distribution in control families was consistently skewed toward low risk.

Twin studies. Twin studies are also aimed at separating the effects of genes and environment. The classical twin method involves identifying twin pairs through affected members and comparing the *concordance* rates of MZ (monozygotic, identical) and DZ (dizygotic, or fraternal) twins. Assuming that MZ and DZ twins share environmental factors to a similar degree but differ in their genetic similarity, this comparison allows the estimation of *heritability*, defined as the proportion of the variance on an underlying *liability* to disease that is due to common genes, and *environmentality*, the proportion due to shared environment. Various extensions of the twin design include comparisons of twins reared apart and twin family studies. For example, Lichtenstein et al. (2000) estimated the heritability of breast cancer in a cohort of 44,799 Scandinavian twin pairs to be only 27%, suggesting that environmental factors played a stronger role in the general population.

Adoption studies. Like studies of twins reared apart, adoption studies aim to separate the effects of genes and environment by comparing individuals who share a common environment but have different ancestry or vice versa. A search of the breast cancer literature yielded no adoption studies, but the approach is well illustrated by a study of relatives of 34 adoptees with schizophrenia and 34 control adoptees. Ingraham and Kety (2000) found a 5% risk (14 cases out of 275) among their biological relatives but only a 0.4% risk (1/253) among biological relatives of controls and no cases among the adoptive relatives of either group.

Inbreeding studies. Offspring of consanguineous matings are more likely to carry two copies of the same allele and hence be at elevated risk of *recessive* diseases (those for which two mutant alleles are necessary). Inbreeding studies can be done as case-control or cohort studies, in either case treating the exposure as some measure of the degree of inbreeding, such as Wright's coefficient of inbreeding F, the probability of carrying two copies of the same allele from a common ancestor (Wright, 1922). Breast cancer does not provide a good example of this type of study, since I will show that it is inherited primarily in a *dominant* fashion (i.e., a single mutant allele is sufficient), although recent evidence suggests that there could be a recessive component after the effects of the *BRCA1* and *BRCA2* genes are removed (Antoniou et al., 2001; Dite et al., 2003). To detect this effect by an inbreeding study would, however, require the use of molecular methods to identify carriers of the dominant genes first.

Segregation analysis

Segregation analysis is the process of fitting formal genetic models to data on phenotypes of family members, often ascertained through affected probands in the case of a dichotomous phenotype. Again, the technique can be applied to continuous, dichotomous, or variable age-at-onset disease traits.

The fitting process uses the method of *maximum likelihood* (Chapter 4). Essentially, the parameters of the model are fitted by finding the values that maximize the probability (likelihood) of the observed data. The construction of genetic likelihoods is very complex and will be discussed only briefly here. The essential elements of the likelihood are (*1*) the penetrance function, (*2*) the population genotype distribution (for a major Mendelian gene, a function of the allele frequency), (*3*) the transmission probabilities within families, and (*4*) the method of ascertainment. The first three items are introduced in Chapter 3. Some form of ascertainment correction is necessary, since families ascertained through affected probands are likely to over-represent the gene frequency relative to the general population. Likewise, families with many cases are more likely to be ascertained than those with just one, which could lead to overestimation of penetrances.

Since the underlying genotypes are unknown, the likelihood of the observed phenotypes is computed by summing over all possible combinations of genotypes that are compatible with the observed data and Mendelian laws. This set of possible genotypes is potentially extremely large—3^N for a single major gene with two alleles, where N is the number of family members, although not every combination is actually possible. Brute force enumeration of all possible genotypes is therefore not feasible, even on the fastest computers, except for very small families. However, a very efficient algorithm for identifying the set of legal genotypes, known as *peeling* (Elston and Stewart, 1971), makes the calculation feasible. This algorithm essentially involves starting at the bottom of a pedigree and computing the probability of the parents' genotypes, given their phenotypes and the offsprings', and working up from there, at each stage using the genotype probabilities that have been computed at lower levels of the pedigree.

Although it is possible to do segregation analysis on nuclear families or small pedigrees, larger pedigrees are more informative. However, it is important that such pedigrees be assembled in a systematic fashion to avoid bias. For example, if one used anecdotal information about cases reported by relatives to decide which branches of a family to pursue, one would tend to overestimate the familial risk. A set of principles by Cannings and Thompson (1977), known as *sequential sampling of pedigrees,* provides the basis for an efficient and unbiased method of developing large, informative pedigrees.

A segregation analysis of the CASH data described above was subsequently conducted by Claus et al. (1991) to determine whether the pattern of inheritance was compatible with a single major gene hypothesis. They found that the data were best explained by a rare dominant gene, with a population allele frequency of 0.3% and a genetic relative risk that declined markedly with age. The lifetime risk in carriers of this mutation was estimated to approach 100%.

Linkage analysis

It is possible to identify the approximate chromosomal location of a major gene as a result of the phenomenon of recombination. The first principle is that genes on different chromosomes segregate independently, so there can be no linkage between them. The second principle is that the probability θ of recombination between two loci on the same chromosome increases with the physical distance between them, eventually reaching the limiting value of 1/2, the same probability as for two separate chromosomes. (Recombination rates are often expressed in units of 1%, called a centiMorgan [cM].) Thus, if a genetic marker is found to have a low recombination rate with a disease gene, one can infer that the disease gene must be close to that marker. The basic idea is then to determine the genotypes of various markers (whose locations are known) for various members of multiple case families. (Laboratory methods for marker typing include the *polymerase chain reaction* [*PCR*] used to magnify a single sequence of DNA into a sufficient quantity to be typed and *restriction fragment length polymorphisms* [*RFLP*] and *variable number of tandem repeats* [*VNTR*] assays for typing markers.) For this purpose, large families with many cases still alive are highly informative, and concerns about their representativeness are less important. Other approaches require only sib pairs or small pedigrees. It may be convenient to identify such pedigrees through a systematic population-based search for cases, followed by the application of sequential sampling principles, but this is not essential.

Suppose that both the disease gene and the marker gene are diallelic; let us continue to denote the disease gene alleles as d and D and let us denote the marker alleles as m or M. (Most modern markers have many alleles, however.) A *doubly heterozygous* individual's genotype then might be represented as $dm \mid DM$ or $dM \mid Dm$, distinguishing their *phase*. In principle, we would therefore look for parent-offspring pairs (meioses) in which the parent is doubly heterozygous and count the number of occasions for which the transmitted haplotype is a recombinant or a nonrecombinant. The proportion of recombinants out of all meioses is then a direct estimate of the recombination fraction (hence, this is known as the *direct counting* method). The difficulty is that unless the disease gene is fully penetrant, with no phenocopies, we cannot unambiguously determine the genotypes of the individuals, and even if we could, we might not always be able to figure out the phase. In practice, linkage analysis therefore uses one of two basic techniques: lod score methods or affected sib pair methods.

Lod score methods. The term *lod score* simply refers to the logarithm of the likelihood ratio, but taken to base 10 rather than base e. In linkage analysis, the ratio that is of interest is between the likelihood at the null value $\theta = 0.5$ and its maximum at $\hat{\theta}$. The lod score is calculated using the peeling method described under "Segregation Analysis," now summing likelihood contributions over all possible combinations of marker and disease genotypes (including phases of the double heterozygotes). Because there are many more possible combinations than there are in segregation analysis, this is usually done by fixing the segregation parameters (penetrances and allele frequencies) at values determined by an earlier segregation analysis and then evaluating the lods over an array of values of θ. (The other reason the segregation parameters are fixed in this way is that linkage analysis is often done on a selected subset of highly informative families, for which it would be impossible to obtain valid estimates of segregation parameters. This selection, however, does not necessarily bias estimates of the θ, because the marker data were not used to select the subset.)

So far, we have discussed linkage to a single marker locus (*two-point linkage*). Greater power can be obtained (at the cost of a more complex analysis) using *multi-point linkage,* in which two or more marker loci are used simultaneously. The primary aim of such analyses is to identify *flanking markers,* which are on opposite sides of the disease locus and thus help localize that locus.

The first convincing linkage of breast cancer to chromosome 17q was reported by Hall et al. (1990), who found stronger evidence for linkage in young breast cancer families. Pooling 214 families from many groups, the Breast Cancer Linkage Consortium (Easton et al., 1993) was able to localize the gene down to about a 13 cM region of chromosome 17q21. Extensive analysis revealed that only 45% of these multiple-case breast cancer families were linked to this gene, although the proportion linked was somewhat higher in families with many cases or with young mean age at onset. In contrast, all families with at least one ovarian cancer patient appeared to be linked to this gene. The cumulative risk of either breast or ovarian cancer up to age 70 in carriers of the gene was estimated to be 82%.

Affected sib pair methods. Because calculation of disease likelihood is complex and requires an assumed genetic model, sib pair methods are often favored as a nonparametric procedure. Sib pairs would be expected by chance to share two alleles *identical by descent (IBD)* (i.e., derived from the same grandparent) one-fourth of the time, to share one allele IBD one-half of the time, and to share neither allele one-fourth of the time. If two sibs are both affected by the disease and the disease is linked to a particular marker, then one would expect to see more sharing of marker alleles IBD than expected by chance. One therefore simply tabulates the number of alleles shared IBD by all pairs of affected sibs and compares that distribution to the expected distribution using a standard chi-square test. This procedure provides a test of the null hypothesis but no estimate of θ. It is often used as a simple screening test for linkage before proceeding to the more complex lod score method. Variants of this approach are applicable to continuous traits (the *sib pair* method) or to more distant relatives (the *affected relative pair* method).

As part of the pooled analysis of the Breast Cancer Linkage Consortium data, Easton et al. (1993) summarized the data on IBD sharing by affected relatives. Unfortunately, the number of affected sib pairs in these extended pedigrees was very limited, but showed a pattern consistent with the lod score analysis: among sib pairs both of whom were under age 45 at diagnosis, the number sharing zero, one, or two haplotypes spanning the linked region were 7, 10, and 3 (compared with an expected 5, 10, and 5), whereas among older sib pairs, the corresponding numbers were 10, 22, and 10 (compared with 10.5, 21, and 10.5 expected). Although not significant, this difference supports the stronger linkage among younger pairs.

Fine mapping and cloning

Once a set of markers close to the disease susceptibility locus have been identified, the chances of finding more recombinants in the same families that would further pinpoint the location of the disease gene become very small. However, the closer markers are to the disease locus, the more likely their alleles are to be associated with the disease. This is the basis for a fine mapping technique known as *linkage disequilibrium mapping.* Other fine mapping techniques involve the creation of *haplotypes,* a series of alleles at closely linked marker loci that reside on the same chromosomal copy and tend to be transmitted intact. Overlapping segments of haplotypes that are shared by cases (within or between families) can help localize the region where the gene is most likely to be located. The observation of *loss of heterozygosity (LOH)* or *cytogenetic rearrangement* in a single case may also help pinpoint the gene. Ultimately, however, it may be necessary to sequence an entire region, looking for coding regions (which comprise only about 2%–4% of the genome), and then look for polymorphisms in cases that are not seen in controls. This can be a very labor-intensive process, particularly if the region is large or the causal variant occurs in a regulatory region rather than a coding sequence. This process has been considerably expedited by the completion of the draft sequence of the entire human genome, thereby allowing investigators to query genomic databases to identify known genes, coding sequences, fragments, and, increasingly, even available polymorphism data. Still, however, a great deal of genetic testing might need to be done to identify the causal variant in a large region.

BRCA1 was cloned in the 17q21 region in 1994 (Miki et al., 1994), followed in short order by the cloning of a second gene, *BRCA2,* on 13q (Wooster et al., 1995). The original report described five distinct mutations in *BRCA1,* including an 11 base-pair deletion, a 1 base-pair insertion, a stop codon, a missense substitution, and an inferred regulatory mutation, which were not seen in any of over 100 controls. Subsequently, over 300 distinct mutations scattered throughout the gene were identified (Shattuck-Eidens et al., 1995). The gene is very large, comprising 5592 nucleotides spread over approximately 100,000 bases of genomic DNA, in 24 exons, producing a protein consisting of 1863 amino acids. It is not clear whether all mutations have the same effect on penetrance. Preliminary data suggest that the location of the mutation may influence whether it has a larger effect on the risk of breast or ovarian cancer. In addition to major mutations, numerous missense mutations and neutral polymorphisms have been reported; their phenotypic effects are still unclear.

Candidate gene association studies

Usually a region identified by linkage analysis will contain a number of genes that have already been identified. Of these, one or more might have some known function that is plausibly related to the disease under study and might be the gene one is looking for. This would be called a *candidate gene*. Studies of candidate gene *associations* provide a direct test of the hypothesis that it is the gene being sought. Typically these studies might use a standard case-control design with population-based cases and unrelated controls. One could then array the results in the usual 2×2 table and test the association using a chi-square test. However, an appropriate choice of controls is essential to ensure the validity of this method. Ethnic origin is probably the biggest concern, since racial groups have different distributions of many genes, and spurious results can easily occur if cases and controls are not carefully matched on this factor. This is not easily done, however, since even among Asians and Caucasians, there are strong differences between various ethnic subgroups.

One method for developing a control series that is not affected by ethnic stratification is to use family members as controls. Most commonly, either siblings or parents are used for this purpose. A *case-sibling design* can be thought of as a standard case-control study but matched on sibship, although there are some subtleties in the handling of families with multiple cases or multiple controls that will be discussed in Chapter 9. In *case-parent trio* designs, the parents themselves are not used as controls, but rather the set of alleles carried by the parents of the case that were not transmitted to the case. Thus, each case has two *transmitted* alleles and the control has the two *non-transmitted* alleles. The data are arranged in the usual fashion for matched case-control studies, cross-tabulating the alleles that each parent transmitted to the case versus those not transmitted. The standard McNemar test (or its generalization to multiple alleles) is used to test whether a particular allele is transmitted more frequently than expected by chance. This is known as the *transmission/disequilibrium test* (*TDT*).

A significant association does not necessarily imply that the gene has a causal effect on the disease due to the phenomenon of *linkage disequilibrium*. If a disease gene and a marker gene are closely linked, their alleles may not be independently distributed in the population; that is, carriers of the D allele may also be more likely to carry a particular marker allele. This can occur, for example, as a result of a fairly recent mutation that has not yet had time to reach equilibrium among descendants or as a result of some selective pressure that causes a particular combination of disease and marker alleles to persist. Thus, association does not necessarily imply causation, but may reflect either linkage to a nearby gene or simply a spurious result due to an inappropriate choice of controls.

Because breast cancer is primarily a disease of relatively late onset, it is difficult to enroll the parents of cases, a high proportion of whom are likely to have died (although this would be easier if one restricted the study to very young cases). Candidate gene associations with this disease have therefore tended to use case-control designs with unrelated or sister controls. Here attention has focused on two main classes of genes—those related to hormone synthesis pathways and those related to DNA repair. As an example of the former, Cui et al. (2003b) used a family-based case-control design to study a polymorphism in the *CYP17* gene, which regulates an early step in the estrogen synthesis pathway, and found a recessive effect of the *T* allele, with a relative risk of about 1.5. Heterozygous mutations in the *ATM* gene have also been suggested on the basis of population-based case-control studies to be associated with cancer generally and breast cancer in particular, for which a meta-analysis of several studies yielded a pooled relative risk of 3.9. In its homozygous form, this gene produces the neurologic disease *ataxia-telangiectasia,* which has as one of its features an extreme sensitivity to ionizing radiation. Since it is known that *ATM* encodes a protein that forms a complex with several others (including BRCA1) responsible for repair of double-strand breaks (that are caused by radiation), the hypothesis that *ATM* and radiation might interact in breast cancer is of particular interest and currently is the subject of both population-based and family-based studies.

Characterizing the effects of cloned genes

Once a gene has been identified, the final challenge is to understand how it works. In part, this is a job for the molecular biologist, who must determine its normal function and the effects of each mutation on that function. This is a particularly labor-intensive process, typically involving direct sequencing of many samples to search for point mutations. Once a mutation has been discovered, it may be possible to develop a rapid screening test to detect it in future samples. However, a gene may have many different mutations, so a negative screening test for selected mutations does not necessarily imply that the individual has the wild type, and further sequencing may be needed to confirm this.

Having identified some mutations, the genetic epidemiologist can contribute by providing population-based data on the frequency of each mutation and characterizing the effects of each mutation on disease rates, including any interaction with environmental or host factors. The first step in the process is usually case-based, aimed at simply identifying all mutations that occur among cases of the disease. Bear in mind, however, that (*1*) mutations may be very rare, so random samples of cases could have a very low yield, and (*2*) not all cases are necessarily caused by a mutation in that gene, so some comparison is needed to infer that a particular mutation has an effect on disease risk. Perhaps the first comparison that one might want to make is therefore between sporadic and familial cases (especially cases in linked families), since the latter are more likely to be due to the particular gene, and in any event, the yield of mutations is likely to be larger in familial cases.

Two main approaches are used to estimate penetrance and allele frequencies. The first is to conduct a population-based case-control study using unrelated cases. Conventional case-control analyses can then allow one to estimate the relative risk associated with each mutation and any interactions with host or environmental factors. The control series also provides a direct estimate of the population allele frequencies. If mutations are relatively common (as in many of the metabolic genes), then this is the obvious way to proceed, but not if they are rare.

The alternative is a family-based cohort study, with families identified through affected probands. Once the specific mutation carried by the proband has been identified, a simple screening test can be used to identify other family members who carry the same mutation. The relative risk for each mutation can be estimated using a case-control design in which relatives are used as matched controls, thereby avoiding the difficulties of matching on ethnicity. Alternatively, the penetrance can be estimated directly by standard person-years methods. Allele frequencies can be estimated from the distribution of genotypes in founders and marry-ins after the proband's alleles are removed. Further efficiency can be gained by restricting the families to multiple-case families, but then some correction for the method of ascertainment is needed.

Since the cloning of *BRCA1* and *BRCA2,* there have been extensive efforts to characterize these two genes. It has become apparent that mutations in both genes are more common in Ashkenazi Jews. The first population-based estimate of penetrance was based on a familial cohort study in Ashkenazi Jewish volunteers in the Washington, D.C., area (Struewing et al., 1997). By comparing the incidence of cancer in relatives of carriers and relatives of noncarriers, the investigators estimated a cumulative risk to age 70 of 56% for breast cancer and 16% for ovarian cancer, significantly lower than the rates derived from the Breast Cancer Linkage Consortium data. Subsequent estimates from the general population of Australia (not restricted to Ashkenazi Jews) were as low as 40% (Hopper et al., 1999b).

Ursin et al. (1997) used a case-only design to study the interaction between *BRCA1/2* mutations and use of oral contraceptives (OCs) in young

Ashkenazi Jewish breast cancer cases. They found a 7.8-fold higher risk in carriers who had used OCs for at least 5 years than would be expected based on the main effects of the two factors. This was a small study, but preliminary reports from several confirmatory studies indicate similar findings. In contrast, OCs appear to be protective against ovarian cancer in carriers, as they are in the general population (Narod et al., 1998). Given these intriguing findings relating to possible interactions with hormonal factors and the strong role that hormonal factors play in these cancers in the general population, there is doubtless some role for the various genes in the estrogen metabolism pathway (*CYP17*, *CYP19*, *17HSD1*, and *ER*). Whether these genes also interact with *BRCA1/2* remains to be seen. These and related questions involving the joint effects of *BRCA1/2* mutations with other risk factors are a major thrust of research by such international collaborations as the U.S. National Cancer Institute's Cancer Family Registries for Breast Cancer Studies and the Cancer Genetics Network.

Conclusions

This brief summary of the process of genetic epidemiology illustrates how the different approaches can each shed light on the etiology of a disease from a different perspective.

Descriptive epidemiology revealed a 10-fold variation in breast cancer rates worldwide and significant variation by race, ethnicity, and social class within countries. These variations suggest the possibility that genetic factors play a role, although environmental factors could also be part of the explanation, as indicated by the changes in disease rates in migrants.

Familial aggregation studies, using case-control and cohort methods, clearly indicated a tendency for breast cancer to run in families and also showed that this tendency is strongest for early-onset disease. This familial clustering could also, of course, be interpreted as either a genetic or shared environmental effect, and twin studies suggested that both play a role, since the risk was higher in MZ than DZ twins, but not as much as would be expected with a purely genetic hypothesis.

Segregation analysis of various population-based family studies strongly rejected purely environmental or purely polygenic models in favor of a major gene, with a dominant mode of inheritance fitting best. The mutant allele appeared to be very rare (0.3% in the general population) and to confer a large relative risk that declined with age, yielding a lifetime risk in carriers approaching 100%.

Linkage analyses localized the gene to the region 17q21, where *BRCA1* was found in 1994. These analyses suggested that nearly all families containing one or more ovarian cancers, but fewer than half of those with only breast cancer, were linked to this gene, families with many breast cancers being more likely to be linked. Another breast cancer gene, *BRCA2*, was identified on chromosome 13q a year later. Many different mutations have since been found in both genes, most of them being rare, although three are relatively common in Ashkenazi Jews.

Population-based family studies have shown the penetrance of these genes to be substantially lower than that estimated from the high-risk families used to locate the genes, perhaps about 50% for breast cancer and 16% for ovarian cancer by age 70, but with substantial variation from study to study. Among the environmental factors known to be involved in breast cancer, hormones and reproductive events are perhaps the most important. Preliminary data suggests that use of OCs might interact with *BRCA1/2* mutations to increase the risk of breast cancer in a more than multiplicative manner, while at the same time reducing the risk of ovarian cancer.

Association studies also suggested that a polymorphism in *CYP17* (one of the genes on the estrogen synthesis pathway) may increase the risk of breast cancer, and other genes on this pathway are currently under study. Although the relative risk is much smaller than for *BRCA1/2*, the much higher prevalence of these polymorphisms could translate into a larger population attributable risk. *BRCA1* produces a protein that combines with ATM and other proteins to produce a complex that is known to be involved in the repair of double-strand breaks, such as those caused by ionizing radiation, an established risk factor for breast cancer. For this reason, evidence from both case-control and family studies of ataxia-telangiectasia probands suggesting that heterozygous mutations in *ATM* also confer an increased risk of breast cancer and may interact with ionizing radiation are intriguing and the subject of ongoing research.

Reanalyses of family studies after removal of those known to carry mutations in *BRCA1/2* suggest that there may be other major genes still to be identified, perhaps acting in a recessive manner. Either linkage or association studies could be used to find them.

While breast cancer provides an opportunity to illustrate most of the steps in the process of genetic epidemiology, we will see in the concluding chapter, on colorectal cancer, that research often does not proceed in such a simple linear fashion. There is enormous scope for creativity in the search for causes of disease, and many different disciplines must be brought to bear. Nevertheless, the basic thought process outlined here should be applicable to elucidating the genetic epidemiology of almost any complex disease.

2

Basic Concepts of Molecular Genetics

SUE INGLES

The study of genetic epidemiology and the statistical tools it uses requires at least a rudimentary understanding of the principles of molecular biology on which the phenomena of transmission of genes are based. This chapter provides a general survey of the structure of DNA, chromosomes, and genes, their reproduction by mitosis in somatic cell division and by meiosis in the creation of the gametes that are transmitted from parents to offspring, their expression in proteins, and the types of polymorphisms that can occur. Readers interested in more detail are encouraged to read one of the excellent textbooks on molecular biology, such as that of Strachan and Read (1999) or Lewin (1997). Research in genetic or molecular epidemiology inevitably involves collaboration with laboratory scientists, and some understanding of the methods they use to obtain, amplify, and store DNA and to detect polymorphisms or mutations is also essential. Since these techniques are in a rapid state of evolution, I do not attempt to describe them here, but rather encourage readers to consult with their molecular science colleagues about how best to gain this experience.

Chromosomes

The normal human genome is composed of 23 *chromosomes:* 22 *autosomes* (numbered 1–22) and 1 *sex chromosome* (an X or a Y). Cells that contain one copy of the genome, such as sperm or unfertilized egg cells, are said to be *haploid.* Fertilized eggs and most body cells derived from them contain two copies of the genome and are said to be *diploid.* A diploid cell contains 46 chromosomes: 22 *homologous pairs* of autosomes and a pair of fully homologous (XX) or partially homologous (XY) sex chromosomes. The members of a chromosome pair are referred to as *homologs*.

Chromosomes can be seen under the microscope only during cell division. By stimulating cells to divide and then treating them with chemicals that block the last stages of cell division, one can observe and photograph individual chromosomes. Homologous chromosomes are matched up and arranged by size, from largest (chromosome 1) to smallest (chromosomes 21 and 22), followed by the sex chromosomes to form a display called a *karyogram*. A precise description of the chromosomes (including the overall count, identification of any extra or lost chromosomes, identification of regions of a chromosome that may have been deleted or inverted or moved to another chromosome, etc.) is called the *karyotype*. The normal complement of chromosomes is designated as 46,XY (male) or 46,XX (female).

Variations from the normal chromosome number are occasionally inherited and present in all body cells, but more commonly are seen in cancer cells from chromosomally normal individuals. Cells that contain one or more extra sets of chromosomes are called *polyploid*. If there are three complete sets, the cells are *triploid;* four sets is *tetraploid*. If individual chromosomes are in excess or are missing, the cell is said to be *aneuploid*. If a single chromosome (say chromosome 21) is lost, the state is referred to as *monosomy* 21. If there are three of chromosome 21, it is *trisomy* 21 (the abnormality that gives rise to Down's syndrome).

Chromosomes are often depicted as they would appear during cell division: as two duplicate chromosomes, joined to each other at the middle, looking something like an *H* (Fig. 2.1). The joined chromosomes are *not* the two chromosomes in the diploid pair, nor are they the double strands of DNA that make up a single chromosome (described in the section "DNA" below). They are the result of chromosome duplication in preparation for cell division. The point at which the two copies or *chromatids* are joined is called the *centromere*. The position of the centromere (*metacentric*, meaning "in the middle," or *acrocentric*, meaning "near the end") aids identification of each of the 23 chromosomes.

The centromere divides the chromosome into two arms, designated *p* (French *petit*) for the shorter of the two and *q* (French *queue*) for the longer. Within each arm, staining produces characteristic *bands*, which are grouped into regions and numbered, counting outward from the centromere. For example, the band referred to as 11q23 is the third band of the second region of the long arm of chromosome 11. Note that band 23 is referred to as *two-three*, not *twenty-three*. Depending on the resolution of the staining procedure, sub-bands (labeled 11q23.1, 11q23.2, etc.) and sub-sub-bands (11q23.11, 11q23.12, etc.) may be distinguished. Using cytogenetic

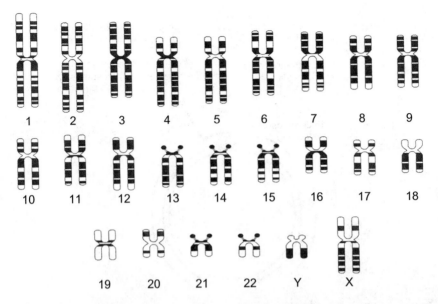

Figure 2.1 Ideogram of human chromosomes showing the Giemsa banding patterns, arranged and numbered according to the Paris classification of 1971. (Reproduced with permission from Moody, 1975)

banding, the smallest structural defects (loss or gain of chromosomal material) that can be distinguished are about 4 megabases of DNA.

Cell Division

Cell cycle

The sequence of events that occurs between two cell divisions is called the *cell cycle* and consists of four phases (Fig. 2.2): *G1 phase* (gap 1), *S phase* (DNA synthesis), *G2 phase* (gap 2), and *M phase* (mitosis). Sometimes nondividing cells are said to be in G0, a modified G1 resting phase.

Normal cells spend most of their time in G1 phase. During G1, the chromosomes are relatively diffuse and open, allowing transcription to take place. This is the stage when cells produce the proteins needed to carry out their normal functions. When cell division is required, either for growth, development, repair, or replacement of worn-out cells, cells progress from G1 to S phase. Since S phase (DNA replication) commits the cell to dividing, this step must be undertaken only if resources are available to allow the cell to complete the cell cycle successfully. If conditions are not favorable, biochemical signals will stop the cell cycle at the *G1 checkpoint*, preventing entry into S phase.

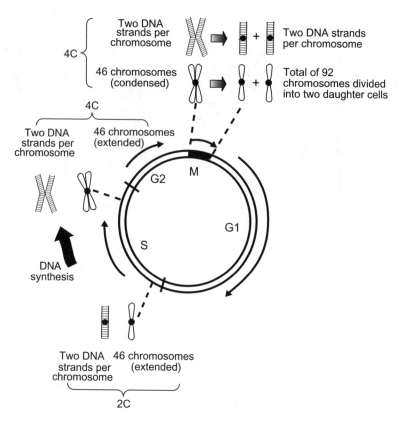

Figure 2.2 Cell cycle. (Reproduced with permission from Lewin, 1997)

If conditions are favorable, cells progress to *DNA synthesis* or replication. The two strands of the double-stranded DNA separate, and each strand is used as a template for synthesis of another (complementary) strand. It is important that the enzyme that synthesizes the new strand (*DNA polymerase*) does so with very high fidelity, since mistakes may introduce a mutation. At the end of DNA synthesis, each cell contains two (it is hoped) identical copies of the 46 chromosomes. For human cells in culture, the S phase is completed in about 8 hours. The cell then enters G2 phase, a brief period of cell growth, and passes through the *G2 checkpoint* to ensure that DNA replication has indeed been completed before mitosis begins.

Mitosis

During mitosis (Fig. 2.3), the chromosomes become compacted into short structures, less than 1/10,000th of the stretched-out chromosomal length,

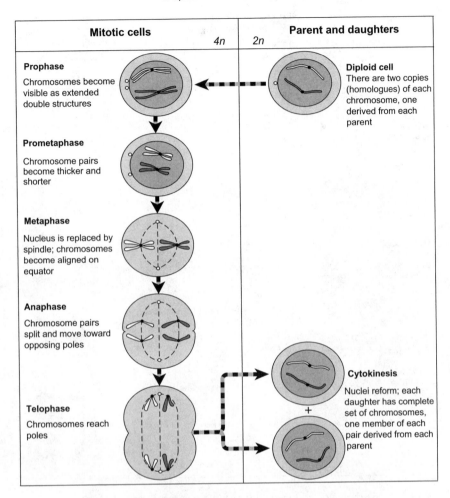

Mitotic cells		
	4n	2n

Prophase

Chromosomes become visible as extended double structures

Prometaphase

Chromosome pairs become thicker and shorter

Metaphase

Nucleus is replaced by spindle; chromosomes become aligned on equator

Anaphase

Chromosome pairs split and move toward opposing poles

Telophase

Chromosomes reach poles

Parent and daughters

Diploid cell

There are two copies (homologues) of each chromosome, one derived from each parent

Cytokinesis

Nuclei reform; each daughter has complete set of chromosomes, one member of each pair derived from each parent

Figure 2.3 Mitosis. (Adapted with permission from Lewin, 1997)

and become visible under the microscope. The two sister chromatids of each chromosome can be seen to segregate, and the cell divides into two identical diploid daughter cells. Mitosis can itself be divided into several phases based on the appearance of the cell when observed under the microscope. During *metaphase* the chromosomes align and the fibers needed to draw the duplicate pairs apart are formed; in *anaphase* this separation occurs; and in *telophase* the nucleus itself divides. The fourth phase of mitosis, *interphase*, is actually the sum of all of the nonmitotic phases, G1 + S + G2. Mitosis is the usual form of cell division seen in *somatic cells* (cells other than germ cells). Mitosis produces identical daughter cells, and the normal diploid chromosome number is maintained.

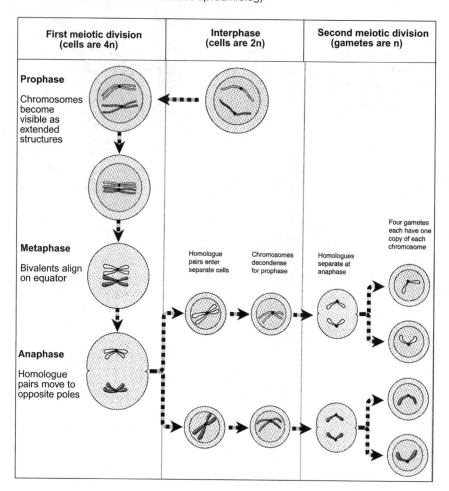

Figure 2.4 Meiosis. (Reproduced with permission from Lewin, 1997)

Meiosis

A second kind of cell division, *meiosis* (Fig. 2.4), results in reduction of chromosome number from diploid to haploid. Meiosis occurs only in germ cells (*primary oocytes* and *primary spermatocytes*) and produces *gametes, sperm* and *ova* that are genetically different from the parent cells. Like mitosis, meiosis is preceded by a round of DNA synthesis, but in meiosis this is followed by two rounds of cell division, called meiosis I and II. *Meiosis I* differs from mitosis in that it is not the sister chromatids that separate but rather the maternal and paternal homologs. Maternal and paternal homologs, each consisting of two sister chromatids, pair up, forming a *bivalent*, a structure consisting of four chromosomes of the same type. When the nucleus divides, both chromatids of the maternal chromosome go one way, while the two chromatids of the paired paternal chromosome go the other way. Mendel's law of *independent assortment* states that segregation of maternal and paternal homologs to the two daughter cells is independent from chromosome to chromosome. Thus, there are at least 2^{23} (approximately 8.4 million) possible types of sperm or ova that can be produced by one person. As we will see below, this number is actually much larger when we consider meiotic recombination.

Meiosis I results in two daughter cells, each having 23 duplicated chromosomes. In males, these cells are the same size and both progress to the second round of cell division. In females, uneven division of cytoplasm during meiosis I results in one large cell and a small *polar body* that does not divide further. *Meiosis II* is identical to cell division in mitosis (again, except for uneven division of the cytoplasm in females). The two chromatids of each chromosome separate, and cell division results in two haploid cells. Meiosis can take a long time: in women, meiosis I *begins* during embryogenesis and is completed many years later at the time of ovulation. If this were the full description of meiosis, each of the 22 autosomes in a gamete would be an exact copy of one of the two parental homologs. In fact, a process called *meiotic recombination* mixes the genetic material of the homologs during meiosis, so that each chromosome present in the gamete has contributions from both parents.

Genetic Recombination

Meiotic recombination

In the bivalent complexes of meiosis I, homologous chromatids pair up and form physical connections called *chiasmata* (singular, *chiasma*). Chiasmata are essential for correct chromosome alignment and segregation and thus are thought to perform a role in meiosis I similar to the role of centromeres in mitosis and meiosis II. Each chromosome arm normally forms at least one chiasma, and females form approximately 50% more chiasmata than do males. In males, the X and Y chromosomes, which are very different in size and in genetic makeup, pair up at a region near the end of the short arms, known as the *pseudoautosomal region*. As the name suggests, genes in this region behave as if they were autosomal. They are present on both X and Y chromosomes, they exhibit crossing-over (described below), and in the female they escape X inactivation, the random inactivation of one X chromosome in each cell early in development (see Chapter 12).

Meiotic recombination or *crossing-over* occurs at the chiasmata (Fig. 2.5). Specific enzymes break the DNA strands and repair the break in a way that

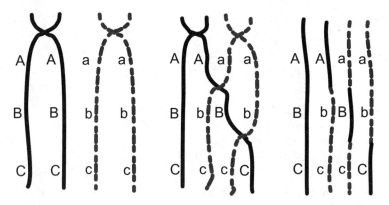

Figure 2.5 Crossing-over. (Reproduced with permission from Ott, 1999)

swaps material from one chromosome with material from another. The most important consequence of meiotic recombination is that gametes receive contributions from both homologs of a chromosome pair (thus from both grandparents). Two alleles that are linked (on the same chromosome) in the parent may or may not be linked in the offspring. As a result, a single person can produce essentially an infinite number of genetically different gametes.

Mitotic recombination

Recombination is not a normal feature of mitosis, since paternal and maternal homologs do not associate during mitosis. It can occur, however, usually in cancer cells. Unbalanced mitotic recombination is one mechanism for loss of DNA from one chromosome. If the region lost contains a tumor suppressor gene and the retained allele is inactive (through mutation), the recombination results in loss of the only functioning allele of the tumor suppressor gene. This process is referred to as *loss of heterozygosity (LOH)*. Cancer epidemiologists often compare a patient's *germline DNA* (DNA that the patient inherited from his or her parents and is found in all of the normal body cells) and *tumor DNA* to look for LOH. If the germline DNA is heterozygous for some marker and the tumor is homozygous for the same marker, then it is likely that a tumor suppressor gene, located somewhere near the marker, was important in the development of the cancer.

Sister chromatid exchange. Recombination between sister chromatids during mitosis is called *sister chromatid exchange (SCE)*. Since sister chromatids are identical, an SCE has no functional effect at all. However, since SCEs arise from breaks in the DNA strands, counts of SCEs have been used by epidemiologists as markers of exposure to DNA-damaging agents.

DNA

Each chromosome is made up of two *strands* of *deoxyribonucleic acid (DNA)* held together by weak hydrogen bonds and coiled into a *double helix* (Fig. 2.6). Each strand of DNA is a single (very long) molecule with a *deoxyribose backbone* (Fig. 2.7). The backbone consists of deoxyribose sugars covalently bound together into a long chain. Phosphates act as the "glue" between the sugars, linking the 3′ carbon of one sugar to the 5′ carbon of the next sugar in the strand. The terminal sugar at one end of the DNA strand has a free 5′ carbon, and the sugar at the other end has a free 3′ carbon. The convention is to distinguish the two ends of a DNA strand by referring to the *5′* or *3′ end*. Attached to each sugar is a *base*. Four different bases are found in DNA: two *purines: adenine (A)* and *guanine (G); and two *pyrimidines: cytosine (C)* and *thymine (T)*. Sugar-base units are referred to as *nucleosides (deoxyadenosine, deoxyguanosine, deoxycytidine, and deoxythymidine)* and the corresponding sugar-base mono-phosphates as *nucleotides* (denoted *dAMP, dGMP, dCMP,* and *dTMP*). The linear sequence of nucleotides or bases encodes the genetic information needed to create proteins. Each cell contains

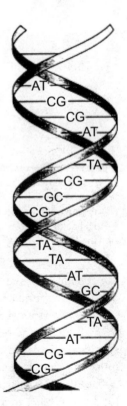

Figure 2.6 Double-stranded DNA. (Reproduced with permission from Strachan and Read, 1999)

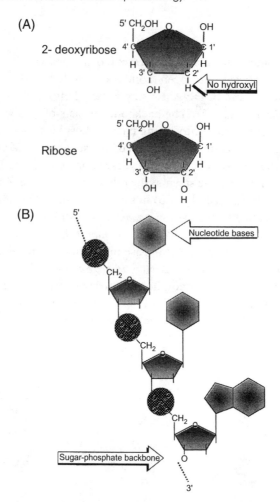

Figure 2.7 2-Deoxyribose, a polynucleotide chain. (A) 2-Deoxyribose is the sugar in DNA and ribose is the sugar in RNA. The carbon atoms are numbered as indicated for deoxyribose. The sugar is connected to the nitrogenous base via position 1. (B) A polynucleotide chain consists of a series of 5'–3' sugar-phosphate links that form a backbone from which the bases protrude. (Reproduced with permission from Lewin, 1997)

the genetic information, coded as nucleotide sequences, to create any protein that might be needed by any type of cell in the body (Fig. 2.8).

The two strands of a double-stranded DNA molecule are held together by hydrogen bonding between opposing bases (Fig. 2.7). Bonding occurs specifically between A and T and between G and C; thus the two strands must be *complementary* (e.g., 5'-ATTCATCGGA-3' on one strand and 3'-TAAGTAGCCT-5' on the other; Fig. 2.9). Note that the two strands bind (or *anneal*) in an *anti-parallel* manner; that is, one strand runs in the

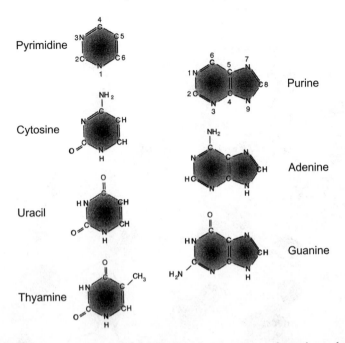

Figure 2.8 Purines and pyrimidines providing the nitrogenous bases in nucleic acids. The purine and pyrimidine rings show the general structures of each type of base; the numbers identify the positions on the ring. (Reproduced with permission from Lewin, 1997)

5′ to 3′ direction and the other in the 3′ to 5′ direction. Since the sequence of one strand can be easily inferred from that of the other strand, sequences are usually specified by writing only a single strand (by convention, in the 5′ to 3′ direction).

Each base, along with its complementary base on the opposite strand, is called a *base-pair*. To describe neighboring bases on the same strand, it is usual to denote the phosphate between the nucleosides. For example, CpG means that C and G are on the same strand, whereas CG means that C and G are base-paired and are on opposite strands. Since the human genome is made up of 3 billion base-pairs, each chromosome is, on average, 125 million base-pairs in length.

Gene Expression

By various estimates, there are 30,000 to 50,000 *genes* in the human genome. A typical gene spans 1 to 200 kilobases (kb), and some genes span over 2000 kb of DNA; however, only a small proportion of this sequence codes for protein. The coding sequence of a gene is spread across several relatively

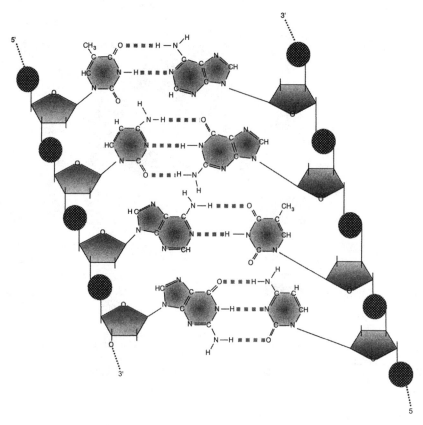

Figure 2.9 The double helix maintains a constant width because purines always face pyrimidines in the complementary A-T and G-C base pairs. (Reproduced with permission from Lewin, 1997)

small sequence blocks called *exons*. Interspersed between the exons are long intervening sequences called *introns*. Exons and introns are distinguished by the fact that exonic (but not intronic) sequences are represented in the mature mRNA (see below). In addition to exons and introns, genes contain regulatory sequences lying upstream (in the 5′ direction) of the first exon. The structure of a gene is often represented schematically by several boxes (exons) connected by lines (introns), as shown in Figure 2.10. A line to the left (upstream) of the first box represents the region containing untranscribed regulatory sequences.

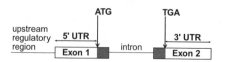

Figure 2.10 Simplified structure of a gene.

The following sections give an overview of the process of gene expression, that is, the transfer of genetic information from DNA to RNA (transcription) and from RNA to protein (translation).

Transcription

Messenger RNA (mRNA) is a transitory molecule that moves genetic information from the nucleus of the cell, where information is stored (as DNA), to the cell cytoplasm, where that information is translated into protein. RNA is very similar to DNA, except that (*1*) the backbone is made of the sugar ribose (rather than of deoxyribose), (*2*) the base *uracil* (U) is used in place of thymine, and (*3*) it is present in single-stranded form only. RNA molecules are also much shorter than DNA molecules since an RNA molecule is transcribed from a single gene.

For a segment of DNA to be transcribed into RNA, the two DNA strands must separate over a short distance, so that a single strand of RNA can be synthesized against the *template,* the strand of DNA that encodes the protein sequence. Transcription is initiated on the template by binding of transcription factors that in turn attract the enzyme *RNA polymerase.* RNA polymerase adds nucleotides to the 3′ end of the growing RNA chain. Base pairing (U to A, A to T, C to G, G to C) ensures that the RNA sequence is complementary to the DNA template. Because the growing strand of RNA has the same direction and base sequence (except U for T) as the nontemplate DNA strand, the nontemplate strand is called the *sense strand* and the template strand is called the *antisense strand.* When reporting DNA sequences, it is customary to report the sequence of the sense strand. Not all genes on the same chromosome are transcribed off of the same physical strand of DNA. The sense strand for one gene may be the antisense strand for another.

Some genes, called *housekeeping genes,* are transcribed in nearly all cells. In general, however, different types of cells transcribe different sets of genes according to their needs. Red blood cell precursor cells, for example, transcribe globin genes at a high level to produce large amounts of hemoglobin. This is an example of a permanent change in gene expression that occurs with cell differentiation. In addition, the RNA content or *transcriptome* (i.e., the set of genes transcribed and the level of transcription) of a given cell can be temporarily altered by extracellular signals. Signaling molecules such as steroid hormones and growth factors activate intracellular signaling pathways that culminate in the activation of *transcription factors.* The amounts and types of transcription factors available in a cell can dramatically alter gene expression.

A given transcription factor recognizes a specific DNA sequence and acts only on those genes that contain the specific regulatory sequence. The regulatory sequences are called *cis-acting* elements because they are located on the same DNA strand (cis) as the template to be transcribed, whereas the transcription factors are said to be *trans-acting* because they are products of remotely located genes and must migrate to their sites of action.

Initiation of gene transcription is regulated by a cluster of cis-acting regulatory sequences called the *promoter,* which usually lies just upstream (at the 5′ end) of the transcription start site (Fig. 2.10). Core promoter elements usually include an *initiator element (PyPyCAPuPu* or variant, where *Py* = pyrimidine and *Pu* = purine) and a *TATA box* (TATAAA or variant) surrounded by a GC-rich sequence. Some promoters lack a TATA box and are said to be *TATA-less.* These promoters have an alternate sequence element called the *downstream promoter element (DPE)* located approximately 30 base-pairs downstream from the transcription start site. Transcription factors that recognize these core promoter elements are present in all cells and are sufficient to confer a basal or *constitutive* level of transcription.

Basal transcription can be either increased or turned off by additional transcription factors acting on positive or negative regulatory elements (enhancers or silencers, respectively) located either in the promoter region or farther upstream or downstream, often at a considerable distance from the coding region. After binding regulatory proteins, the DNA strand may loop back so that the transcription factor complexes can interact with the promoter region to alter the rate of transcription. The transcription factors that recognize enhancer and silencer elements are often restricted in their expression, either by tissue type or by developmental stage. In this way, different subsets of genes are transcribed by different tissues at different stages of development. Obviously, mutation or polymorphism in cis-acting sequences could have important functional consequences, even though most of these elements do not lie within protein-coding sequences.

RNA processing

Since transcription proceeds from the beginning of the first exon (the transcription start site), through all of the exonic and intronic sequences, to the end of the last exon, the *RNA primary transcript,* known as *heterogeneous nuclear RNA (hnRNA),* contains much more sequence than is needed to code the protein or polypeptide. The introns are immediately removed from the hnRNA by a process called *RNA splicing.* Splicing is controlled by more than 60 different trans-acting factors (more than 55 polypeptides and 5 *small nuclear RNAs (snRNAs)* that recognize and bind weakly conserved intronic cis-elements in a developmental and tissue-specific manner. It is now recognized that at least 50% of genes display *alternative splicing*, with certain exons being spliced out in certain tissues. In this way, several variant proteins can be created from a single gene.

After removal of introns, the resulting mRNA still includes two noncoding regions. The exonic sequences between the transcription start site and the translation start site, comprising at least the beginning of exon 1 and sometimes the entire first exon or even several exons, is called the *5' untranslated region* (*5' UTR*). The 5' UTR contains cis-elements that regulate transcription. Similarly, the exonic region downstream of the stop codon is called the *3' UTR*. The 3' UTR also contains cis regulatory elements, the most well understood being sequence elements that control mRNA stability.

The array of cis regulatory elements in the 5' UTR of an mRNA of a given gene can vary from tissue to tissue. Many genes contain multiple untranslated first exons, each having its own promoter and transcription start site. Through tissue-specific alternative splicing, different 5' UTRs, containing different regulatory elements, can be utilized in different tissues. In this way, tissue-specific responsiveness to various transcription factors is conferred.

In addition to splicing, two additional processing steps are necessary for formation of *mature mRNA*. A 7-methylguanosine is added to the 5' end of the RNA. This 5' cap protects the mRNA from degradation. Finally, the 3' end of the mRNA is formed by cleavage at a specific site in the 3' UTR (usually signaled by AAUAAA), with the addition of approximately 200 A residues at this site. This *poly-A tail* is thought to stabilize the mRNA and possibly facilitate transport of the mRNA from the nucleus to the cytoplasm.

Translation

Translation of mRNA into protein is carried out in the cytoplasm on large protein-rRNA (ribosomal RNA) complexes called *ribosomes*. Binding of mRNA to ribosomes is the controlling step in the regulation of translation. Both the 5' and 3' UTRs of the mRNA contain cis-acting sequences important for ribosome recruitment. The 3' UTR also has sequences important for translational regulation and for mRNA stability and localization. Thus, mutation or polymorphism in UTR sequences could have important functional consequences.

After attachment to the ribosome, the mRNA coding region is translated into a sequence of *amino acids* (the building blocks of proteins) according to the *genetic code* (Table 2.1). The genetic code is a three-letter code: a sequence of three bases (a *codon*) specifies one amino acid. In this way the

Table 2.1 The Genetic Code

First Position (5' End)	Second Position	Third Position (3' End)			
		U	C	A	G
U	U	Phe	Phe	Leu	Leu
	C	Ser	Ser	Ser	Ser
	A	Tyr	Tyr	STOP	STOP
	G	Cys	Cys	STOP	Trp
C	U	Leu	Leu	Leu	Leu
	C	Pro	Pro	Pro	Pro
	A	His	His	Gln	Gln
	G	Arg	Arg	Arg	Arg
A	U	Ile	Ile	Ile	Met
	C	Thr	Thr	Thr	Thr
	A	Asn	Asn	Lys	Lys
	G	Ser	Ser	Arg	Arg
G	U	Val	Val	Val	Val
	C	Ala	Ala	Ala	Ala
	A	Asp	Asp	Glu	Glu
	G	Gly	Gly	Gly	Gly

four types of bases, combined into $4 \times 4 \times 4 = 64$ types of codons, can uniquely specify the 21 types of amino acids. Because several codons can specify the same amino acid, the genetic code is said to be *degenerate*. The degeneracy is often in the third position of the codon; for example, UUC and UUU both specify the amino acid phenylalanine.

To initiate translation, the ribosome must first identify the correct *reading frame* and the *start codon*. Since the bases could be grouped in three different ways to form codons and since either strand could be encoding a gene, there are actually six possible reading frames. The correct reading frame is identified by scanning for the first AUG (specifying methionine) as the ribosome travels down the mRNA strand. However, AUG is efficiently recognized as a start codon only when it is embedded in a *Kozak sequence* (GCCPuCCAUGG). In a few genes, ACG, CUG, or GUG is used as the start codon.

Once the start codon has been identified, the ribosome travels down the mRNA strand, codon by codon, incorporating amino acids into a polypeptide chain (Fig. 2.11). Decoding of the mRNA sequence is accomplished by base-pairing between mRNA codons and complementary *anticodon* sequences of *transfer RNA (tRNA)* molecules. Each tRNA molecule transports a specific amino acid to the ribosome. For example, tRNA molecules bearing a TTT anticodon (complementary to UUU) carry phenylalanine. Pairing of the anticodon with the complementary mRNA codon exposed on the active site of the ribosome allows the amino acid to be added to

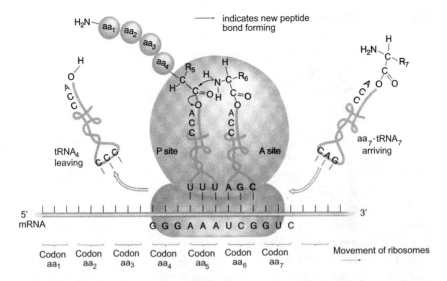

Figure 2.11 Translation. (Reproduced with permission from Griffiths et al., 2000)

the growing polypeptide chain. Translation proceeds until the ribosome encounters a *stop codon* (UAA, UAG, or UGA). It should be noted that these three sequences account for approximately 5% of codons in a random sequence of bases. Therefore, if the reading frame has not been correctly established and maintained, stop codons are frequently encountered. It is possible for two different reading frames of the same DNA sequence to encode overlapping genes, however; this situation is rare in eukaryotic genomes, and frameshift mutations usually result in premature termination of translation.

Post-translational modification

The final step in gene expression involves *post-translational modification* of the newly synthesized polypeptide to produce a mature, functional protein. Carbohydrates or lipids may be added to specific amino acids of many proteins. Proteins that must be secreted or transported across a membrane undergo cleavage to remove localization sequences. Some polypeptides are cleaved to produce two or more polypeptide chains with different functions. Thus a single gene may encode multiple polypeptides. Finally, some polypeptides function as protein subunits of *multimeric proteins;* hence, multiple genes may be required to encode the polypeptides that make up a single functional protein.

DNA Polymorphism

Despite the wide range of phenotypes observed in the human race, our DNA has surprisingly little variability. More than 99% of the nucleotides in DNA are the same in all humans. Those DNA locations, or loci, that vary from person to person are said to be *polymorphic*. The alternate sequences found at a polymorphic locus are called *alleles*. At some highly polymorphic loci, most persons are *heterozygous* (have different alleles on the two chromosomes). Persons with two copies of the same allele are said to be *homozygous*. The mean heterozygosity of the human genome is 0.1%–0.4%; that is, one in every 250 to 1000 bases is polymorphic.

Technically, the term *polymorphism* is generally restricted to those variations that are relatively common (present in at least 1% of individuals) and that do not have highly deleterious consequences. Highly deleterious rare variants are usually referred to as *mutations*. See Cotton and Scriver (1998) for further clarification of this nomenclature. While some common polymorphisms are thought to contribute to the etiology of disease (the *common disease–common variant* hypothesis), common polymorphisms are also of interest to the genetic epidemiologist for another reason. A large number of DNA markers are needed to follow the inheritance of specific regions of a chromosome in a family.

The most common type of polymorphism in the human genome is the *single nucleotide polymorphism* (*SNP*) or *point mutation*. *Transitions,* the substitution of one purine for another ($A \leftrightarrow G$) or one pyrimidine for another ($C \leftrightarrow T$), are the most common type of SNP. *Transversions,* in which a purine is replaced by a pyrimidine, or vice versa, are less common. When the SNP occurs in a coding region, it can be classified as *synonymous* (*silent*) or *nonsynonymous,* depending on whether or not it changes the amino acid sequence. Nonsynonymous SNPs may be classified as *missense* (changing one amino acid to another) or *nonsense* (changing an amino acid to a stop codon). Missense SNPs are said to be *conservative* if the two amino acids are functionally similar. *Frameshifts,* resulting from insertions or deletions of one or two (but not three) nucleotides in a coding region, completely change the amino acid sequence downstream of the mutation (Fig. 2.12). This type of DNA variant is one kind of mutation rather than a polymorphism, since it is almost certain to be rare and detrimental. *Insertions* and *deletions* can also occur in noncoding regions, where they likely have no functional consequences.

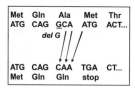

Figure 2.12 Insertions and deletions leading to frameshift mutations.

Another type of polymorphism that is useful as a marker is the *DNA microsatellite*. Microsatellites are short sequences of DNA (usually one to six nucleotides) that are repeated multiple times (usually 10 to 60 times). They belong to the class of DNA called *variable number of tandom repeats* (*VNTRs*). The most commonly used microsatellites are probably the $(CA)_n$ *repeats* (sequences like CACACACACA). Misalignment of the repeated unit during cell division can lead to changes in the number (n) of repeats, creating a high degree of polymorphism in the population. Their high degree of polymorphism, along with their widespread distribution throughout the genome (the human genome contains approximately 50,000 $[CA]_n$ repeats) makes microsatellites an important source of genetic markers.

Conclusions

The basic genetic information is encoded in genes, which reside on chromosomes made up of DNA. In somatic cells, this information is duplicated during each mitotic cell division, yielding two identical daughter cells (except in the rare event of a somatic mutation, which could lead to cell death or a step in some disease process like cancer, as discussed in Chapter 12). Gene expression occurs through the processes of transcription and translation (protein synthesis), which are subject to complex regulatory control mechanisms that depend on the specific type of cell and the environmental or developmental influences on it.

In germ cells, the process of meiosis leads to the creation of gametes (sperm and ova) containing only one copy of each gene for transmission to offspring. During meiosis, independent assortment of chromosomes and recombination between chromosomes allow for creation of an essentially infinite number of genetically different gametes that could be passed on to the next generation. Observation of recombination between generations provides the basic information that permits the geneticist to localize disease genes, using the techniques of linkage analysis described in Chapter 7.

Most genes are polymorphic, and these differences can range from silent polymorphisms that have no effect on the coding sequence through a variety of missense polymorphisms to major mutations that can by themselves lead to disease. The following chapter will discuss parent–offspring transmission of mutations responsible for classical Mendelian disorders, to set the stage for more complex inheritance patterns discussed in later chapters. Use of polymorphisms as tools for finding genes and characterization of the effects of causal mutations will be discussed in the final chapters of this book.

3

Principles of Mendelian Inheritance

This book focuses mainly on statistical methods for studying *complex diseases*, those that do not exhibit simple patterns of inheritance traceable to a single major gene that is both a necessary and a sufficient cause. Such diseases may involve multiple genes, environmental factors, age-dependent risks, and complex interactions between these factors. Before we tackle these complicated situations, however, some basic ideas about simple Mendelian patterns of inheritance need to be presented and some terminology established. I begin with a more formal treatment of such concepts as familiality, heredity, genotype, phenotype, penetrance, transmission, and causation. The rest of this chapter will outline the classical patterns of dominant, recessive, and X-linked inheritance.

Basic Concepts

The belief that a trait "runs in families" is a familiar one. Of course, some family clusters can be expected simply by chance. Assuming, however, that the tendency is systematic, we would refer to such a trait as *familial* until it is determined whether the primary reason for this familial aggregation is environmental or genetic (or some combination of the two). Family members, of course, share many environmental exposures that could be related to the disease under study. They tend to eat together, are exposed to the same household pollutants, and share certain habits like smoking and alcohol consumption. Not all family members, of course, are genetically related (spouses, for example). By studying family groupings, it is often possible to tease apart the environmental and genetic contributions to disease risks.

The terms *familial* and *hereditary* are often used in a somewhat different sense in discussing diseases that have already been shown to have a genetic component. Unless the disease is caused solely by a major mutation, some cases will have been caused by genes, some by environmental factors, and some by both, either by independent mechanisms or by acting in combination. Thus, modern genetic epidemiologists think less in terms of *nature versus nurture* than in terms of the joint action of genetic and environmental factors in determining disease (gene–environment [$G \times E$] interactions). Until the responsible gene has been identified and a test is available, however, it is impossible to know for certain the cause of any particular case, but the family history may provide a clue. We use the word *sporadic* to refer to isolated cases without a family history of the disease and *familial* to refer to cases with a positive family history. (Of course, this concept is itself imprecise—would a single affected cousin constitute a positive family history?) But even among cases with a strong family history, not all may be caused by the gene. Hence, we reserve the term *hereditary* for those cases where there is a clear pattern of inheritance within the family (Chapter 6) or where even stronger evidence is available, such as from linked genetic markers (Chapter 7) or a mutation in a causal gene (Chapters 9 and 11). The opposite of a hereditary case is called a *phenocopy*, that is, a diseased case without a genetic etiology.

Table 3.1 illustrates the difference between familial and hereditary cases using data from a population-based family study of breast cancer (Hopper et al., 1999a) in which probands were genotyped for *BRCA1* and *BRCA2*. (Cui and Hopper, 2000, use computer simulation to explore this distribution in greater detail, based on parameters estimated from this study.) All four possible combinations of familiality and heredity are represented: (*A*) individuals with no family history whose disease is due solely to environmental factors; (*B*) individuals whose disease has a genetic cause but with no evident family history; (*C*) individuals whose disease is solely environmental but with a family history that could be due to shared environment or chance; and (*D*) individuals with a family history that is attributable to a shared genetic cause. Here we see that the vast majority of familial cases of

Table 3.1 Classification of Cases as Familial versus Hereditary: Illustrative Data for Breast Cancer

Family History	Genetic Cause		All
	None	Yes	
Negative	$A = 66.5\%$	$B = 3.5\%$	Sporadic (70%)
Positive	$C = 27.7\%$	$D = 2.3\%$	Familial (30%)
All	Phenocopy (94.2%)	Hereditary (5.8%)	(100%)

Source: Adapted from Hopper et al. (1999a).

breast cancer are actually phenocopies ($27.7/30 = 92\%$), while a majority of hereditary cases are sporadic ($3.5/5.8 = 60\%$).

The important point is that the occurrence of disease results in part from predictable factors, both genetic and environmental, in part from real but unobserved factors, and in part from the operation of chance. Hence, one must distinguish between familial *clusters* that could be entirely coincidental and familial *aggregation*, which is a systematic tendency for disease to cluster in families, for whatever reason.

To make the distinction between sporadic and hereditary cases more rigorous, we need to introduce the concept of *penetrance*. An individual's observable outcome is called his or her *phenotype* or *trait*. Phenotypes can be measured on a continuous scale, such as blood pressure; on categorical or ordinal scales, such as hair color or severity of disease; on a dichotomous scale, such as presence or absence of disease; or as age at onset of a dichotomous disease trait, which may be *censored* in some individuals by death from competing causes, loss to follow-up, or end of the study (i.e., the age at onset, if any, is known only to have been after the last observation time). An individual's (possibly unobserved) genetic status is called his or her *genotype*. For a given trait, the relevant genotypes may consist of

- a *major gene:* a single locus, each individual having two copies, one from each parent; or
- *polygenes:* the cumulative effect of a large number of genetic loci, each having a small effect, the total effect tending to be normally distributed;

or combinations thereof (multiple major genes [*oligogenic*] or a major gene plus polygenic effects [*multifactorial* or *mixed model*]). An individual's *genome* refers to his or her entire genetic constitution. The *penetrance function* is the set of probability distribution functions for the phenotype given the genotype(s). Letting Y denote the phenotype and G the genotype, we write the penetrance as $\Pr(Y \mid G)$. For simplicity, I will restrict attention here to a binary disease trait Y (with $Y = 1$ indicating affected and 0 unaffected) and write the penetrance or risk of disease as a function of genotype, $\Pr(Y = 1 \mid G)$, simply as $\Pr(Y \mid G)$.

Suppose we know that a disease is caused by a single major gene that exists within the population in two distinct forms (*alleles*): d, the *wild type* or normal allele, and D, the *mutant* or *disease susceptibility* allele. (Of course, for many genes there are more than two alleles.) Genotype dd would thus represent the normal genotype, and the penetrance $\Pr(Y \mid G = dd)$ would be the risk of disease (or probability distribution of a continuous phenotype) in *noncarriers*. If $\Pr(Y \mid dd) = 0$, there are no phenocopies; that is, all cases of the disease are caused by the gene (the D allele is a necessary condition for

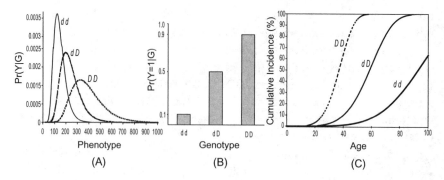

Figure 3.1 Examples of penetrance functions: (A) continuous trait, (B) binary trait, (C) censored age-at-onset trait.

the disease, but other factors may be necessary to complement the allele in order to create a sufficient condition). If $Pr(Y \mid DD) = 1$ [or $Pr(Y \mid dD) = 1$ in the case of a dominant allele], we say that the genotype is *fully penetrant*, meaning that it is sufficient to cause the disease. Aside from classical genetic traits that are manifest at birth, most of the chronic diseases we will use as examples involve genes that have phenocopies and are not fully penetrant; thus $0 < Pr(Y \mid G) < 1$ for all G.

Figure 3.1 provides examples of penetrance functions for three different types of phenotypes. In panel A, the probability densities for individuals with the three genotypes are lognormally distributed, with differing means (but the same geometric standard deviation); such distributions might differ in location, variability, or shape. In panel B, the risk of a binary disease trait is shown as a function of genotype. Panel C shows the cumulative incidence curves for an age-dependent disease trait; in this case, the lifetime risk eventually is 100% for all genotypes (absent death from competing causes), but the distribution of age at onset differs and hence the cumulative risk at any specific age differs as well.

The concept of *dominance* is an inherent part of the penetrance model. For a single major gene with two alleles, there are three possible genotypes: dd, dD, and DD. In many instances, only one copy of the gene is expressed, so that there may be only two distinct penetrance functions. We distinguish the following situations:

- *Dominant:* $Pr(Y \mid dD) = Pr(Y \mid DD)$. A single copy of the mutant allele is sufficient to produce an increase in risk, and we say that allele D is dominant over allele d.
- *Recessive:* $Pr(Y \mid dD) = Pr(Y \mid dd)$. Two copies of the mutant allele are necessary to produce an increase in risk, or equivalently, one copy of the normal allele is sufficient to provide protection; we say that D is recessive to d (or equivalently, d is dominant over D).

- *Codominant:* $\Pr(Y \mid dd) \neq \Pr(Y \mid dD) \neq \Pr(Y \mid DD)$. All three genotypes have different effects on disease risk. In most cases, the heterozygotes have an effect that is intermediate between that of the two homozygotes (e.g., additive, described below), but there are exceptions, such as the protection from malaria conferred by heterozygosity of the sickle cell gene that has led to evolutionary maintenance of the recessive trait of sickle cell anemia in populations where malaria is endemic (Vogel and Motulsky, 1986).
- *Additive* or *Dose-Dependent:* $\Pr(Y \mid dD)$ is midway between $\Pr(Y \mid dd)$ and $\Pr(Y \mid DD)$. Each allele confers an increase in risk. What we mean by midway depends on the scale that is used to model these probabilities. On the natural scale, for example, this would correspond to an additive model, whereas on the logit scale it would correspond to a multiplicative model.

The meaning of dominance can depend on the context. A *tumor-suppressor gene* acts recessively in somatic cells, since both copies of the wild type must be inactivated to cause a cell to become malignant. But the gene is *inherited* in a dominant fashion, because only one mutation is likely to be inherited from a parent, the other usually being *acquired* as a *somatic mutation* in a single cell that goes on to beget a *malignant clone* of cells.

In the previous paragraphs, the word *cause* has been used loosely. In an observational science like epidemiology, experimental guidelines like Koch's postulates (Koch, 1882) used in microbiology, are not available. Epidemiologists have long recognized that most diseases have multiple causes that combine in various ways, so that no single factor is either necessary or sufficient. Instead, they tend to think in terms of a complex *web of causation* (MacMahon and Pugh, 1970). Rothman (1976) formalized this notion in terms of a *sufficient component causes model* in which there may be several alternative pathways, any of which is sufficient to cause the disease and each of which has several components that are all necessary to make the pathway sufficient.

Although this is a useful theoretical framework, in practice epidemiologists study statistical *associations* and rely on a set of well-established but subjective criteria (Hill, 1965)—biological plausibility, dose–response, size of the effect, temporal sequence of cause and effect, consistency across multiple studies, and coherence with evidence from other disciplines—to decide whether the association represents a causal phenomenon or some statistical artifact. Rothman and Greenland (1998) provide a thorough discussion of the general principles of causal inference in epidemiology. Parascandola and Weed (2001) review five basic types of definitions of causation used in epidemiology and advocate a probabilistic concept as a causal factor being one that increases the probability that a disease will occur, all other factors being held constant.

Modern thinking about causation is based on the principle of *counterfactual inference* (Rubin, 1990; Pearl 2000), in which two circumstances are compared: the conditions that actually occurred in a set of individuals and the hypothetical result that would have been expected in these same individuals had their conditions been different. Thus, to assess the effect of an exposure, one might compare the outcomes of exposed individuals to the outcomes they would have experienced had they not been exposed. Diseases that occurred in exposed individuals that would not have occured had they been unexposed are deemed to have been *caused* by the exposure. Those that did not occur when exposed that would have occurred if they had been unexposed are deemed to have been *prevented*. In the other two combinations (affected under both exposure conditions or unaffected under both conditions), the exposure had no effect. Since the counterfactual outcomes in the same individual cannot be observed directly, one must infer their distribution by comparing groups of individuals who differ in exposure but are otherwise comparable in all relevant features. Experimental studies ensure comparability on average by randomization, whereas observational studies rely on such techniques as matching or statistical adjustment to achieve reasonable comparability (Greenland, 1990). For opposing views of the general utility of counterfactuals, see Maldonado and Greenland (2002) and Dawid (2000) and the commentaries following each.

These concepts can be applied to genetic studies as well. In principle, what we mean by a *genetic cause* is that, all other factors being equal, an individual's risk of disease depends on his or her genotype (Khoury and Flanders, 1989; Thomas and Witte, 2002; Cotton and Scriver, 1998). Of course, as in observational epidemiology, the real challenge is ensuring comparability of all other factors, since the genotype under study could be associated with genotypes at many other loci or with ethnic origins that are associated with other risk factors. In terms of counterfactual inference, one would call a gene causal if some affected individuals would not have gotten their disease had they had a different genotype or if some unaffected individuals would have been affected had they had a different genotype. Of course, genotype being an inborn characteristic, the counterfactual condition is difficult to imagine and the parallel life (had the individual had a different genotype) might well differ in many other respects! Page et al. (2003) provide an excellent discussion of concepts of causation in genetics and suggest practical guidelines for distinguishing causation from mere association.

Mendelian Inheritance at a Single Locus

The first coherent description of the inheritance of genes was presented by Gregor Mendel in 1865, based on breeding experiments with pea plants, which he summarized in two principles. First, Mendel postulated that each individual carries two copies of each gene, one inherited from each parent. Alleles at any given gene are transmitted randomly and with equal probability. This principle is known as the *segregation of alleles*. Second, he postulated that the alleles of different genes are transmitted independently, a principle known as *independent assortment*. We now know that this does not apply when loci are located near each other on the same chromosome (*linked*). From these two principles, we can derive the basic probability laws governing Mendelian inheritance.

A third concept, distinct from the two basic Mendelian principles but generally considered part of the Mendelian framework, assumes that the expression of two genes is independent of which parent they came from; that is, heterozygotes have the same penetrance irrespective of whether the D allele came from the father and the d allele from the mother or vice versa. In recent decades, however, exceptions to this principle, such as *imprinting*, and other forms of parent-of-origin effects have been recognized; this is discussed further in Chapter 12.

A final assumption commonly made in calculating probabilities on pedigrees is random mating (or no *assortive mating*), that is, that the probability that any two individuals will mate is independent of their genotype. To some extent, this assumption is clearly violated by the fact that individuals are more likely to mate within their ethnic groups, which differ in terms of many genes but possibly not for a specific gene of interest with respect to a trait under study.

Suppose that there are only two alleles for a single major gene. Let us first consider the probability distribution for gametes transmitted from a single parent to his or her offspring (*transmission probabilities*), as shown in Table 3.2. Obviously, if the parent is homozygous for either the d or the D allele, then that is the only allele he or she can transmit. On the other hand, if the parent is heterozygous, then, following Mendel's principle of segregation of alleles, either the d or the D allele can be transmitted, both with probability 1/2.

Now, consider the joint effect of the two parents' genotypes on the offspring's full genotype (the combination of the two transmitted gametes).

Table 3.2 Probability Distribution for Gametes from One Parent

Parental Genotype	Transmitted Gamete	
	d	D
dd	1	0
dD	1/2	1/2
DD	0	1

Table 3.3 Probability Distribution for Offspring's
Genotype, Conditional on Parental Genotypes

Father's Genotype	Mother's Genotype	Offspring's Genotype		
		dd	dD	DD
dd	dd	1	0	0
dd	dD	1/2	1/2	0
dd	DD	0	1	0
dD	dd	1/2	1/2	0
dD	dD	1/4	1/2	1/4
dD	DD	0	1/2	1/2
DD	dd	0	1	0
DD	dD	0	1/2	1/2
DD	DD	0	0	1

Table 3.3 provides what are called the *transition probabilities*, which form one of the key elements in the specification of a genetic model. For example, if both parents are heterozygotes, either could transmit D alleles with a probability of $1/2$ each, so the resulting offspring probabilities are $1/4$, $1/2$, and $1/4$ for dd, dD, and DD, respectively. In Chapter 6, we will describe some alternative specifications used in testing whether the observed pattern of disease in families really corresponds to Mendelian inheritance. When two or more loci are considered (such as a disease locus and a genetic marker used to try to find the disease gene), the transition probabilities become a function of the joint genotypes at all the loci and the *recombination fractions* between them. These probabilities will be described in Chapter 7.

The other two key elements in a genetic model are the penetrances (discussed above, including dominance) and the *population allele frequencies*. Again, supposing that there are only two alleles segregating in the population, let q denote the prevalence of the D allele and let $p = 1 - q$ denote the prevalence of the d allele. If the two copies of each gene were distributed randomly (following the principle of independent assortment), then the three genotypes would be distributed in the general population as $\Pr(dd) = p^2$, $\Pr(dD) = 2pq$ (since dD and Dd are indistinguishable), and $\Pr(DD) = q^2$. The remarkable fact is that, under appropriate conditions, if one combines these probabilities for parental genotypes with the above transition probabilities, one obtains the exact same probabilities for the offspring. (The necessary conditions include random mating, no migration, no inbreeding, no selective survival factors related to genotype, a large population, and no mutation.) This theorem is known as *Hardy-Weinberg equilibrium*, shown formally in Chapter 8.

It is worthwhile to consider the implications of these mathematical results for the special cases of classical dominant, recessive, and X-linked inheritance for genes that are necessary and sufficient causes of disease.

Classical autosomal dominant inheritance

Most deleterious dominant alleles are rare; otherwise, natural selection would have removed them. As a result, the probability that an individual is a homozygous carrier is extremely small and can be ignored. For the purposes of this discussion, we also assume that the gene is fully penetrant, with no phenocopies ($Pr(Y \mid dd) = 0$ and $Pr(Y \mid dD) = 1$). It follows that a case must be a carrier Dd. Since the disease allele is rare, it is unlikely that two carriers will mate, so the only matings of interest will be $dD \times dd$. Following the Mendelian transition probabilities (Table 3.3), it also follows that one-half of the offspring of such matings will be dd and one-half dD. Assuming complete penetrance and no phenocopies, it further follows that on average, half of the offspring of a case will be affected and half not (obviously this will vary in any specific family due to chance). Other consequences of the above assumptions are as follows:

1. All affected individuals will have at least one affected parent, so the disease will appear in all generations.
2. Males and females will be affected equally.
3. Males and females will both transmit the disease to their offspring.
4. The disease does not appear in the descendants of two normal persons.

These principles are illustrated in Figure 3.2. Note how the disease appears in every generation, with a single affected parent in each mating that has affected offspring and about half of all offspring of such matings being affected. (Following the standard conventions for pedigrees, males are denoted by squares, females by circles, and affected individuals are shaded. Parents are connected by a horizontal line, with their descendants arrayed below them.)

These are the cardinal features that geneticists use to infer that a disease has an autosomal dominant mode of inheritance. However, it must be emphasized that the presence of phenocopies and/or incomplete penetrance will produce exceptions to the above rules. A phenocopy will not transmit the disease to any of his or her descendants, nor will he or she have affected

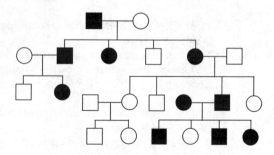

Figure 3.2 Typical pedigree for an autosomal dominant condition.

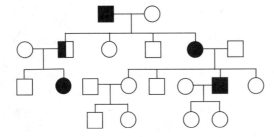

Figure 3.3 An example of reduced penetrance: the left-
shaded individual in the second
generation represents an unaffected carrier.

ancestors (unless they too are phenocopies). Conversely, parents and offspring of a carrier may not themselves be affected, particularly if the disease
is usually not manifest until late in life and the relatives have either died
of other causes or have not yet reached the age of greatest risk. Figure 3.3
illustrates this phenomenon, where individual 2 in generation II is probably
a gene carrier, since he likely was the one who transmitted the mutant allele
to his son but is not himself affected.

Classical autosomal recessive inheritance

We now assume that only the DD genotype is affected, and again assume
full penetrance and no phenocopies. Thus, an affected individual must have
inherited one defective gene from each parent. Most recessive traits are rare,
so parents are unlikely to be homozygotes—the parents are therefore likely
to be $dD \times dD$. Referring again to the transition probabilities in Table 3.3,
we see that $1/4$ of their offspring will be dd, $1/2$ will be dD, and $1/4$ will
be DD. Only the last group will be affected, so $1/4$ of the sibs will also be
affected and $1/2$ will be carriers. If a case marries, it will most likely be
to a dd individual, so none of their offspring will be affected but all will
be carriers. If the trait is rare, carriers are also somewhat uncommon and
$dD \times dD$ matings would be unlikely by chance. Hence, this mating is likely
to have arisen through consanguinity, since family members of a carrier are
more likely than the general population to be carriers themselves. These
principles lead to the following hallmarks of recessive inheritance:

1. Most affected individuals have two normal parents, so the disease appears
   to skip generations.
2. The disease is expressed and transmitted by both sexes.
3. On average, one-quarter of carrier $\times$ carrier offspring will be affected.
4. Consanguinity is more likely among affected families than in the general
   population.
5. Matings between affected and normal individuals yield normal offspring,
   all of whom are carriers.
6. All offspring of affected $\times$ affected matings will be affected.

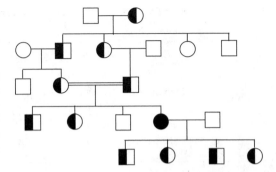

Figure 3.4 Typical recessive pedigree: left-shaded individuals represent unaffected carriers; solid symbols are affected homozygotes; the double horizontal line represents a consanguineous mating.

Again, there are exceptions to these cardinal features if there are phenocopies and/or incomplete penetrance.

These principles are illustrated in Figure 3.4. The double horizontal line in generation III indicates a consanguineous mating between two first cousins, both of whom have inherited the same mutant allele from their grandfather. The half-filled symbols denote carriers who are themselves unaffected. The first affected individual (the fully filled circle) does not appear until generation IV. Note that she has two unaffected carrier siblings and one noncarrier sibling, in accordance with the expected probabilities. If the affected individual in generation IV were to mate with a noncarrier, all her offspring would be unaffected carriers.

Classical X-linked inheritance

Males have one X and one Y chromosome, whereas females have two X chromosomes. In females, only one of the two X chromosomes is expressed, the other being *inactivated* early in development; which copy is inactivated appears to be essentially at random, through the mechanism of DNA methylation (Chapter 12). The mother thus always transmits an X chromosome, whereas the father can transmit either an X or a Y chromosome, thereby determining the sex of the offspring. Now suppose that one of the three parental X chromosomes contains a mutation in a disease-predisposing gene. The result will depend upon three factors:

- Whether the father or the mother was the mutation carrier;
- Whether the offspring was male or female; and
- Whether the gene is dominant or recessive.

The resulting probabilities are shown in Table 3.4. For a dominant X-linked gene, if the mother is affected, she must be a carrier and half of her offspring will be carriers and hence affected, irrespective of their gender, since a single copy of the mutation is sufficient to cause the disease. On

Table 3.4 X-Linked Dominant and Recessive Inheritance

	Dominant Gene			Recessive Gene	
Mother:	Carrier (Affected)	Normal	Mother:	Carrier (Normal)	Normal
Father:	Normal	Carrier (Affected)	Father:	Normal	Carrier (Affected)
Sons:	50% affected	100% normal	Sons:	50% affected	100% normal
Daughters:	50% affected	100% affected	Daughters:	100% normal 50% carriers	100% carriers (normal)

the other hand, if the father is affected, he too must have been a carrier, but he can only transmit the X chromosome to his daughters, all of whom will be affected, while none of his sons will be affected. These patterns are illustrated in Figure 3.5. Note how in the dominant case (A) the affected male transmits the disease to all of his daughters but to none of his sons in generation II. The affected female transmits the disease to half of her sons and half her daughters in generation I.

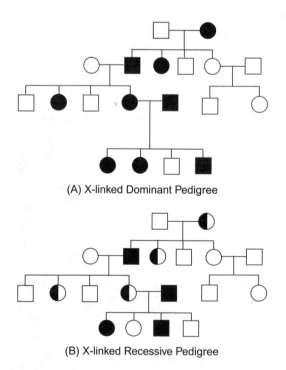

(A) X-linked Dominant Pedigree

(B) X-linked Recessive Pedigree

Figure 3.5 Typical pedigrees for X-linked inheritance: (A) X-linked dominant; (B) X-linked recessive.

For a recessive X-linked gene (Fig. 3.5B) only males are affected. If the mother is a carrier, half of her offspring of either sex will be carriers, but only the males will be affected. An affected father (a carrier) can again transmit the mutation only to his daughters, all of whom will be carriers but unaffected.

Multiallelic loci

Not all genes have only two alleles, while some have very many. An example is the ABO blood group, which has three alleles A, B, and O. Because allele O is dominant over A and B, while A and B are codominant, there are thus four possible phenotypes: O (corresponding to genotype OO), A (genotypes AA and AO), B (genotypes BB and BO), and AB (genotype AB). If we denote the allele frequencies by q_A, q_B, and q_O, then the population prevalances of the four blood groups can be readily computed as:

$$Pr(A) = q_A^2 + 2q_A q_O$$

$$Pr(B) = q_B^2 + 2q_B q_O$$

$$Pr(O) = q_O^2$$

$$Pr(AB) = 2q_A q_B$$

The offspring of O $\times$ AB mating will be equally likely to have blood groups A and B (with genotypes AO and BO, respectively), but the distribution of offspring of other mating types is more complex. For example, an A $\times$ B mating could involve any of the following genotypes

Genotype		Population	Offspring Phenotype Probability			
Father	Mother	Probability	A	B	O	AB
AA	BB	$q_A^2 q_B^2 / S$	0	0	0	1
AA	BO	$2q_A^2 q_B q_O / S$	1/2	0	0	1/2
AO	BB	$2q_A q_B^2 q_O / S$	0	1/2	0	1/2
AO	BO	$4q_A q_B q_O^2 / S$	1/4	1/4	1/4	1/4

where $S = Pr(A)Pr(B)$. Hence, the phenotype probabilities among the off-spring of this mating type would be given by

$$Pr(A | A \times B) = q_A q_B q_O (q_A + q_O)/S$$

$$Pr(B | A \times B) = q_A q_B q_O (q_A + q_O)/S$$

$$Pr(O | A \times B) = q_A q_B q_O^2 / S$$

$$Pr(AB | A \times B) = q_A q_B (q_A + q_O)(q_B + q_O)$$

A similar calculation would apply to the other mating types involving the A or B blood groups.

Mendelian Inheritance at Two Loci

Under Mendel's law of independent assortment, genes at two unlinked loci segregate independently. Thus, an individual who is heterozygous at loci A and B will transmit the four possible combinations of alleles ab, aB, Ab, and AB equally likely. On the other hand, if the two loci are immediately adjacent to each other (tightly linked) so that no recombination is possible, then if one chromosome contains the alleles ab and the other AB, then only the ab or the AB combination will be transmitted (but with equal probability). In between these two extremes, if the two loci are located on the same chromosome but not tightly linked, with recombination fraction is θ, then the ab and AB nonrecombinant haplotypes will be transmitted with probability $(1 - \theta)/2$ each and the recombinanant haplotypes aB and Ab with probability $\theta/2$ each.

Suppose by experimental breeding, we were to cross two inbred lines $aabb$ and $AABB$ to create a generation of double heterozygotes $aAbB$. Suppose as well that the A and B alleles are dominant, so all of this generation would have the A and B phenotypes. If we observed a mating of these AB × AB heterozygotes, we would expect 3/4 of them to have the A phenotype (1/2 with the aA genotype and 1/4 with the AA genotype) and likewise 3/4 of them would have the B phenotype. But the distribution of their *joint* phenotypes would depend upon the recombination fraction, as follows:

Offspring Phenotype	Recombination Fraction		
	1/2	θ	0
ab	1/16	$(1 - \theta)^2/4$	1/4
aB	3/16	$\theta(2 - \theta)/4$	0
Ab	3/16	$\theta(2 - \theta)/4$	0
AB	9/16	$1/2 + (1 - \theta)^2/4$	3/4

Thus, in the case of free recombination (e.g., two loci on the different chromosomes), the probabilities of the two traits are independent; that is, they are the products of the corresponding marginal probabilities. On the other hand, if the two traits are tightly linked, then two traits are always transmitted together.

Conclusions

Few concepts are more central to genetic epidemiology than the complex relationship between genotypes and phenotypes. In this chapter we have illustrated the classical patterns that are easily recognizable in rare Mendelian single-gene disorders with full penetrance and no phenocopies. Most chronic diseases are not like that. Breast cancer, for example, is known to be caused by at least two rare dominant major genes and more common polymorphisms in a number of other genes. Other rare major genes may yet be discovered. Most of these genes have numerous alleles, not just a single mutation. Penetrance is not a single probability for each genotype, but a complex function of age with a relative risk that also varies by age as well as other factors. $G \times E$ and gene–gene ($G \times G$) interactions may well be involved. All these complications make the task of finding genes and characterizing their effects for complex diseases like breast cancer very challenging. These are problems that require the more sophisticated techniques we will consider in the rest of this book.

4

Basic Epidemiologic and Statistical Principles

Throughout this book, we will be relying on a variety of basic epidemiologic concepts and statistical tools that are covered in greater depth in standard textbooks. While it is not essential for the statistical geneticist or genetic epidemiologist to be fully conversant with the mathematical statistics theory underlying these methods, a working knowledge of their use is essential to understand much of what follows. Readers with a strong statistical background can safely skip this chapter, and the applied reader who wishes to delve quickly into the subject might also choose to skip it for now, referring back to it as needed. So that the book can be self-contained, however, the basic tools essential to the material in later chapters are discussed here.

This chapter will cover six basic topics—probability theory, epidemiologic study designs and measures of disease frequency, maximum likelihood, generalized estimating equations, Markov chain Monte Carlo methods, and randomization procedures—as general statistical tools, without at this stage invoking any particular genetic applications. In the chapters that follow, other more specialized statistical methods will be introduced as needed, but the basic approaches are used in many of the methods of familial aggregation, segregation, linkage, and association analysis.

Basic Probability Theory

Before describing the basic approaches to the analysis of epidemiologic data, it is necessary to establish some elementary concepts from probability theory. Let us denote a *random variable* (a quantity that varies between observational units—individuals, times, and so on—in some manner that is not completely predictable) by the symbol Y and use the corresponding lower-case letter y to denote the specific value a particular observation may have. Three kinds of random variables that are particularly important in statistical genetics are binary (dichotomous), count, and continuous variables. A binary variable is one with only two possible values, for example, present ($Y = 1$) or absent ($Y = 0$). A count variable is one that can take any non-negative integer value, such as the number of cases of a binary disease in a group. A continuous variable can take any real value (although possibly over some restricted range, such as only positive numbers).

We refer to the set of probabilities that a random variable can take various values as its *probability density function*. For example, for a binary variable, we might write $p = \Pr(Y = 1)$ and $q = 1 - p = \Pr(Y = 0)$. We say that two random variables, say X and Y, are *independent* if the value of one does not affect the probability distribution for the other. In this case, we can write $\Pr(X = x \text{ and } Y = y) = \Pr(X = x) \Pr(Y = y)$. (From now on, we will write the numerator simply as $\Pr(X = x, Y = y)$, with the comma meaning *and*.) For example, if p is the probability that any random individual in a particular group will have a disease, then the probability that two independent individuals will both have the disease is $p \times p = p^2$. If the disease is infectious, however, and the two individuals were in close contact with each other, then their outcomes would probably not be independent; likewise, if two individuals are genetically unrelated, then their probabilities of carrying a particular mutation or of developing a particular genetic disease are independent, but if they are related to each other, then these probabilities would not be independent. These examples illustrate two different ways dependent data can arise: as a direct causal connection in the case of transmission of an infectious disease or as a result of a shared *latent* (unobserved) variable in the case of a shared ancestry.

For count data, the two most important distributions are the Binomial and Poisson distributions. Suppose that we have a group of $i = 1, \ldots, N$ individuals, each of whom is characterized by a binary random variable Y_i, and let $Y = \sum_i Y_i$ be the number of cases in the group (the number with $Y_i = 1$). Then if each individual's value is independent, with the same probability p, the probability distribution function for Y is given by the binomial distribution, Binom $(Y \mid N, p)$

$$\Pr(Y = y) = \binom{N}{y} p^y (1 - p)^{N-y} = \frac{N!}{y!(N - y)!} p^y (1 - p)^{N-y}$$

where $N! = 1 \times 2 \times \cdots \times (N - 1) \times N$. Now suppose instead that we have some large population in which events (say, disease) occur only rarely at rate λ per unit time, and let Y denote the number of cases over some period of time T. Now the probability distribution function for Y is given by the Poisson distribution:

$$\Pr(Y = y) = e^{-\lambda T}(\lambda T)^y/y!$$

The Poisson distribution can be thought of as the limit of the Binomial distribution as N becomes very large while p becomes very small, converging to $p = \lambda T/N$.

For continuous distributions, the most important probability distribution function is the normal distribution, with density

$$f(y) = \Pr(y \le Y \le y + dy) = \frac{1}{\sqrt{2\pi}\sigma} \exp\left(-\frac{(y-\mu)^2}{2\sigma^2}\right) dy$$

where $\mu = E(Y)$ is the mean and $\sigma^2 = \text{var}(Y) = E(Y - \mu)^2$ is the variance of Y.

Because we are particularly interested in describing the *relationships* between variables that are not independent (or testing hypotheses about whether they are independent), we are frequently interested in their *conditional* probability, $\Pr(Y \mid X)$, that is, the probability of Y given the value of X. For example, we might be interested in the risk of disease Y in the sibling of someone who is affected by the same disease X, $\Pr(Y = 1 \mid X = 1)$. The fundamental law of conditional probability states that

$$\Pr(Y \mid X) = \frac{\Pr(Y, X)}{\Pr(X)}$$

If the two variables were independent, the numerator would become $\Pr(Y)\Pr(X)$, so $\Pr(Y \mid X) = \Pr(Y)$; that is, the probability of Y would not depend on X. By cross-multiplication, the law of conditional probability can also be written as $\Pr(Y, X) = \Pr(Y \mid X)\Pr(X)$. Of course, we could just as well write $\Pr(Y, X) = \Pr(X \mid Y)\Pr(Y)$. Equating these two expressions and solving for $\Pr(Y \mid X)$ leads to the famous *Bayes theorem*,

$$\Pr(Y \mid X) = \frac{\Pr(X \mid Y)\Pr(Y)}{\Pr(X)}$$

which defines the relationship between the two conditional probabilities.

Statistics is the study of the distribution of random variables, of ways of estimating summaries of these distributions, and testing hypotheses about whether the distributions of two or more random variables differ, based on random samples from some larger unobserved population to which we wish to generalize. For example, we might wish to estimate the risk of disease p in some population by obtaining a sample of N individuals from that population and observing the number Y who are affected. The sample proportion Y/N, denoted $\hat{p}$, is an *estimator* of the unknown true population risk p. Likewise, for a continuous variable, the sample average $\bar{Y} = \sum_{i=1}^{N} Y_i/N$ is an estimator of the population mean μ. *Confidence intervals* describe the likely range of possible estimates that could be generated by hypothetical replication of the observations using the same procedures (e.g., with the same sample size and method of sampling).

Generally, we are particularly interested in testing a hypothesis about some particular *null hypothesis* value of a population parameter, again based on some finite sample of observations. For example, we might want to know whether the risk of disease p_1 in a particular subgroup of the population (say, individuals carrying a particular mutation) differs from that in the general population p_0. Then we would write the null hypothesis as $H_0 : p_1 = p_0$. We would then compute some summary statistic (such as the chi-square statistic $(Y - E)^2/E$, where $E = Np_0$) for the observed data and compare that value to the distribution of possible values of the statistic that would be expected in hypothetical replications of the study if the null hypothesis were true. If the observed value is quite unlikely—say, fewer than 5% of these hypothetical replications would be expected to lead to more extreme values—then we would call the result *statistically significant* and quote as the p-value the probability of obtaining by chance a result as extreme as or more extreme than that observed. Note that the p-value should not be interpreted as the probability that the null hypothesis is true. The latter would require agreement on the *prior* probability that the null hypothesis was true (the probability we would have assigned before seeing the data), a consensus on which would be difficult to achieve. Therein lies the difference between classical (*frequentist*) and Bayesian statistics, which we will discuss further below. These basic concepts of probability and statistics are explained in greater detail in virtually any elementary statistics textbook, but this cursory treatment of the subject should be sufficient for the particular applications in genetic epidemiology discussed below.

Basic Epidemiologic Principles

Although continuous phenotypes are occasionally discussed in later chapters, our main focus is on dichotomous disease traits with variable age at onset. Whereas continuous traits are often studied with simple random samples, using standard linear models for normally distributed random variables (possibly after some appropriate transformation), disease traits require the use of specialized sampling designs and methods of survival analysis. This section provides a brief introduction to these principles as they apply to the study of independent individuals in conventional epidemiology rather than to families (the primary focus of the rest of this book). It is necessarily terse, and the reader who wants a more in-depth treatment of these topics might refer to standard epidemiology (Klienbaum et al., 1982; Rothman and Greenland, 1998) and biostatistics (Breslow and Day, 1980, 1987) textbooks.

Study designs

Epidemiologists distinguish two basic types of studies—*descriptive* and *analytical*. Descriptive studies include examination of routinely collected disease rates in relation to basic demographic characteristics (age, gender, race/ethnicity, place of residence, etc.) in the hope of getting clues to possible risk factors. A commonly used approach is the *ecologic correlation* study, in which groups rather than individuals are the unit of analysis and one studies the correlation between disease rates and the prevalence of some characteristic of interest. Examples were discussed in Chapter 1 with regard to the genetic epidemiology of breast cancer. Such studies are often useful for generating hypotheses but are subject to numerous sources of bias and cannot provide rigorous tests of hypotheses. In genetic epidemiology there are relatively few routinely collected characteristics, other than race or ethnicity, that would shed much light on a possible genetic etiology. Even family history is seldom collected in a systematic manner on death certificates or disease registries. Hence, genetic epidemiology, like most other branches of epidemiology, typically relies on analytical studies involving collection of original data on individuals in order to test specific hypotheses in a controlled manner.

The two principal analytical study designs used in traditional risk-factor epidemiology are the *cohort* and *case-control* designs. (We defer discussion of family-based designs to the next chapter.) These are distinguished primarily by the direction of inference: cohort studies reason forward in time from an exposure to disease (in this chapter, we use the word *exposure* in a generic sense to encompass any risk factor—environmental agent, family history, genotype, etc.); in contrast, case-control studies reason backward in time from disease back to possible causes. It is important to understand that it is this direction of inference, not the temporal sequence of data collection, that is conceptually important. Either cohort or case-control studies can be conducted *retrospectively* (using records from the past) or *prospectively* (collecting new observations as they occur in the future). Some authors have used the terms prospective and retrospective to refer to cohort and case-control designs, leading to a confusion we shall try to avoid by restricting these terms to the direction of data collection, not inference.

Cohort study design. Conceptually, the fundamental design in epidemiology (if not the most commonly used one) is the cohort study, in which a cohort of at-risk individuals (currently free of the disease under study) is identified, characterized in terms of their baseline risk factors, and followed over time to identify the subjects who develop disease and thereby estimate the risk of disease in relation to previously measured risk factors. During the follow-up period, changes in risk factors might also be recorded, but this is not an essential element; the important element is that exposure is recorded before disease occurs. This design is generally believed by epidemiologists to be less subject to the selection and information biases to which case-control studies are prone, as discussed below. Nevertheless, for studies of anything but the most common diseases, a cohort study is an ambitious undertaking, generally requiring enrollment of a large cohort (sometimes hundreds of thousands of individuals) and follow-up for many years, with the consequent difficulties of tracing subjects over time and completely ascertaining disease outcomes. For these reasons, the preferred design for most rare diseases is the case-control design discussed in the following paragraph. Use of historical records (retrospective data collection) avoids one of the fundamental challenges of cohort studies, namely, the long period of observation needed. The feasibility of this option depends on the availability of a suitable sampling frame for defining the cohort members in the past, as well as mechanisms for tracking the current status of individuals (including those who have died or moved away in the interim).

Case-control study design. The case-control design begins with ascertainment of a representative series of cases of the disease and a comparable group of individuals from the same population who are free of the disease, and inquires into aspects of their past history that might account for their different outcomes. Frequently controls are selected by being individually matched to each case on established risk factors that are not of particular interest, such as age, gender, and race. The inquiry into possible risk factors might be done by a structured questionnaire or retrieval of medical records, designed in such a way as to avoid any lack of comparability between the quality of information for the two groups, for example by blinding interviewers to whether subjects are cases or controls.

One of the major expenses of a cohort study involves assembling the exposure information on the entire cohort when perhaps only a very small portion of the cohort will develop the disease. For example, in a genetic cohort study, obtaining genotype information on a large cohort can be very expensive indeed. To minimize these costs, an efficient compromise is to obtain this information only on the cases that develop and on a random sample of the rest of the cohort. There are two principal variants of this idea. In the *nested case-control design*, controls are individually matched to each case by random sampling from the set of subjects who are at risk at the time that case occurred; the data are then analyzed as a matched case-control study. (In this scheme, it is possible for a subject to be sampled as a control for more than one case and for a case to serve as a control for an earlier case. Lubin and Gail [1984] show that this scheme leads to unbiased estimation of the relative risk parameter β, while the alternative of excluding cases from eligibility to serve as controls for other cases would lead to a bias away from the null.) In the *case-cohort design* (sometimes known as a *case-base design*), the controls are a random sample of the entire cohort (the *subcohort*) at the time of enrollment, irrespective of whether or not they later became cases; the analysis compares the cases as a group to the controls using a variant of the standard Cox regression model for survival data described below (Prentice, 1986). Advantages of the case-cohort approach are that the same control group can be used for comparison with multiple case groups and that the baseline data on the subcohort can be obtained early in the study while the cases are accumulating (e.g., blood specimens could be obtained and genotyping started without waiting to see who should be sampled as controls). The main disadvantages are that a more complex analysis is required and it can be less efficient than a nested case-control study for long-duration studies with many small strata (Langholz and Thomas, 1990).

Measures of disease frequency and association

Measures of absolute risk. *Risk* is defined as the probability of new disease occurring during some defined time period among a group of individuals free of the disease at the start of the period. Denoting the time period $[0, t]$, we might write the risk as $F(t) = \Pr[Y(t) = 1 \mid Y(0) = 0]$. (Any of a number of time scales might be relevant, such as age, time since the start of observation, or calender year. In etiologic research, age is usually taken as the primary time scale, with year of birth and year of start of the observation being treated as covariates.) Being a probability, risk is a dimensionless quantity between 0 and 1. If in a random sample of N observations from some population at risk we observe Y cases developing during the at-risk period, then we would treat the random variable D as having a binomial distribution

$$\Pr(Y \mid N, F) = \binom{N}{Y} F^Y (1 - F)^{N-Y}$$

and estimate the risk by the sample proportion $\hat{F} = Y \mid N$ with variance $\mathrm{var}(\hat{F}) = Y(N - Y)/N^3$. The chi-square distribution can be used to test the significance of the departure of the observed frequency from some null value $H_0 : F = F_0$ (say, the population risk, for comparison with that observed in the cohort)

$$\frac{(Y - F_0 N)^2}{F_0(1 - F_0)N} \sim \chi_1^2$$

In contrast, a *rate* is based on a probability density, expressed in units of person-time at risk (typically as a rate per 100,000 person-years). The probability density of disease occurrence at any instant of time within the period of observation among individuals free of the disease the instant before is defined as

$$\lambda(t) = \lim_{dt \to 0} \Pr[Y(t + dt) = 1 \mid Y(t) = 0]/dt \tag{4.1}$$

Viewed as a function of time, $\lambda(t)$ is known as a *hazard function*. Incidence and mortality rates used in epidemiology are forms of a hazard rate, often expressed as step functions, constant over some arbitrary grid of age and time intervals. *Incidence* is thus the rate at which new cases are developing in a population previously free of the disease and is distinguished from *prevalence*, which is the proportion of cases in the population at any particular point in time. (Prevalence combines the incidence of the disease and its average duration—for a chronic disease, the average survival time. It is thus not a very useful measure for etiologic research because a risk factor could be associated with prevalence by having an effect on case fatality without having any effect on incidence.) Now suppose that the $i = 1, \ldots, N$ individuals have each been observed from time 0 to t_i (where t_i denotes the time of disease occurrence, loss to follow-up, or termination of the study, whichever comes first), and let $T = \sum_i t_i$ be the total person-time of observation. Now the number of events has a Poisson distribution

$$Y \sim \text{Poisson}(\lambda T) = e^{-\lambda T}(\lambda T)^Y / Y!$$

and we would estimate the incidence or hazard rate as $\hat{\lambda} = Y/T$ with variance $\text{var}(\hat{\lambda}) = Y/T^2$.

Risks and rates are related by the fundamental relationships:

$$S(t) = \exp\left(-\int_0^t \lambda(u) \, du\right) \tag{4.2}$$

$$\lambda(t) = -\frac{dS(t)/dt}{S(t)}$$

where $S(t) = 1 - F(t) = \Pr[Y(t) = 0 \mid Y(0) = 0]$ is known as the *survival function*. The survival function can be estimated in a number of ways. Using individual data, the *Kaplan-Meier* or *product-limit* estimator of the survival curve is given by $\hat{S}(t) = \prod_{i \mid t_i < t}(1 - Y_i/R_i)$, where Y_i is an indicator of whether subject i developed the disease and R_i is the number of subjects who are still at risk (free of disease and under observation) at age t_i. This estimate is a step function, with discontinuous drops at the observed event times. Alternatively, one could start with a grouped time estimator of the incidence rate $\hat{\lambda}_k = Y_k/T_k$ for some categorization of the time axis (say, 5-year intervals Δ_k) and compute the survival function as $\hat{S}(t_k) = \exp(\sum_{j \le k} \hat{\lambda}_k \Delta_k)$. Both of these approaches estimate the probability of remaining free of disease absent *competing risks*, that is, assuming that one does not die of some unrelated cause first. To estimate the lifetime risk of disease or the probability of developing disease at any specific age, allowing for competing risks, the *lifetable* method is used. Let $\mu(t)$ denote the risk of dying of causes other than the disease of interest and assume that the two causes *compete independently*. Then the probability of developing the disease at age t is $f(t) = \lambda(t) \exp(- \int_0^t [\lambda(u) + \mu(u)] \, du)$ and the cumulative risk of disease to age T is $F(T) = \int_0^T f(t) \, dt$. Thus, the lifetime risk is $F(\infty)$. These calculations are illustrated for breast cancer mortality in Table 4.1.

Table 4.1 Calculation of Age-Specific and Lifetime Risk of Dying of Breast Cancer Using the Lifetable Method

Age Interval	Mortality Rate per 100,000 Breast	All Other	Probability of Surviving Interval	Cumulative	Risk of Breast Cancer During	Cumulative
0–4	0.0	256.3	0.9873	0.9873	0.00000	0.00000
5–9	0.0	23.5	0.9988	0.9861	0.00000	0.00000
10–14	0.0	22.6	0.9989	0.9850	0.00000	0.00000
15–19	0.0	50.4	0.9975	0.9825	0.00000	0.00000
20–24	0.2	58.2	0.9971	0.9796	0.00001	0.00001
25–29	1.3	65.8	0.9967	0.9764	0.00006	0.00007
30–34	4.9	82.6	0.9956	0.9721	0.00024	0.00031
35–39	11.8	114.7	0.9937	0.9660	0.00057	0.00088
40–44	22.2	80.5	0.9949	0.9610	0.00107	0.00195
45–49	37.3	267.8	0.9849	0.9465	0.00177	0.00371
50–54	54.6	424.3	0.9763	0.9241	0.00252	0.00624
55–59	70.4	665.7	0.9639	0.8907	0.00314	0.00937
60–64	83.6	1044.9	0.9451	0.8418	0.00352	0.01289
65–69	95.7	1592.0	0.9191	0.7737	0.00370	0.01659
70–74	110.2	2517.9	0.8769	0.6784	0.00374	0.02033
75–79	125.4	4022.2	0.8127	0.5514	0.00346	0.02379
80–84	146.4	6750.5	0.7083	0.3906	0.00286	0.02665
85–89	185.7	14339.7	0.4837	0.1889	0.00175	0.02840

Source: U.S. females, all races, 1969–1999, from http://www.seer.cancer.gov.canques/

Observe that by age 90, the cumulative risk of dying of breast cancer is about 2.8%; continuing the calculations beyond this age (assuming that the death rates remain constant), the lifetime risk eventually converges to 3.0%. This is substantially smaller than the estimated 12% lifetime risk of developing breast cancer.

In genetic epidemiology, we are primarily concerned with rates and risks in individuals classified by genotype. These are the penetrances. In particular, the probability that an individual with genotype $G = g$ has remained free of disease until age t would be $S_g(t)$, and the probability that an individual develops disease at age t would be $\lambda_g(t)S_g(t)$.

Measures of relative risk. The term *relative risk* (*RR*) is used in a variety of ways, depending on the context, but generally refers to the ratio of risks or rates between groups differing with respect to some risk factor. For example, in the next chapter, we define the *familial relative risk* (the ratio of risks between those with and without a family history) and the *genetic relative risk* (the ratio of risks between those carrying and not carrying a susceptible genotype). In its simplest form, *RR* might be defined as a ratio of risks, $F_1(T)/F_0(T)$, comparing individuals with or without some risk factor, or as a ratio of rates (*hazard ratio*) $\lambda_1(t)/\lambda_0(t)$. A constant *RR* model assumes that these quantities do not vary over time, although there are numerous examples in which they do—for example, the decline in the genetic and familial relative risks of breast cancer with age mentioned in Chapter 1. In many contexts, a more useful measure of association between some risk factor and disease is the *odds ratio* (*OR*)

$$OR = \frac{F_1(T)/[1 - F_1(T)]}{F_0(T)/[1 - F_0(T)]}$$

or the ratio of the *odds* of disease between those with and without the risk factor. For a rare disease, the *OR* approximates the risk ratio, but more important, under appropriate circumstances, it provides an estimator of the hazard ratio even without the rare disease assumption (Greenland and Thomas, 1982).

Epidemiologic data from cohort or case-control studies are frequently presented in the form of a 2×2 contingency table, as in Table 4.2. Using these data, a test of the null hypothesis $H_0 : OR = 1$ is given by the chi-square test

$$X^2 = \frac{[A - \mathrm{E}(A)]^2}{\mathrm{E}(A)} + \frac{[B - \mathrm{E}(B)]^2}{\mathrm{E}(B)} + \frac{[C - \mathrm{E}(C)]^2}{\mathrm{E}(C)} + \frac{[D - \mathrm{E}(D)]^2}{\mathrm{E}(D)}$$

$$= \frac{(AD - BC)^2 N}{(A + B)(A + C)(B + D)(C + D)}$$

Table 4.2 Presentation of Data from a Cohort Study or an Unmatched Case-Control Study of a Binary Risk Factor

Risk	Disease Status	
Factor	Unaffected ($Y = 0$)	Affected ($Y = 1$)
Absent ($Z = 0$)	A	B
Present ($Z = 1$)	C	D

where $E(A) = (A + B)(A + C)/N$ and so on. Under the null hypothesis, X^2 has asymptotically (i.e., in large samples) a chi-square distribution on 1 degree of freedom (df) (henceforth, we write statements like this as $X^2 \sim \chi_1^2$). A continuity correction of $-N/2$ is usually added to $|AD - BC|$ in the numerator to allow for the discreteness of the possible values of the chi-square test for a given sample size. In small samples, a more appropriate procedure for significance testing is *Fisher's exact test,* which takes the form

$$\Pr(X > A \mid A + B, A + C, N) = \sum_{X=A+1}^{\min(A+B, A+C, A-D)} \Pr(X \mid A + B, A + C, N)$$

where

$$\Pr(X \mid A+B, A+C, N) = \frac{A! \; B! \; C! \; D!}{X! \, (A + B - X)! \, (A + C - X)! \, (D - A + X)! \, N!}$$

The *OR* is estimated as AD/BC and its asymptotic variance as

$$\mathrm{var}(\ln OR) = \frac{1}{A} + \frac{1}{B} + \frac{1}{C} + \frac{1}{D}$$

A confidence interval with $100 - \alpha$ percent coverage is then given by

$$\exp[\ln OR \pm Z_{\alpha/2}\sqrt{\mathrm{var}(\ln OR)}]$$

Of course, there could be more than two categories of exposure, for example, zero, one, or more than one affected first-degree family member in a study of familial aggregation or the three possible genotypes in a gene association study; the relevant degrees of freedom of the chi-square test would then be one fewer than the number of categories.

For pair-matched case-control studies, the data presentation needs to keep the matched pairs intact rather than tabulate independent individuals, as shown in Table 4.3. Here the McNemar estimator of the *OR* is given by b/c with asymptotic variance

$$\mathrm{var}(\ln(OR)) = \frac{1}{b} + \frac{1}{c}$$

Table 4.3 Presentation of Data from a Matched Case-Control Study of Familial Aggregation

Control	Case Risk Factor		
Risk Factor	Absent	Present	Total
Absent	a	b	C
Present	c	d	D
Total	A	B	N

and significance test under H_0

$$\frac{(b-c)^2}{b+c} \sim \chi_1^2 \tag{4.3}$$

Here the appropriate continuity correction to $|b - c|$ in the numerator is $-1/2$. The corresponding exact test would be

$$\Pr(X > B \,|\, B + C) = \sum_{X=B+1}^{B+C} \text{Binom}\left(X \,|\, N, \frac{1}{2}\right)$$

$$= \sum_{X=B+1}^{B+C} \frac{(B+C)!}{X! \, (B+C-X)! \, 2^{B+C}}$$

For a cohort study, in which individuals might be followed over a long and variable length of time and a range of ages, the standard method of data analysis is the *standardized incidence ratio* (SIR, or, for mortality, the *standardized mortality ratio, SMR*). One begins by tabulating each individual's time at risk over a two-dimensional array of ages and calendar years (e.g., 5-year intervals), known as a *Lexis diagram* (Fig. 4.1) to obtain the total person-time T_{zs} in each age-year stratum s and exposure category z. Next, one tabulates the number of observed cases Y_z in each exposure category and compares them with the corresponding numbers expected E_z on the basis of a set of standard age-year specific incidence rates λ_s by multiplying these rates by the total person-time and summing over strata, $E_z = \sum_s \lambda_s T_{zs}$. (Standard rates might come from some external source, like national death rates or incidence rates from a disease registry, or from the cohort under study as a whole, ignoring the exposure classification.) The data are typically displayed as shown in Table 4.4. The SIR for each exposure category is defined as the ratio of observed to expected events and the standardized *RR* as the ratio of SIRs between exposure categories.

Measures of interaction. By *interaction* or *effect modification* we mean a variation in some measure of the effect of an exposure on disease risks across the levels of some third variable W, known as a *modifier* (Fig. 4.2). For

Table 4.4 Presentation of Data from a Cohort Study Using the Standardized Incidence Ratio (*SIR*) Method

Exposure Status	Cases		Incidence Rate Ratio	SRR
	Observed	Expected		
Unexposed	Y_0	$E_0 = \sum_s \lambda_s T_{0s}$	$SIR_0 = Y_0/E_0$	1
Exposed	Y_1	$E_1 = \sum_s \lambda_s T_{1s}$	$SIR_1 = Y_1/E_1$	SIR_1/SIR_0

SRR, standardized relative risk.

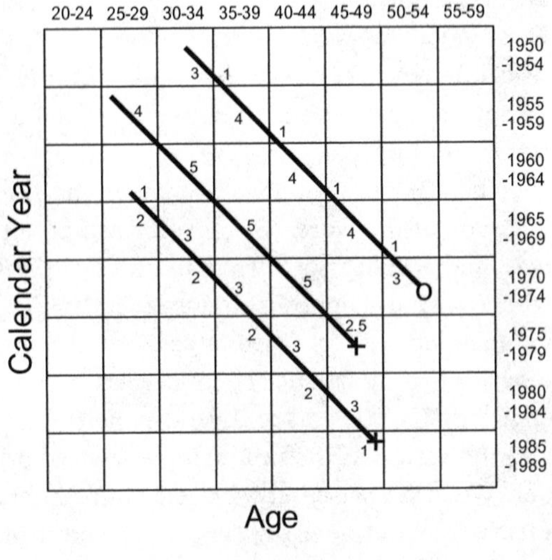

Figure 4.1 Lexis diagram illustrating the calculation of events and person-time at risk in a cohort study. Diagonal lines represent periods of time and ages of individuals at risk, terminating in either an event (denoted by a +) or censoring (denoted by o).

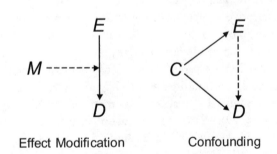

Effect Modification   Confounding

Figure 4.2 Schematic representation of effect modification (left panel) and confounding (right panel). *E* denotes exposure, *D* disease, *M* a modifier, and *C* a confounder. In effect modification, the variable *M* modifies the strength of the true relationship between *E* and *D*. In confounding, the variable *C* induces a spurious association between *E* and *D* or distorts the strength of that relationship by being associated with both.

73

example, the relative risk of breast cancer for being a *BRCA1* mutation carrier varies from over 50 in women under age 40 to less than 10 in women over 70 (Claus et al., 1991), so we would call age a modifier of the effect of carrier status. The definition of interaction depends on the measure of association used. As we will see in Chapter 6, the *excess* risk (the difference in annual incidence rates between carriers and noncarriers) is nearly constant across the age range. Hence, age is a modifier of the *RR* but not of the excess risk. In general, the absence of interaction on a scale of *RR* corresponds to a multiplicative model for the joint effect of the two factors, that is, $R(Z, W) = R_0 \times RR_Z \times RR_W$, whereas the absence of interaction on a scale of excess risk corresponds to an additive model $R(Z, W) = R_0 + ER_Z + ER_W$, where $R(Z, W)$ represents some measure of risk (lifetime risk, hazard rate, etc.), R_0 the risk in the absence of exposure to both factors, RR the relative risk for the indicated factor, and ER the corresponding excess risk.

There is a philosophical debate in the epidemiologic literature about the meaning of the word *synergy;* some reserve this term for any joint effect of two factors that is greater than additive (Rothman and Greenland, 1998), whereas others apply it to any departure from some biological model for independent effects (Siemiatycki and Thomas, 1981). In genetic epidemiology, we are particularly concerned with two kinds of interaction: gene–environment ($G \times E$) and gene–gene ($G \times G$), although, of course, we are also interested in the modifying effects of other variables like age and gender. We distinguish between *qualitative* interaction, where the effect of one variable is completely absent in one stratum or the other or even goes in the opposite direction, and *quantitative* interaction, where the effect is in the same direction in all strata but varies in magnitude. These issues are discussed further in Chapter 11.

Simple descriptive analyses of interaction effects can be accomplished by stratifying the analysis into categories of the modifier, estimating the association and its variance in each stratum, and comparing the magnitudes of the two strata. For example, if, in a case-control study, the odds ratios in two strata of the modifier were OR_1 and OR_2, with the variances of $\ln OR$ being V_1 and V_2, respectively, then we might take the ratio of the two ORs, $\psi = OR_1/OR_2$, as a measure of interaction. The variance $\mathrm{var}(\ln \psi) = V_1 + V_2$, so we could test the null hypothesis of no interaction (constancy of the OR) $H_0 : \psi = 1$ by testing $\ln \hat{\psi}/\sqrt{\mathrm{var}(\ln \hat{\psi})}$ against a normal distribution. Confidence limits on ψ would be obtained in the usual way as $\exp[\ln \hat{\psi} \pm \sqrt{\mathrm{var}(\ln \hat{\psi})}]$ for large enough sample sizes (i.e., *asymptotically*). Note, however, that the finding of a significant effect in one stratum but not in another does not necessarily imply interaction: the sample size in one or both subgroups might simply be too small to attain significance even though the magnitude of the effects did not differ by much; or differences might appear large but might be quite unstable due to inadequate sample sizes. Hence a claim of an interaction should be reserved for situations where the two estimates actually differ from each other in an appropriate significance test.

Multivariate models for disease risk. Disease risks are seldom describable by a single number, but depend in complex ways on age and a variety of risk factors, genetic or environmental. Letting $\mathbf{Z} = (Z_1, \ldots, Z_k)$ denote a vector of k measurable risk factors (which could include genotype(s)) and $\boldsymbol{\beta} = (\beta_1, \ldots, \beta_p)$ a vector of corresponding regression coefficients, two widely used multivariate models are the *logistic model* for binary traits

$$\Pr(Y = 1 \mid \mathbf{Z}) = \frac{\exp(\beta_0 + \mathbf{Z}'\boldsymbol{\beta})}{1 + \exp(\beta_0 + \mathbf{Z}'\boldsymbol{\beta})} \tag{4.4}$$

or equivalently

$$\text{logit } \Pr(Y = 1 \mid \mathbf{Z}) = \ln\left(\frac{\Pr(Y = 1 \mid \mathbf{Z})}{\Pr(Y = 0 \mid \mathbf{Z})}\right) = \beta_0 + \mathbf{Z}'\boldsymbol{\beta}$$

and the *proportional hazards model* for censored age-at-onset traits

$$\lambda(t \mid \mathbf{Z}) = \lambda_0(t) \exp(\mathbf{Z}'\boldsymbol{\beta}) \tag{4.5}$$

where $\lambda_0(t)$ can be an arbitrary function of time. These models are generally fitted using the technique of maximum likelihood, described below. In later chapters, we will discuss how these models can be used to describe joint effects of age, genes, and environmental factors, including $G \times E$ and $G \times G$ interactions.

Multivariate models are particularly flexible ways of examining interaction effects. For example, suppose that we are interested in a $G \times E$ interaction, where we have coded both G and E as binary variables (carrier vs. noncarrier, exposed vs. unexposed). Then we need only replace the exponential terms in Eq. (4.4) or (4.5) by $\exp(\beta_0 + \beta_1 G + \beta_2 E + \beta_3 GE)$ (in the proportional hazards model, the term β_0 would be replaced by the $\lambda_0(t)$ factor). Here β_1 is the ln OR for the effect of genotype in the absence of exposure, β_2 is the ln OR for the effect of exposure in noncarriers, and $\beta_3 = \ln(\psi)$ is the logarithm of the interaction effect. Thus, the OR in exposed carriers (relative to unexposed noncarriers) would be $\exp(\beta_1 + \beta_2 + \beta_3)$. Of course, more complex patterns of interaction (say, among continuous or multi-level categorical variables or three-way or higher-order interactions) can easily be added by appropriate specification of the covariates $\mathbf{Z}$ to be included in the model. In practice, however, epidemiologic studies seldom offer much power for testing more than two-way interactions.

Interpretation of epidemiologic associations

As practitioners of an observational science, epidemiologists do not generally have the opportunity to test hypotheses by conducting controlled experiments relying on randomization to ensure comparability of the groups compared. Hence, the associations between risk factors and disease found in epidemiologic studies are subject to a wide range of potential biases and do not necessarily indicate causation (see pp. 49–50). Epidemiologists have developed a series of criteria for judging when an inference of causality is warranted from an observed association, of which the most famous are those outlined by Sir Austin Bradford Hill (1965) and incarnated in most modern epidemiology textbooks. Most relevant to genetic epidemiology is freedom from bias, which is generally divided into three types:

- *Selection bias:* any of a number of study design aspects that would tend to make the groups sampled not representative of their respective source populations (e.g., using hospital controls to represent the population of unaffected individuals);
- *Information bias:* any of a number of study design aspects that would tend to make the quality of the information obtained on subjects noncomparable between the groups compared (e.g., recall bias in a case-control study, where cases might tend to recall past exposures differently from unaffected individuals); and
- *Confounding:* distortion of a true relationship by the action of another variable that is associated with exposure in the source population and, conditional on exposure, is also an independent risk factor for disease. (We emphasize that confounding is a very different phenomenon from effect modification, discussed above, although both involve the joint relationship among two determinants of disease risks; see Fig. 4.2).

Generally, cohort studies are believed to be less susceptible to selection and information bias than case-control studies, because the cohort is enrolled as a single group and everyone is followed in the same way, and because the exposure information is obtained prior to the onset of disease. But cohort studies are not immune to bias; for example, usually some individuals are lost to follow-up, and the probability of being lost may depend on exposure or disease status. These issues must be considered as carefully in designing a genetic epidemiology study as any other.

Probably the most important confounders in genetic studies are race and ethnicity. Many genes have substantial variation in allele frequencies between different ethnic groups (Cavalli-Sforza et al., 1994), and there can also be substantial variation in baseline risks of disease that are unrelated to the gene of study (recall, for example, the data on international and ethnic variation in breast cancer rates in Figs. 1.1 and 1.2; similar data on colorectal cancer will be presented in Chapter 12). The relation of both genotypes and disease risks to ethnicity can easily produce spurious associations that are a reflection of some other aspect of ethnicity (e.g., diet, environmental exposures, cultural practices). Epidemiologists attempt to control confounding by matching, stratified analysis (e.g., the SIR discussed earlier), covariate adjustment (e.g., the logistic model), or restriction to homogeneous populations. We will discuss this issue further in Chapter 9, including ways of using family studies or molecular methods to get around this problem.

Maximum Likelihood

Many methods in genetics are based on the principle of maximum likelihood, a very general approach to fitting any kind of statistical model. By a *model*, we mean a probability density function $f(Y \mid \Theta)$ for a set of observations Y_i in relation to a vector of parameters Θ. For example, in ordinary linear regression, one might write $f(Y_i \mid \mathbf{Z}_i; \Theta) = \mathcal{N}(Y_i - \mathbf{Z}_i' \boldsymbol{\beta}, \sigma^2)$, where $\mathbf{Z}_i$ is a vector of covariates for the ith subject, $\Theta = (\boldsymbol{\beta}, \sigma^2)$ are the regression coefficients and residual variance one wishes to estimate, and $\mathcal{N}$ denotes the normal density function. Then if a set of $i = 1, \ldots, N$ observations are independent, one would form the *likelihood function* as the product of these probabilities,

$$\mathcal{L}(\Theta) = f(\mathbf{Y} \mid \mathbf{Z}, \Theta) = \prod_{i=1}^{N} \mathcal{N}(Y_i - \mathbf{Z}_i' \boldsymbol{\beta}, \sigma^2)$$

which is now viewed as a function of the parameters Θ conditional on the observed data, rather than the reverse.

For example, consider a sample of observations of a continuous phenotype $Y_i (i = 1, \ldots, N)$ that is normally distributed, with unknown mean μ and unknown variance σ^2. The likelihood is

$$\mathcal{L}(\mu, \sigma^2) = \frac{1}{(\sqrt{2\pi}\sigma)^N} \exp\left(-\sum_{i=1}^{N} \frac{(Y_i - \mu)^2}{2\sigma^2} \right)$$

We will see shortly that this yields an estimator of $\hat{\mu} = \sum_i Y_i / N$ and $\hat{\sigma}^2 = \sum_i (Y_i - \hat{\mu})^2 / N$.

In the problems we typically encounter in genetics, the observations on family members are *dependent*, requiring more complex likelihood functions, perhaps based on multivariate distributions or summations of distributions of unobserved *latent* variables, such as genotypes. For example, in Chapter 5, we will introduce a variance components model for a vector $\mathbf{Y}_i = (Y_{i1}, \ldots, Y_{i\mathcal{J}_i})$ of phenotypes of the $\mathcal{J}_i$ members of family i of the form

$$\mathcal{L}(\boldsymbol{\Theta}) = \prod_{i=1}^{N} \mathcal{N}_{\mathcal{J}_i}[\mathbf{Y}_i - \mu, \mathbf{C}_i(\boldsymbol{\Theta})]$$

where $\mathcal{N}_{\mathcal{J}}(,)$ denotes the $\mathcal{J}$-dimensional multivariate normal density and $\mathbf{C}_i(\boldsymbol{\Theta})$ represents a covariance matrix composed of various environmental and genetic variance components that are to be estimated. In Chapter 6, we will introduce the basic segregation analysis likelihood for a major gene model of the form

$$\mathcal{L}(\boldsymbol{\Theta}) = \prod_{i=1}^{N} \sum_{\mathbf{g}} \Pr(\mathbf{Y}_i, \mathbf{G} = \mathbf{g} \mid \boldsymbol{\Theta})$$

where $\boldsymbol{\Theta}$ now comprises such parameters as the population allele frequency q in $\Pr(G)$ and the penetrances in $\Pr(Y \mid G)$. In Chapter 7, the parameter of primary interest will be the recombination fraction, denoted θ. I will defer further discussion of the specification of these likelihood functions until the later chapters and here concentrate on their general uses for testing hypotheses about the parameters and for point and interval estimation. Thus, in the remainder of this section, we simply let $\mathbf{Y}$ denote the observed data and Θ a generic parameter (or vector of parameters) to be estimated.

The principle of maximum likelihood states that for any model, we prefer the value of Θ for which it is most likely that we would have observed the data (i.e., which maximizes the likelihood function; this value is known as the *maximum likelihood estimate (MLE)* and is denoted $\hat{\Theta}$. This is not the most likely value of Θ, given the data, *unless all parameter values were equally likely before the data were seen*. The value that would maximize the posterior probability given the data, $\Pr(\Theta \mid \mathbf{Y})$, is called the *posterior mode;* its calculation would require specification of a prior distribution for parameters $\Pr(\Theta)$. Then by the Bayes formula, the posterior distribution is proportional to

$$\Pr(\Theta \mid \mathbf{Y}) = \frac{\Pr(\mathbf{Y} \mid \Theta)\,\Pr(\Theta)}{\Pr(\mathbf{Y})} \propto \mathcal{L}(\Theta)\,\Pr(\Theta)$$

I shall return to this approach to estimation when we explore Bayesian methods later, but for now, I shall focus on to maximum likelihood methods.

In most cases, it turns out to be more convenient to work with the logarithm of the likelihood rather than the likelihood itself. Because the log transformation is monotonic, it follows that the value $\hat{\Theta}$ that maximizes the loglikelihood function $\ell(\Theta) = \ln[\mathcal{L}(\Theta)]$ will also maximize the likelihood function $\mathcal{L}(\Theta)$. Since most likelihood functions are products of contributions from a set of independent observations, the loglikelihood becomes a sum of independent contributions, whose derivatives are more easily found than the derivative of a product. Furthermore, since often these contributions are members of the *exponential family* of distributions, their loglikelihood contributions are simple in form. The maximum of a function is found by setting its slope equal to zero. The slope of the loglikelihood is known as the *score function*, denoted $U(\Theta)$, and the expression

$$U(\Theta) \equiv \frac{\partial \ell(\Theta)}{\partial \Theta} = 0$$

is called an *estimating equation*. In the example of the normally distributed phenotype, to find the MLE of μ we would solve this equation as follows:

$$\ell(\mu, \sigma^2) = -n \ln \sqrt{2\pi}\sigma - \sum_{i=1}^{N} \frac{(Y_i - \mu)^2}{2\sigma^2}$$

$$U_\mu(\mu, \sigma^2) = \frac{\partial \ell}{\partial \mu} = 2 \sum_{i=1}^{N} \frac{Y_i - \mu}{2\sigma^2} = 0$$

$$\sum_{i=1}^{N} Y_i - N\mu = 0$$

$$\hat{\mu} = \sum_{i=1}^{N} Y_i / N$$

the familiar sample mean estimator of the population mean. Similarly, setting $U_\sigma(\mu, \sigma^2)$ to zero yields the MLE for σ^2 given earlier, with the sum of squares divided by N rather than the unbiased estimator using $N - 1$ in the denominator. (MLEs are theoretically *Fisher consistent*, meaning that they converge to the true value as the sample size goes to infinity but are not guaranteed to be unbiased in small samples.)

Finding the MLE usually requires iterative methods because the estimating equations cannot usually be solved in closed form (at least for the complex genetic likelihoods we will be concerned with). The most commonly used technique is the *Newton-Raphson method,* which basically constructs a better estimate at each cycle by moving along a straight line in the direction of increasing likelihood, as viewed from the perspective of the current estimate. The Newton-Raphson method uses the *Fisher information,* the negative of the expectation of the matrix of second derivatives,

$$\imath(\Theta) = -E_Y[\partial^2 \mathcal{L}(\Theta)/\partial\Theta^2]$$

replacing the current estimate of Θ by a new estimate

$$\Theta' = \Theta + U(\Theta)\,\imath^{-1}(\Theta)$$

and continues by computing new values of $\mathbf{U}(\Theta')$ and $\imath(\Theta')$ and repeating this updating procedure until no further changes result. This process is illustrated in Figure 4.3. Starting with an initial guess θ_0, we fit a tangent line through the curve $U(\theta)$ at that point, which has a height $U(\theta_0)$ and a slope $\imath(\theta_0)$. This tangent line crosses the θ-axis at the point θ_1. Drawing a

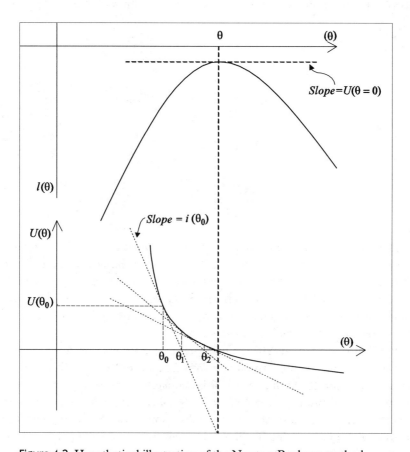

Figure 4.3 Hypothetical illustration of the Newton-Raphson method.

new tangent line at θ_1 and extending it back to the axis yields a new estimate θ_2 and so on.

Unfortunately, unlike most of the likelihoods used in epidemiology, genetic likelihoods may have multiple maxima, and the Newton-Raphson method may converge to a local maximum rather than the global maximum. Hence, it may be desirable to perform the maximization several times from different starting values to see if the values converge to the same maximum. Finding the global maximum requires more sophisticated methods that are beyond the scope of this book (see, e.g., Press et al., 1992, for computational algorithms).

Having found the MLE, we wish to put confidence bounds around it and to test the statistical significance of various hypotheses. Confidence limits are usually determined in one of two ways. The first is based on assuming that asymptotically the likelihood function is approximately normal and uses the asymptotic variance derived from Fisher information, specifically,

$$\operatorname{var}(\hat{\Theta}) = \imath^{-1}(\hat{\Theta}) \tag{4.6}$$

and the standard error of the pth component is $SE(\hat{\Theta}_p) = \sqrt{\imath^{pp}(\hat{\Theta})}$, the pth diagonal element of the inverse of the $\imath$ matrix. For a one-parameter model, this standard error is simply $1/\sqrt{\imath(\hat{\Theta})}$. Thus, the asymptotic $(1 - \alpha)$ confidence limits on $\hat{\Theta}_p$ are simply

$$\hat{\Theta}_p \pm Z_{\alpha/2} SE(\hat{\Theta}_p) = \hat{\Theta}_p \pm Z_{\alpha/2} \sqrt{\imath^{pp}(\hat{\Theta})} \tag{4.7}$$

(see Fig. 4.4A). These are commonly known as *Wald confidence limits* because of their connection with the Wald test described below; by construction they are always symmetric around the MLE. *Likelihood-based limits* are defined as those values for which the likelihood ratio test (given below) is exactly significant, are superior to those based on the asymptotic variance, but require further iterative search and are not widely used in genetics because of their computational difficulty. In multiparameter models, it may be important to show the full confidence region if the components are highly correlated (Fig. 4.4B), but this is difficult to do in more than two dimensions.

Hypothesis testing is done to compare alternative models where one is a special case of the other. Thus, for a given model form, we view the specific models generated by different values of the parameters as a family of models and wish to determine whether we can reject a specific null hypothesis H_0: $\Theta = \Theta_0$. For example, in linkage analysis we are interested in testing the null hypothesis $H_0: \theta = 0.5$, where θ denotes the recombination fraction. There are three tests available to do this based on likelihood theory: the *likelihood*

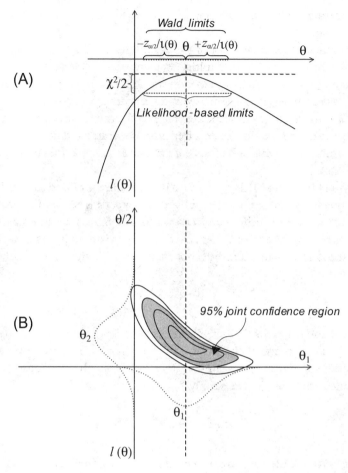

Figure 4.4 Hypothetical illustration of confidence limits based on the likelihood function. (A) A one-parameter model showing Wald limits (dashed interval) and likelihood ratio limits (dotted interval). (B) A two-parameter model showing the joint confidence region.

ratio (LR) test, the *score test,* and the *Wald test:*

$$G^2 = 2\ln[\mathcal{L}(\hat{\Theta})/\mathcal{L}(\Theta_0)] = 2[\ell(\hat{\Theta}) - \ell(\Theta_0)] \quad \text{LR test}$$

$$X^2 = \mathbf{U}(0)'\, \imath^{-1}(0)\, \mathbf{U}(0) \qquad\qquad\qquad \text{Score test}$$

$$Z^2 = \hat{\Theta}'\, \imath(\hat{\Theta})\, \hat{\Theta} \qquad\qquad\qquad\quad \text{Wald test}$$

All three are asymptotically equivalent—not in the sense that they give identical answers on any individual data set, but in the sense that in large enough samples (*asymptotically*) they will have the same test size and power. The LR test is generally the best behaved in small samples and is the most widely used in genetics. The score test generally converges to its asymptotic distribution faster than the Wald test, which can be seriously misleading when the likelihood is highly skewed. However, the Wald test has the appeal that there is a one-to-one correspondence between the significance test and confidence limits based on Eq. (4.7). Most simple chi-square tests based on a comparison of observed and expected events can be derived as score tests from the appropriate likelihood. These include the tests of familial aggregation and association (Chapters 5 and 9), as well as the nonparametric tests of linkage based on IBD (Chapter 7).

All three tests are distributed as a chi square with df equal to the difference in dimensions between Θ and Θ_0. For example, suppose that we wished to test a null hypothesis of dominant inheritance against the more general codominant model. The general model would have three penetrance parameters $\mathbf{f} = (f_0, f_1, f_2)$ plus an allele frequency q, for four parameters in all. The dominant submodel would constrain $f_1 = f_2$ for a total of three parameters. Thus, the LR test for dominant versus codominant inheritance would have $4 - 3 = 1$ df. On the other hand, suppose that we wanted to test the null hypothesis of no genetic inheritance: then the null hypothesis would be $f_0 = f_1 = f_2$, so the LR test of this hypothesis versus the general codominant model would in principle have 2 df. (It is actually a bit more complicated than this because under this null hypothesis there is no major gene, so the allele frequency q becomes meaningless.)

In some circumstances, the null hypothesis value of a parameter is located on the boundary of the permissible parameter space. An example of this arises in linkage analysis, where the parameter of interest is the recombination fraction θ with $H_0 : \theta = 1/2$ and the admissible range is $0 \leq \theta \leq 1/2$. In this case, the usual asymptotic distribution theory does not apply, and typically the null distribution of the LR and other tests is a mixture of chi-square distributions with differing df (Self and Liang, 1987).

The chi-square distribution is appropriate only for comparing *nested* models, meaning that one of these models is a subset of a more general model. For example, in linear regression, model $M_1 : Y = \alpha + \beta_1 X_1 + \epsilon$ is more general than model $M_0 : Y = \alpha + \epsilon$ and $M_2 : Y = \alpha + \beta_1 X_1 + \beta_2 X_2 + \epsilon$ is even more general; hence, we can compare the likelihood ratio statistics for M_1 with M_0 or M_2 with M_1 as chi squares on 1 df or M_2 with M_0 directly as a chi square on 2 df. However, we cannot directly compare M_2 with $M_3 : Y = \alpha + \beta_1 X_2 + \beta_3 X_3$ because they are not nested—neither is a submodel of the other. In order to make such a comparison, we generally nest both models to be compared in an even more general one that includes both as submodels, for example, $M_4 : Y = \alpha + \beta_1 X_1 + \beta_2 X_2 + \beta_3 X_3 + \epsilon$.

Now all the models M_0–M_3 are submodels of M_4, so in particular we could compare M_2 and M_3 separately to M_4 as 1 df tests. If, for argument's sake, we were to reject M_2 and fail to reject M_3, we could then conclude that M_3 fits significantly better.

Nevertheless, we frequently wish to compare nonnested models to each other directly, without having to compare each of them separately against some more general alternative. This is often done in a descriptive way using the *Akaike Information Criterion: AIC* $= 2\ln(\mathcal{L}) - 2p$ (Akaike, 1973), where p is the number of free parameters in the model. The subtraction of p is intended to reward more parsimonious models, since obviously, with each additional parameter, the likelihood can only increase. We therefore prefer the model with the highest AIC value. A number of alternative criteria have been suggested, including Mallows' (1973) C_p, the *Bayes Information Criterion BIC* $= 2\ln(\mathcal{L}) - \ln(n)p$ (Schwartz, 1978), and the *Risk Inflation Criterion RIC* $= 2\ln(\mathcal{L}) - 2\ln(p)$ (Foster and George, 1994), each of which has certain theoretical advantages (see George and Foster, 2000, for a review), but the AIC remains the most widely used one in genetics.

For historical reasons, geneticists often use a transformation of the LR test known as the *lod score* or *lods*. The lod score is simply the LR test computed using base 10 rather than natural logarithms and without multiplying by 2; hence

$$\text{lods} = \log_{10}[\mathcal{L}(\hat{\theta})/\mathcal{L}(\theta = 0.5)] = \frac{G^2}{2\ln(10) = 4.6}$$

Thus, the 5% significance level for a 1 df test corresponds to an LR test of 3.84 or a lods of 0.83. A lods of 3, widely used as the criterion for considering a linkage *established*, corresponds to a LR chi square of 13.82 or a p-value of 0.0002. The rationale for adopting this value will be discussed in Chapter 7.

Application to disease risk models. We conclude this section with a brief discussion of the use of maximum likelihood to fit the multivariate models for disease risks and rates described earlier. For the logistic model, we would write the likelihood as

$$\mathcal{L}(\boldsymbol{\beta}) = \prod_{i=1}^{N} \frac{\exp[(\beta_0 + \mathbf{Z}_i'\boldsymbol{\beta})Y_i]}{1 + \exp(\beta_0 + \mathbf{Z}_i'\boldsymbol{\beta})}$$

which leads to the score equation

$$\mathbf{U}(\beta) = \sum_i [Y_i - \Pr(Y = 1 \mid \mathbf{Z}_i)]\mathbf{Z}_i$$

where $\Pr(Y = 1 \mid \mathbf{Z}_i)$ is the logistic function of $\boldsymbol{\beta}$ given in Eq. (4.4). Solution of this equation requires use of the Newton-Raphson method.

Matched case-control studies require a matched analysis. Using the logistic model, the *conditional likelihood* for 1:1 matched case-control pairs i (with the second subscript 1 indicating the case and 0 the control) takes the form

$$\mathcal{L}(\boldsymbol{\beta}) = \prod_{i=1}^{N} \Pr(Y_{i1} = 1 \mid \mathbf{Z}_{i0}, \mathbf{Z}_{i1}, Y_{i0} + Y_{i1} = 1)$$

$$= \prod_{i=1}^{N} \frac{\Pr(Y_{i1}=1 \mid \mathbf{Z}_{i1}) \; \Pr(Y_{i0}=0 \mid \mathbf{Z}_{i0})}{\Pr(Y_{i1}=1 \mid \mathbf{Z}_{i1}) \; \Pr(Y_{i0}=0 \mid \mathbf{Z}_{i0}) + \Pr(Y_{i1}=0 \mid \mathbf{Z}_{i1}) \; \Pr(Y_{i0}=1 \mid \mathbf{Z}_{i0})}$$

$$(4.8)$$

$$= \prod_{i=1}^{N} \frac{\left(\frac{\exp(\alpha_i+\mathbf{Z}_{i1}\boldsymbol{\beta})}{1+\exp(\alpha_i+\mathbf{Z}_{i1}\boldsymbol{\beta})}\right)\left(\frac{1}{1+\exp(\alpha_i+\mathbf{Z}_{i0}\boldsymbol{\beta})}\right)}{\left(\frac{\exp(\alpha_i+\mathbf{Z}_{i1}\boldsymbol{\beta})}{1+\exp(\alpha_i+\mathbf{Z}_{i1}\boldsymbol{\beta})}\right)\left(\frac{1}{1+\exp(\alpha_i+\mathbf{Z}_{i0}\boldsymbol{\beta})}\right) + \left(\frac{1}{1+\exp(\alpha_i+\mathbf{Z}_{i1}\boldsymbol{\beta})}\right)\left(\frac{\exp(\alpha_i+\mathbf{Z}_{i0}\boldsymbol{\beta})}{1+\exp(\alpha_i+\mathbf{Z}_{i0}\boldsymbol{\beta})}\right)}$$

$$= \prod_{i=1}^{N} \frac{\exp(\mathbf{Z}_{i1}'\boldsymbol{\beta})}{\exp(\mathbf{Z}_{i0}'\boldsymbol{\beta}) + \exp(\mathbf{Z}_{i1}'\boldsymbol{\beta})}$$

which does not involve the intercept terms α_i. Thus, each matched pair could have a separate baseline risk, reflecting their matching factors. This conditional likelihood can be extended to general $N : M$ matching by replacing the exponential terms by their products over all N cases and summing in the denominator over all subsets of size N from the set of $N + M$ members (Breslow and Day, 1980).

For variable age-at-onset data, the full likelihood is given by

$$\mathcal{L}(\lambda_0, \boldsymbol{\beta}) = \prod_{i=1}^{N} \lambda(t_i \mid \mathbf{Z}_i)^{Y_i} S(t_i \mid \mathbf{Z}_i)$$

where we recall that $S(t \mid \mathbf{Z})$ is the function of $\lambda(t \mid \mathbf{Z})$ given in Eq. (4.2). A specific model, such as the proportional hazards model, Eq. (4.5), could be used with a parametric function for $\lambda_0(t; \boldsymbol{\alpha})$, where $\boldsymbol{\alpha}$ is a set of parameters to be estimated along with $\boldsymbol{\beta}$. Generally, we are more interested in estimating the relative risk parameters $\boldsymbol{\beta}$ than the baseline hazard $\lambda_0(t)$. The Cox (1972) partial likelihood provides an efficient way to estimate $\boldsymbol{\beta}$ without having to make any assumptions at all about the form of the baseline hazard by comparing each case i to the *risk set* R_i comprising all subjects who were at risk at the same time (including the case). The likelihood is given by

$$\mathcal{L}(\beta) = \prod_{i=1}^{N} \left(\frac{\exp(\mathbf{Z}_i' \beta)}{\sum_{j \in R_i} \exp(\mathbf{Z}_j' \beta)} \right)^{Y_i}$$

This likelihood does not even involve the baseline hazard. Again, maximization of the likelihood requires iterative methods.

Generalized Estimating Equations

Generalized estimating equations (GEEs) are a broad class of techniques for the analysis of dependent data based on fitting the moments of the distribution (e.g., means, variances, covariances) of the observed data to their predicted values under the model without having to specify the entire distribution. Essentially, the method is based on a matrix generalization of weighted least squares. Suppose that we let $\mathbf{Y}_i = (Y_{i1}, \ldots, Y_{i\mathcal{J}_i})$ denote a vector of correlated outcomes for observation i. These might represent longitudinal observations on a single individual, but in the genetics context, they might be the phenotypes for the $\mathcal{J}_i$ members of family i. We postulate a model for the expectation $\boldsymbol{\mu}_i(\beta) = \mathrm{E}(\mathbf{Y}_i \mid \beta)$. For example, if Y is a continuous variable and $\mathbf{Z}_i$ denotes a matrix of covariates, we might write $\mu_{ij} = \mathbf{Z}_{ij}'\beta$, whereas if Y is binary, we might use a logistic model, $\mathrm{logit}(\mu_{ij}) = \mathbf{Z}_{ij}'\beta$. We then solve the estimating equation

$$\sum_i [\mathbf{Y}_i - \boldsymbol{\mu}_i(\beta)]' \, \mathbf{W}_i^{-1} \, \mathbf{D}_i = 0$$

where $\mathbf{W}_i$ is a *working matrix* of covariances among the Y_i and $\mathbf{D}_i = \partial \boldsymbol{\mu}_i / \partial \beta$ (Liang and Zeger, 1986). The beauty of this method is that it ensures robust estimates of the parameters and their asymptotic variances even when the working covariance matrix $\mathbf{W}$ is misspecified. The *sandwich estimator* of the variance is given by

$$\mathrm{var}(\hat{\beta}) = \left(\sum_i \mathbf{D}_i' \mathbf{W}_i^{-1} \mathbf{D}_i \right)' \left(\sum_i \mathbf{D}_i' \mathbf{W}_i^{-1} \mathbf{Y}_i \mathbf{Y}_i' \mathbf{W}_i^{-1} \mathbf{D}_i \right)^{-1} \left(\sum_i \mathbf{D}_i \mathbf{W}_i^{-1} \mathbf{D}_i' \right)$$

Hence one often adopts a quite simple form for $\mathbf{W}$, such as independence ($\mathbf{W} = \sigma^2 \mathbf{I}$) or exchangeability (all off-diagonal elements equal) out of convenience, even if one suspects that it may not be correct, because one is nevertheless assured that the resulting estimates will be unbiased and the sandwich estimator will also be unbiased. Of course, using a working co-variance matrix that is closer to the correct form will lead to more efficient estimators (smaller variance).

What was described above is sometimes called *GEE-1*. For genetics, the parameters of real interest generally concern the covariances among the $\mathbf{Y}_i$, requiring an extension of this equation to higher moments, known as *GEE-2* (Lee et al., 1993). This is done by simultaneously modeling $\mu_i = \mathrm{E}(\mathbf{Y}_i)$ and $\Sigma_i = \mathrm{E}(\mathbf{Y}_i \mathbf{Y}_i')$. Now we consider the empirical covariances of each possible pair of subjects j and k within family i, namely, $C_{ijk} = (Y_{ij} - \mu_{ij})(Y_{ik} - \mu_{ik})$. Now let $\mathbf{C}_i = (C_{i12}, C_{i13}, \ldots, C_{ij_i - 1, j_i})$ and let $\Sigma_i(\alpha) = \mathrm{E}(\mathbf{C}_i \,|\, \alpha)$ denote a model for these covariances, possibly involving additional covariates relating to the pairs of components with parameters α. For example, one might model $\Sigma_{ijk} = \alpha_0 \exp(-\alpha_1 R_{ijk})$, where R_{ijk} is the degree of relationship between members j and k of family i. Then we would set up the GEEs as a pair of vector equations of the form

$$\sum_i (\mathbf{Y}_i - \mu_i(\beta))' \mathbf{W}_i^{-1} \frac{\partial \mu_i}{\partial \beta} = 0$$

$$\sum_i (\mathbf{C}_i - \Sigma_i(\alpha))' \mathbf{V}_i^{-1} \frac{\partial \Sigma_i}{\partial \alpha} = 0$$

so as to estimate both the parameters β in the means model and α in the covariances model. Details of this approach to jointly modeling means and covariances are described by Prentice and Zhao (1991). In a genetic context, it is often these covariances that are of primary interest. For example, in the model described above, the parameter α tests whether familial correlations decay as a function of the degree of relationship. We will revisit other genetic applications of GEE methods in the following chapters (see, e.g., Lee et al., 1993, for an application to segregation analysis and Thomas et al., 1999, for an application to linkage analysis).

Markov Chain Monte Carlo Methods

An attractive alternative that will be developed further in later chapters is the class of Markov chain Monte Carlo (MCMC) methods, the simplest case of which is known as *Gibbs sampling*. This is a general technique for fitting highly structured stochastic systems, such as those with several component submodels comprising many parameters and/or many latent variables. The basic approach involves successive updating of each of the unknown quantities in the model—unobserved latent variables and model parameters—conditional on the observed data and on the current assignment of the other unknowns. Although the approach has its roots in Bayesian statistics, it can also be used as a means of approximating likelihood ratios for frequentist inference.

A generic problem might involve some data Y and a model involving three unknowns, A, B, and C. At the nth iteration of the process, we would sample from the following distributions:

$$\Pr(A_n \mid B_{n-1}, C_{n-1}, Y)$$
$$\Pr(B_n \mid A_n, C_{n-1}, Y)$$
$$\Pr(C_n \mid A_n, B_n, Y)$$

and so on for the $n + 1$st iteration, and so on. After an initial *burn-in* period to allow for convergence, a general theorem (Geman and Geman, 1984) shows that further realizations of this process generate (dependent) samples from the joint posterior distribution $\Pr(A, B, C \mid Y)$, which can be summarized in various ways. For a general background on MCMC methods, see the excellent textbook by Gilks et al. (1996).

Let us consider the specific example of a random effects regression model involving random slopes and intercepts, such as might be used in longitudinal data analysis, where Y_{ij} denotes an observation on subject i at time j, with X_{ij} being a covariate value at that observation. (In a genetic application, i might denote family and j individuals within families.) What makes this more complex than a simple regression problem is that we wish to allow each individual to have a unique intercept a_i and slope b_i, which we will assume have some common normal distributions across individuals. We will also allow each individual to have a unique residual variance s_i^2, which is assumed to have an *inverse gamma* distribution (IG). Thus

$$Y_{ij} \sim \mathcal{N}\left(a_i + b_i X_{ij}, s_i^2\right)$$
$$a_i \sim \mathcal{N}(\alpha, \tau^2)$$
$$b_i \sim \mathcal{N}(\beta, \omega^2)$$
$$s_i^2 \sim IG(S, \sigma)$$

Here the unknowns are the random intercepts, slopes, and residual variances $\{a_i, b_i, s_i^2\}$ (treated as latent variables) and the parameters $\{\alpha, \tau^2, \beta, \omega^2, S, \sigma\}$. Applying the Bayes formula, the *full conditional* distribution of a_i is given by

$$\Pr\left(a_i \mid \{Y_{ij}\}, b_i, X_{ij}, s_i^2, \alpha, \tau^2\right) \propto \left(\prod_j \Pr\left(Y_{ij} \mid a_i + b_i X_{ij}, s_i^2\right)\right) \Pr(a_i \mid \alpha, \tau^2)$$

$$= \mathcal{N}\left(\frac{\dfrac{\sum_j (Y_{ij} - b_i X_{ij})}{s_i^2} + \dfrac{\alpha}{\tau^2}}{\dfrac{N_i}{s_i^2} + \dfrac{1}{\tau^2}}, \frac{1}{\dfrac{N_i}{s_i^2} + \dfrac{1}{\tau^2}}\right)$$

and likewise for the other latent variables b_i, s_i^2.

The full conditionals for the parameters are estimated conditional on the latent variables. For example, for (α, τ^2), the full conditionals are

$$\Pr(\alpha \mid \{a_i\}, \tau^2) \propto \left(\prod_i \Pr(a_i \mid \alpha, \tau^2)\right) \Pr(\alpha) = \mathcal{N}(\bar{a}, \tau^2/I)$$

$$\Pr(\tau^2 \mid \{a_i\}, \alpha) \propto \left(\prod_i \Pr(a_i \mid \alpha, \tau^2)\right) \Pr(\tau^2) = IG\left(\sum_i (a_i - \bar{a})^2, I\right)$$

In genetics, a typical problem involves the distribution of a vector of phenotypes $\mathbf{Y}$ given a set of model parameters Θ that is defined in terms of a vector of unobserved genotype vectors $\mathbf{G}$. Because the space of possible $\mathbf{G}$ vectors can be very large, direct enumeration of all possible combinations may be impractical, but the probability distribution of a single component G_j given all the others $\mathbf{G}_{-j}$ is often quite simple. For example, a typical genetic model might assume

1. that individuals' phenotypes depend only on their own genotypes and are conditionally independent of each other given their genotypes: $\Pr(Y_j \mid \mathbf{Y}_{-j}, \mathbf{G}) = \Pr(Y_j \mid G_j)$ and
2. that individuals' genotypes depend only on their parents' genotypes, and are conditionally independent of their siblings' genotypes and their ancestors' genotypes, given their parents' genotypes, $\Pr(G_j \mid \mathbf{G}_{-j}) = \Pr(G_j \mid G_{m_j}, G_{f_j})$, where $\mathbf{G}_{-j}$ denotes the vector of everyone else's genotypes except that of individual j. (However, if individual j has offspring, their genotypes must also be taken into account, together with the genotype of j's spouse(s), as shown below.)

These relations are illustrated graphically in the form of a directed acyclic graph (DAG) shown in Figure 4.5, where the directions of each arrow indicate which variables depend upon which. The full conditional distribution for each unknown variable can be inferred by the set of all variables that are

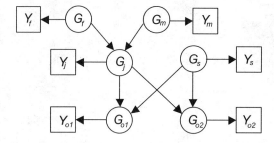

Figure 4.5 A portion of a Directed Acyclic Graph (DAG) for updating the genotype G_j of subject j conditioned on the subject's phenotype Y_i and his immediate family members.

connected to it, either upstream or downstream of an arrow, including the other "parents" of any downstream arrows of that variable. For example, in this figure, the relevant conditioning variables for G_j include Y_j (and any parameters in the penetrance function), the parental genotypes G_{m_j}, G_{f_j}, and the genotypes of all of subject j's offspring (together with j's spouse(s), needed to complete the specification of their genotype probabilities). Hence, the full conditional distribution

$$\Pr(G_j \mid \mathbf{Y}, \mathbf{G}_{-j}, \Theta) \propto \Pr(Y_j \mid G_j) \times \Pr\left(G_j \mid G_{m_j}, G_{f_j}\right) \times \prod_k \Pr\left(G_{o_{jk}} \mid G_j, G_{s_{jk}}\right)$$

is very easy to compute and hence easy to sample from. In this approach, one thus successively samples from each of these distributions, conditional on the observed data and the current assignments of all the other genotypes.

Sometimes these conditional distributions are not easy to sample from. For example, some of the latent variables may have continuous rather than discrete distributions (e.g., a polygene), and there may be no closed-form solution for their full conditional distribution. Alternatively, it may be desirable to sample not a single variable at a time, but rather clusters of closely related variables jointly. In such situations, a variant of this approach known as the *Metropolis-Hastings algorithm* can be used. Letting $\mathbf{X}$ represent the unknown quantities and $\pi(X'_j \mid \mathbf{Y}, \mathbf{X}_{-j})$ the true full conditional one wishes to sample from, one might propose a new value X'_j from some distribution $Q(X_j \to X'_j \mid \mathbf{Y}, \mathbf{X}_{-j})$ that is more convenient to sample from and then decide whether to accept the proposed value using the *Hastings ratio*

$$R = \frac{\pi(X'_j \mid \mathbf{Y}, \mathbf{X}_{-j})}{\pi(X_j \mid \mathbf{Y}, \mathbf{X}_{-j})} \Big/ \frac{Q(X_j \to X'_j \mid \mathbf{Y}, \mathbf{X}_{-j})}{Q(X'_j \to X_j \mid \mathbf{Y}, \mathbf{X}_{-j})}$$

Specifically, the new value X_j is accepted with probability min$(1, R)$; otherwise, one retains the previous value X_j and moves on to the next component. (This approach could just as well be applied to sampling $\Pr(\Theta \mid \mathbf{Y}, \mathbf{X})$;

indeed, it is often the case that these distributions are more difficult to sample from, since they are continuous.) Two special cases are of particular interest:

- In Gibbs sampling X_j, the proposal distribution is exactly the full conditional distribution, $Q(X_j' \mid X_j, \mathbf{Y}, \mathbf{X}_{-j}) = \pi(X_j' \mid \mathbf{Y}, \mathbf{X}_{-j})$, irrespective of the current assignment X_j. In this case, the terms in the numerator and denominator cancel out, so that R is always 1 and the proposal is always accepted.
- In a *random walk*, the proposal is symmetric in the sense that $Q(X_j \to X_j' \mid \mathbf{Y}, \mathbf{X}_{-j}) = Q(X_j' \to X_j \mid \mathbf{Y}, \mathbf{X}_{-j})$. For example, if X_j is continuous, one might propose $X_j' = X_j + U(-\delta, \delta)$ or $X_j' = X + \mathcal{N}(0, \delta^2)$ for some suitable choice of δ. Choices of this form are convenient, because then the proposal portions of the Hastings ratio cancel out, leaving

$$R = \Pr(X_j' \mid \mathbf{Y}, \mathbf{X}_{-j}, \Theta) / \Pr(X_j \mid \mathbf{Y}, \mathbf{X}_{-j}, \Theta)$$

which is generally very easy to compute.

The art in using any of these Metropolis-Hastings approaches is to choose a suitable proposal density: a proposal that is too different from the current state will stand little chance of being accepted, and consequently the chain will tend to stay in the same state for a long time before making a large jump; a proposal that is not different enough will usually be accepted, but will move by such a small amount that the chain will take a long time to explore the entire state space. A rule of thumb is that an optimal proposal should be accepted approximately 25%–50% of the time.

For fully Bayesian analysis, one would specify a prior distribution for Θ and alternately sample from $\Pr(\mathbf{Y} \mid \mathbf{X}, \Theta)$ (as described above) and from $\Pr(\Theta \mid \mathbf{Y}, \mathbf{X}) \propto \Pr(\mathbf{Y}, \mathbf{X} \mid \Theta) \Pr(\Theta)$. Following the same general theoretical results, this process would (after a suitable burn-in period) sample from the posterior distribution, $\Pr(\Theta \mid \mathbf{Y})$. This might be summarized, for example, in terms of its posterior mean and variance, a Bayes p-value, $\Pr(\Theta > \Theta_0 \mid \mathbf{Y})$, or what is known as a *Bayes factor* (Kass and Raftery, 1995)

$$BF(\Theta : \Theta_0) = \frac{\Pr(\Theta \mid \mathbf{Y}) / \Pr(\Theta_0 \mid \mathbf{Y})}{\Pr(\Theta) / \Pr(\Theta_0)}$$

By construction, Bayes factors have a very similar interpretation to likelihood ratios but do not have the same asymptotic distribution theory grounded on the principles of repeated sampling used in frequentist inference. Kass and Raftery suggest the following subjective interpretations: $BF < 1$, evidence against Θ; 1–3, barely worth a mention; 3–20, positive evidence; 20–150, strong evidence; >150, very strong evidence. While the posterior densities needed for computing means and variances, Bayes factors, or Bayes p-values can be estimated from the empiric distribution of sampled values of Θ, a more stable estimator is computed as the mean of the conditional distributions across all the samples $\mathbf{X}^{(s)}, s = 1, \ldots, S$, that is,

$$\Pr(\Theta \mid \mathbf{Y}) = (1/S) \sum_{s=1}^{S} \Pr(\Theta \mid \mathbf{Y}, \mathbf{X}^{(s)})$$

For frequentist inference, MCMC methods can be used to provide a Monte Carlo estimate of the likelihood ratio function using a sample of $\mathbf{X} \mid \mathbf{Y}, \Theta_0$ for some fixed value of Θ_0 (Thompson and Guo, 1991). The reasoning is as follows:

$$
\begin{aligned}
LR(\Theta : \Theta_0) &= \frac{\Pr(\mathbf{Y} \mid \Theta)}{\Pr(\mathbf{Y} \mid \Theta_0)} = \frac{1}{\Pr(\mathbf{Y} \mid \Theta_0)} \sum_{\mathbf{X}} \Pr(\mathbf{Y}, \mathbf{X} \mid \Theta) \\
&= \frac{1}{\Pr(\mathbf{Y} \mid \Theta_0)} \sum_{\mathbf{X}} \left(\frac{\Pr(\mathbf{Y}, \mathbf{X} \mid \Theta)}{\Pr(\mathbf{Y}, \mathbf{X} \mid \Theta_0)} \right) \Pr(\mathbf{Y}, \mathbf{X} \mid \Theta_0) \\
&= \sum_{\mathbf{X}} \left(\frac{\Pr(\mathbf{Y}, \mathbf{X} \mid \Theta)}{\Pr(\mathbf{Y}, \mathbf{X} \mid \Theta_0)} \right) \Pr(\mathbf{X} \mid \mathbf{Y}, \Theta_0) \\
&\approx (1/S) \sum_{\mathbf{X}^{(s)} \mid \mathbf{Y}, \Theta_0} \left(\frac{\Pr(\mathbf{Y}, \mathbf{X}^{(s)} \mid \Theta)}{\Pr(\mathbf{Y}, \mathbf{X}^{(s)} \mid \Theta_0)} \right)
\end{aligned}
\tag{4.9}
$$

In other words, one evaluates the likelihood ratio over a grid of values of Θ relative to Θ_0 for each realization of $\Pr(\mathbf{X}^{(s)} \mid \mathbf{Y}, \Theta_0)$ and then simply averages these likelihood ratio contributions.

Importance sampling methods, like MCMC, involve generating realizations from the distribution of interest, but instead construct independent samples from some approximating distribution that is easier to sample from than the real distribution, and then reweights these realizations according to the ratios of the true and approximating distributions to estimate the marginal summaries of interest.

Randomization Procedures

For many of the models arising in genetic epidemiology, the calculation of the true likelihood (reflecting the complex patterns of dependencies within families, for example) is either computationally intractable or involves questionable assumptions. A variety of statistical approaches to this problem have been developed that rely on randomizing or resampling the data in various ways.

A *randomization test* is a nonparametric test of the null hypothesis based on comparing the observed value of some test statistic S_0 to a distribution of values $\{S_r\}_{r=1\ldots,R}$ obtained by randomly permuting the observed data in such a manner that the variables whose association is being tested ought to be unrelated while keeping the basic data structure intact. If the observed test statistic is found to be among the most extreme in the randomization distribution, the association is claimed to be significant; specifically, the p-value is defined as the proportion of randomized test statistics that exceed the observed value. The form of the test statistic depends on the specific hypothesis being tested. For example, a nonparametric test of whether two samples differ in location might be obtained by using the difference in means as the test statistic or perhaps the number of pairs (x, y) of observations from the two groups for which $x > y$. If one wants to test $H_0 : \beta = 0$ in the regression $Y_i = \alpha + \beta X_i + e_i$ and is reluctant to assume that the e_i are normally distributed, one could take as $S_0 = \hat{\beta}$ from the ordinary least squares regression and then randomly permute the Y_i's, holding the X_i's fixed, recomputing $\hat{\beta}$ on each permutation. The test would then be based on comparing the estimate of $\hat{\beta}$ from the observed data to its randomization distribution. The standard nonparametric tests, such as the Wilcoxon signed rank tests for differences in location or the Spearman rank correlation, are based on this general idea, but because ranks are used, it is possible to develop analytical expressions for the relevant null distributions of the test statistics.

Randomization can be used to obtain a robust test of the null hypothesis, but it does not provide any means of estimating confidence intervals. For this purpose, resampling methods are often used. The *jacknife* entails reanalyzing the data, each time omitting one observation, using the variation in the results to obtain a robust estimate of the mean and its sampling variance (Miller, 1074). The *bootstrap* entails repeatedly drawing samples of the data, with replacement for the same total sample size, and again using the variation in results to estimate a confidence region (Efron and Tibshirani, 1994).

Conclusions

Genetic epidemiology is a very mathematically sophisticated field, relying heavily on probability and statistics. Many of the statistical techniques and study design principles outlined in this chapter will be familiar to readers with experience in epidemiology, but they are reviewed here for completeness. The standard cohort and case-control designs of traditional risk factor epidemiology are useful for studies of familial aggregation (Chapter 5) and candidate gene associations (Chapter 9), but segregation and linkage analyses require the use of family designs, which will be discussed in Chapters 6 and 7. The central machinery that will be used in fitting almost any genetic model is maximum likelihood. However, the calculations required for some kinds of models, such as multipoint linkage analysis in large or complex pedigrees, are so computationally intensive as to be intractable, even on the most powerful computers presently available. Generalized estimating equations (GEEs) and MCMC methods provide promising alternatives for such situations. Their applications to familial aggregation, segregation, and linkage analysis will be discussed in the following three chapters. Even where a relatively simple statistic can be computed, such as for familial aggregation or family-based tests of associations with specific genes, standard asymptotic theory may not be applicable because of small effective sample sizes or complex dependency structures. In this case, randomization procedures may be needed to provide a test of the null hypothesis or to construct valid confidence limits.

5

Familial Aggregation

The first step in the study of a potentially genetic trait is to see whether it tends to aggregate in families, without at this stage having any specific genetic model in mind. We begin by considering a continuous trait (e.g., cholesterol level, blood pressure), for which all family members are informative. One might well study such a trait with a simple random sample of families from the population and look at the correlation in phenotypes between relatives of different types. (For greater statistical efficiency, however, one might still prefer to focus on families with unusually high values of the trait.)

Next, we consider relatively rare dichotomous disease traits. Random samples of families are unlikely to yield many cases, with such traits, particularly the multiple-case families that are the most informative, so these studies are generally done by ascertaining families through affected probands. Standard case-control and cohort analysis techniques can then be used to estimate the *familial relative risk* (*FRR*), although we also consider a range of more sophisticated techniques for analyzing dependent data.

Finally, we consider three special designs: a randomization procedure, twin studies, and adoption studies.

First, however, it is worthwhile to pause in order to introduce some basic concepts about genetic relationships and gene identity.

Genetic Relationships and Gene Identity

Genetic relationships are defined by the probability that two members of a pedigree share one or two alleles from the same source at any autosomal locus. Consider two individuals, j and k, in family i. Since each has two

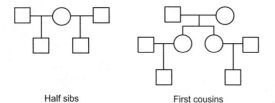

Half sibs   First cousins

Figure 5.1 Examples of unilineal relationships.

alleles, they can share neither, one, or both of them. This sharing can be assessed either by state or by descent.

- Two alleles are *identical by descent (IBD)* if they are derived from a common ancestor.
- Two alleles are *identical by state (IBS)* if they are identical in terms of their DNA composition and function but do not necessarily come from a common ancestor.

Genetic relationships depend on *IBD* status. We defer discussion of *IBS* until observable markers are used in Chapter 7.

Unilineal relatives are related through one side of the family (e.g., half-sibs, parent-offspring, first cousins [Fig. 5.1]); they can share only zero or one allele *IBD*. Bilineal relatives are related through both maternal and paternal lines (e.g., full sibs, double first cousins [Fig. 5.2]); hence they can share zero, one, or two alleles *IBD*.

Consider the *IBD* status of a pair of siblings. Suppose that we label the parents' alleles a,b and c,d. Some of these might be *IBS*, but without knowing their ancestors' genotypes, we cannot determine whether they are *IBD*, so we distinguish them for this purpose. The possible configurations of *IBD* status for two offspring are listed in Table 5.1. Since each of these 16 possible genotype pairs is equally likely, we can see by simply tabulating the number of possibilities by the number of alleles shared *IBD* (Z) that the probability π of sharing zero, one, or two alleles *IBD* is $\pi_0 = 1/4$, $\pi_1 = 1/2$, and $\pi_2 = 1/4$, respectively. The expected number of alleles shared *IBD* is $\pi_1 + 2\pi_2 = 0.5 \times 1 + 0.25 \times 2 = 1$, or equivalently, the expected *proportion $\bar{\pi}$* of alleles shared *IBD* is $1/2$ (since each individual has two alleles). This proportion, called the *coefficient of relationship*, equals 2^{-R}, where R is the *degree*

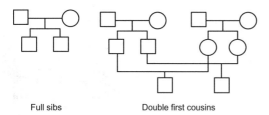

Full sibs   Double first cousins

Figure 5.2 Examples of bilineal relationships.

Table 5.1 Possible Genotypes of a Sib Pair by Identical by Descent (*IBD*)
Status, Given That Their Parents Have Genotypes *ab* and *cd*

Number of Alleles Shared *IBD*	Offspring Genotypes	Probability
0	(*ac,bd*) (*ad,bc*) (*bc,ad*) (*bd,ac*)	1/4
1	(*ac,ad*) (*bc,bd*) (*ac,bc*) (*ad,bd*)	
	(*ad,ac*) (*bd,bc*) (*bc ac*) (*bd ad*)	1/2
2	(*ac,ac*) (*ad,ad*) (*bc,bc*) (*bd,bd*)	1/4

of relationship, that is, 0 for identical (MZ) twins, 1 for first-degree relatives
(sibs or parent-offspring pairs), 2 for second-degree relatives (grandparents,
half-sibs, aunt/uncle), and 3 for third-degree relatives (first cousins, etc.).

The coefficient of relationship is also double the Malécot (1948) *kinship
coefficient*, φ, defined as the probability that a randomly selected pair of
alleles, one from each individual, is *IBD*. For example, for a parent-offspring
pair, there is a 50% probability that a randomly selected offspring allele came
from that parent, and if so, a further 50% probability that it was the same as
a randomly selected parental allele; hence, $\varphi = 1/4$ for the pair. Likewise,
for a sib pair, there is a 50% probability that two randomly selected alleles,
one from each sib, came from the same parent, and if so, a further 50%
probability that they both inherited the same allele from that parent; hence,
$\varphi = 1/4$. Thus, for both relationships, $\bar{\pi} = 2\varphi = 1/2$. We develop this idea
more formally for any type of relationship below.

These quantities are listed for various kinds of relationships in Table 5.2,
together with the probability $\pi_2 \equiv \Delta$ of sharing two alleles *IBD*. The kinship
coefficient is most easily derived by the *path* method. First, identify all the
paths p from the pair of individuals to a common ancestor and let M_p denote
the number of meioses along that path; for example, for a pair of siblings
there are two paths, one to the father and one to the mother, each with two
meioses. Then $\varphi = \sum_p (1/2)^{M_p+1}$. Wright's (1922) *coefficient of inbreeding F*
is computed in a similar way, but for a single individual (or for a mating type,
depending on the application). For example, for a first-cousin mating, there
are two paths, one to each common grandparent with $M_p = 4$, so $F = 1/16$.
We will discuss later the use of the nongenetic quantity γ reflecting the
chances of environmental sharing.

Formal derivation of φ and Δ

The following section, describing the general calculation of *IBD* probabilities
that will be used in later chapters, is somewhat technical and can be skipped
by those less mathematically inclined.

Table 5.2 Degree of Relationship (R), Probability of Sharing Zero, One, or Two Alleles Identical by Descent (*IBD*) (π), Expected Proportion of Alleles Shared *IBD* (φ), and Index of Environmental Sharing (γ) for Different Relative Types

| Type of Relative | R | Probability of IBD Sharing | | | $2\varphi = \pi_1/2 + \pi_2$ $= 2^{-R}$ | γ |
		π_0	π_1	$\Delta = \pi_2$		
Monozygotic twins (living together)	0	0	0	1	1	γ_1
Dizygotic twins (living together)	1	1/4	1/2	1/4	1/2	γ_1
Full sibs (living together)	1	1/4	1/2	1/4	1/2	γ_1
Full sibs (living apart)	1	1/4	1/2	1/4	1/2	0
Parent-offspring (living together)	1	0	1	0	1/2	γ_2
Half-sibs (living together)	2	1/2	1/2	0	1/4	γ_1
Grandparent-grandchild	2	1/2	1/2	0	1/4	0
Aunt/uncle-niece/nephew	2	1/2	1/2	0	1/4	0
First cousins	3	3/4	1/4	0	1/8	0
First cousins once removed	4	7/8	1/8	0	1/16	0
Second cousins	5	15/16	1/16	0	1/32	0
Double first cousins	(2)	9/16	3/8	1/16	1/4	0
Spouse-spouse	∞	1	0	0	0	γ_3
Random unrelated individuals	∞	1	0	0	0	0

In general, we derive the probabilities shown in Table 5.2 by considering all possible vectors of *parental source indicators* (or *segregation indicators*) $\mathbf{S} = (S_{1m}, S_{1f}, \ldots, S_{\mathcal{J}m}, S_{\mathcal{J}f})$, where $\mathcal{J}$ is the number of members of the pedigree who have parents in the pedigree (*nonfounders*) and S_{jp} indicates which grandparent of subject j the allele from the subject's parent p came from; that is, $S_{jm} = m$ if the maternal allele came from the maternal grandmother and $S_{jm} = f$ if the maternal allele came from the maternal grandfather (Fig. 5.3). Thus, a sib pair shares two alleles *IBD* if $S_{jm} = S_{km}$ and $S_{jf} = S_{kf}$ and one allele if only one of these conditions holds. A parent-child pair always shares exactly one allele (irrespective of which grandparent it came from). A grandparent-grandchild pair can share either one or zero alleles but not both: for example, a paternal grandfather share one if $S_{jf} = f$ and zero if $S_{jf} = m$. Determination of the *IBD* status of more distant relative types may involve the source indicators for some of their intermediate relatives. For example, paternal cousins share one allele if $S_{jf} = S_{kf}$ and $S_{f_j S_{jf}} = S_{f_k S_{kf}}$; the first condition requires that paternal alleles for each cousin be descended from the same grandparent; the second condition requires that the two parents have the same allele from that grandparent. Let $Z_{jk}(\mathbf{S})$ denote the number

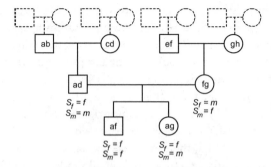

Figure 5.3 Representation of genotypes in a family by means of parental source indicators and founder alleles. Alleles are shown by the letters a–h inside the symbols, arranged so that the allele inherited from the father is displayed on the left and that from the mother is displayed on the right. The parental source indicators are shown below the symbols for each nonfounder.

of alleles shared *IBD* by individuals j and k under source vector $\mathbf{S}$. Then the probability of sharing n alleles *IBD* is simply

$$\Pr(Z_{jk} = n) = \sum_{\mathbf{s}} \Pr(\mathbf{S} = \mathbf{s})\ I[Z_{jk}(\mathbf{s}) = n] \tag{5.1}$$

where $I(-)$ is an indicator variable taking the value 1 if the condition "–" is true, zero otherwise. But since each of the source vectors is equally likely, $\Pr(\mathbf{S} = \mathbf{s}) = 2^{-2J}$, so this probability is simply the number of $\mathbf{S}$ vectors with $IBD_{jk}(\mathbf{S}) = n$ divided by 2^{2J}. For example, for sib pairs there are $2^4 = 16$ possible segregation indicators:

mmmm, mmmf, mmfm, mmff,
mfmm, mfmf, mffm, mfff,
fmmm, fmmf, fmfm, fmff,
ffmm, ffmf, fffm, ffff.

Of these, four have both sources in common—mmmm, mfmf, fmfm, ffff—so the probability of sharing two alleles *IBD* is $4/16 = 1/4$. Even though the probability of specific combinations of alleles that the individuals at the top of the pedigree (the *founders*) carry will differ, the probabilities of each possible transmission are equal.

Familial Correlations of Continuous Phenotypes

For a continuous trait, one might simply enroll a random series of families and look at the pattern of correlations in the phenotype between different types of relatives (sib-sib, parent-offspring, etc.). In principle, standard Pearson correlation coefficients could be computed for each relative type, but there are two subtleties. First, consider twins: if the twins were randomly selected (i.e., not selected through a particular proband), then which member should we designate twin 1 and which twin 2? For some relative types, such as parent-offspring, there may be a natural ordering, but for other types, the members might be more appropriately considered as replicates. Second, consider sibships: if there are three sibs, then there are three sib pairs; if there are four sibs, then there are six pairs. But these pairs are not independent, and treating them as such would inflate the effective sample size, leading to liberal significance tests and unduly narrow confidence limits. For these reasons, familial correlations are more appropriately estimated as *intraclass correlations* from analysis of variance. The model is

$$Y_{ij} = \mu + X_i + E_{ij}$$
$$X_i \sim \mathcal{N}\left(0, \sigma_B^2\right)$$
$$E_{ij} \sim \mathcal{N}\left(0, \sigma_W^2\right)$$

where $i = 1, \ldots, I$ denotes the sibship (or family contributing the particular relative type being estimated), $j = 1, \ldots, \mathcal{J}_i$ the members of the sibship, X_i a random effect corresponding to the deviation of the family from the overall mean μ, and E_{ij} the deviation of member j from the family mean, assumed to be independent of X_i. One then constructs the usual analysis of variance table, shown in Table 5.3, where $\bar{Y}_{i.}$ is the mean of Y for family i, $\bar{Y}_{..}$ is the mean of all I families, MS_B is the between-sibships mean square, and MS_W is the within-sibships mean square. From this analysis of variance (ANOVA) table, one can then derive the variance estimators $\hat{\sigma}_W^2 = MS_W$ and $\hat{\sigma}_B^2 = (MS_B - MS_W)/\mathcal{J}$.

Proof: Substitute the model for Y_{ij} into the expression for SS_B to obtain the expression $E(SS_W) = \sum_{ij}(E_{ij} - \bar{E}_{i.})^2 = I(\mathcal{J} - 1)\sigma_W^2$. (The multiplier is $\mathcal{J} - 1$ because each squared deviation has expectation σ_B^2, but one degree

Table 5.3 Analysis of Variance Table for Computing Components of Variance for a Continuous Phenotype in Sibships

Effect	Sum of Squares	Degrees of Freedom	Mean Square	Parameter Estimator
Between sibships	$SS_B = \sum_{ij}(\bar{Y}_{i.} - \bar{Y}_{..})^2$	$df_B = I - 1$	$MS_B = SS_B/df_B$	$\sigma_W^2 + \mathcal{J}\sigma_B^2$
Within sibships	$SS_W = \sum_{ij}(Y_{ij} - \bar{Y}_{i.})^2$	$df_W = \sum(\mathcal{J}_i - 1)$	$MS_W = SS_W/df_W$	σ_W^2

of freedom must be subtracted for each family because of the subtraction of $\bar{E}_{i\cdot}$.) In a similar way, we can derive that $\mathrm{E}(SS_B) = \mathcal{J}\sum_i(X_i - \bar{X})^2 + \mathcal{J}\sum_i \bar{E}_i^2 = (I - 1)\mathcal{J}\sigma_B^2 + (I - 1)\mathcal{J}(\sigma_W^2/\mathcal{J})$, since the variance of $\bar{E}_i$ is $\sigma_W^2/\mathcal{J}$. Dividing these expressions by the corresponding degrees of freedom, we obtain $\mathrm{E}(MS_W) = \sigma_W^2$ and $\mathrm{E}(MS_B) = \sigma_W^2 + \mathcal{J}\sigma_B^2$, as shown in the last column of Table 5.3. Solving for the σ^2s, we obtain the variance estimators given above.

The intraclass correlation is then estimated as

$$r_I = \frac{\sigma_B^2}{\sigma_B^2 + \sigma_W^2} = \frac{MS_B - MS_W}{MS_B + (\mathcal{J} - 1)MS_W}$$

If the sibships vary in size, then this expression can be used, replacing $\mathcal{J}$ by $[\sum \mathcal{J}_i - (\sum \mathcal{J}_i^2/\sum \mathcal{J}_i)]/(I - 1)$.

The results of these calculations might then be arrayed in a table, giving the observed correlations for different types of relationship. The next task is to try to fit these observed correlations to the expected correlations from some model for hidden environmental and genetic factors that are producing the correlations. (The effects of any measured covariates are generally eliminated before beginning this analysis using regression; the familial correlation analysis is then done on the residuals from the regression model.) The conceptual model for this analysis is a linear model of the form

$$Y_{ij} = \mu + G_{ij} + C_{ij} + E_{ij}$$

where G, C, and E represent unobservable random variables for genotype, shared environment, and independent environment, respectively. This implies that the variance of Y can be written

$$\mathrm{var}(Y) \equiv \sigma^2 = \sigma_G^2 + \sigma_C^2 + \sigma_E^2$$

since by definition, G, C, and E are independent. We then define *broad sense heritability* h^2 as the proportion of variance due to genotype, σ_G^2/σ^2. (What is called *independent environment* includes both true interindividual variability and phenotype measurement error. Hence, h^2 should be interpreted as the heritability of *measured* phenotypes and will be an underestimate of the heritability of *true* phenotypes.)

The genetic variance, in turn, can be subdivided into components σ_A^2, representing the additive effects of the individual alleles (the *additive genetic variance*); σ_D^2, the interaction between alleles at the same locus (the *dominance variance*); and σ_I^2, the interaction between different loci (the *epistatic variance*). (Actually, the term for the epistatic variance relates only to the interaction between the additive components of the two loci; additional terms could be added to allow for additive–dominance or dominance–dominance interactions, and so on for three-way or higher-order interactions.) *Narrow sense* heritability refers just to the additive component, that is, σ_A^2/σ^2. These variance components do not distinguish between a single major gene, a few moderately strong genes, or many genes with small effects (polygenes), but merely reflect their aggregate contributions (we will revisit such questions in the following chapter). These various variance components can be estimated from the covariances between relative pairs of different types

$$\text{cov}(Y_{ij}, Y_{ik}) = 2\varphi_{jk}\sigma_A^2 + \Delta_{jk}\sigma_D^2 + \varphi_{jk}^2\sigma_I^2 + \gamma_{jk}\sigma_C^2 + \delta_{jk}\sigma_E^2$$

where γ_{jk} is the proportion of environmental influences they share in common (fixing $\gamma_1 = 1$ for identifiability [Table 5.2]) and $\delta_{jk} = 1$ if $j = k$, 0 otherwise. A number of possibilities are available for defining γ_{jk}; for example, we might want to distinguish sharing in childhood (e.g., among sibs) from sharing in adulthood (e.g., among parents). Care must be taken to avoid overparameterizing the model, however; for example, if only twins are available, attempting to distinguish environmental sharing in MZ and DZ pairs (although likely to differ) would be indistinguishable from their genetic difference.

Techniques for fitting the model are complex and described in Khoury et al. (1993, § 7.3). The covariances can be conveniently arrayed in a matrix to display the expected correlation structure of an entire pedigree. For a nuclear family with two offspring, for example, the matrix would look as follows:

$$\mathbf{C} = \begin{pmatrix} \sigma_G^2 + \sigma_C^2 + \sigma_E^2 & \gamma_3\sigma_C^2 & \sigma_G^2/2 + \gamma_2\sigma_C^2 & \sigma_G^2/2 + \gamma_2\sigma_C^2 \\ \gamma_3\sigma_C^2 & \sigma_G^2 + \sigma_C^2 + \sigma_E^2 & \sigma_G^2/2 + \gamma_2\sigma_C^2 & \sigma_G^2/2 + \gamma_2\sigma_C^2 \\ \sigma_G^2/2 + \gamma_2\sigma_C^2 & \sigma_G^2/2 + \gamma_2\sigma_C^2 & \sigma_G^2 + \sigma_C^2 + \sigma_E^2 & \sigma_G^2/2 + \gamma_1\sigma_C^2 \\ \sigma_G^2/2 + \gamma_2\sigma_C^2 & \sigma_G^2/2 + \gamma_2\sigma_C^2 & \sigma_G^2/2 + \gamma_1\sigma_C^2 & \sigma_G^2 + \sigma_C^2 + \sigma_E^2 \end{pmatrix}$$

where the four rows and columns refer to father, mother, sib 1, and sib 2, respectively. Hence, one approach to fitting such a model is to treat the data as a multivariate normal with this covariance matrix, that is, to maximize the likelihood

$$\mathcal{L}(\sigma^2) = \prod_{i=1}^{n} \mathcal{N}_{\tilde{J}_i}(\mathbf{Y}_i - \mu\mathbf{1}, \mathbf{C}_i)$$

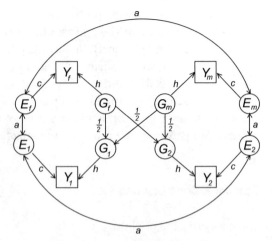

Figure 5.4 Simplified path model for familial correlation of a single phenotype. (Reproduced with permission from Khoury et al., 1993)

where $\mathcal{N}_{\mathcal{J}}(,)$ represents the $\mathcal{J}$-dimensional multivariate normal density, $\mathcal{J}_i$ being the number of members in pedigree i. General methods of inference using maximum likelihood were described in the previous chapter and will be elaborated in the following chapters.

Path diagrams are a convenient way of visualizing the linear model and inferring the expected correlations as a function of the various shared factors. The path model is generally represented in terms of a path diagram, as illustrated for a simple family with two parents and two offspring in Figure 5.4. The circles represent the unobserved genetic and environmental factors, and the arrows indicate the relationships between them. The expected correlations between any pair of observable variables are given by the sum over all paths connecting them of the products of the various path coefficients along each path; hence:

$$E[\mathrm{corr}(Y_f, Y_m)] = c^2 a$$

$$E[\mathrm{corr}(Y_f, Y_i)] = E[\mathrm{corr}(Y_m, Y_i)] = \frac{1}{2}h^2 + c^2 a \text{ for } i = 1, 2 \quad (5.2)$$

$$E[\mathrm{corr}(Y_1, Y_2)] = \frac{1}{2}h^2 + c^2 a$$

For further details about fitting methods, see Khoury et al. (1993, §7.4) and Neale and Cardon (1992).

One might also identify families through *probands* with elevated values of the phenotype or some correlate thereof (e.g., melanoma for a study of nevi or heart disease for a study of lipid levels or hypertension). In this case, the analysis needs to allow for the way the families were ascertained. This can be done using a conditional likelihood, computed by dividing the likelihood for the observed data by the probability that the family was ascertained. For threshold ascertainment (i.e., all families with at least one member having $Y > T$, where T is the ascertainment threshold), this corresponds to the integral of a multivariate normal distribution with the corner $Y_j < T$ for all j removed (e.g., cells A and B in Fig. 5.7B for the liability model discussed below). A much simpler method, however, is just to omit the proband from the analysis, since the correlation structure of the remaining relatives is not influenced by the way the proband was selected.

Familial Risk of Disease

The concept of familial risk

Familial risk is defined as the probability that an individual will be affected by a disease, given that he or she has an affected family member. *Familial relative risk* (*FRR*) is the ratio of that risk to the risk in the general population or perhaps to the risk given no affected family members. Familial risk obviously depends on a number of factors, including

- the age, gender, and year of birth of the individual in question;
- other risk factors (race, environmental factors, host factors, etc.);
- the number and type(s) of relatives affected;
- the number and ages of relatives at risk.

Implicit in the definition of *FRR* is that the two risks being compared are comparable on these factors. The magnitude of the relative risk might also be modified by some or all of the above factors. Thus, a more appropriate comparison than lifetime risks might be of age-specific incidence (or mortality) *rates*. Methods for making such comparisons will be discussed later.

It is important to distinguish the concept of familial risk from *genetic risk*, which is the probability that an individual will be affected by a disease, given his or her genotype. Again, this can be defined in terms of lifetime risks or age-specific incidence rates, as can relative risks comparing, say, genotypes *AA* and *aa* for a single major locus.

It is instructive to consider the relationship between these two measures of risk. For simplicity, we consider the case of a single major gene with two alleles, although a similar analysis is possible for polygenic models (see Chapter 6). In the next few paragraphs, we describe in some detail the calculation of the familial risk for a major gene model, justifying each step in the derivation. The casual reader might wish to skip some of the details, but be warned that these ideas will prove central to segregation analysis and likelihoods on pedigrees, as developed more extensively in Chapters 6 and 7.

Derivation of familial risk. For simplicity, we describe the calculations for a single genetic locus, but in principle, similar calculations could be done for multiple loci, possibly interacting, or for polygenic models (see Chapter 6). Consider the pedigree shown in Figure 5.5A, where we wish to compute the risk to subject j given that k is affected. To conceptualize the calculations which follow, consider the DAG shown in Figure 5.5B, where squares represent observed random variables and circles represent unobserved random variables or model parameters.

Genetic models are expressed in terms of three components: (*1*) the population genotype probabilities for unrelated individuals, (2) the *transition* probabilities for the relationship between parental and offspring genotypes, and (*3*) the penetrances. These three components are represented in the top, middle, and bottom portions of the DAG shown in Figure 5.5B. Let q denote the frequency of the A allele, $p = 1 - q$ the frequency of the a allele, and Q_g the genotype probabilities under Hardy-Weinberg equilibrium,

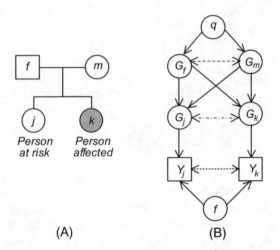

(A)   (B)

Figure 5.5 (A) Simple nuclear family with two offspring affected, for which the familial risk of the other offspring is to be computed. (B) Directed Acyclic Graph for this pedigree: squares represent observed quantities; circles represent unobserved latent variables or model parameters. The dotted line between G_f and G_m indicates the assumption of no assortive mating, the one between G_j and G_k indicates the assumption of independent segregation of offspring genotypes given the parental genotypes, and the dotted line between Y_j and Y_k indicates the assumption of conditional independence of phenotypes given the genotypes.

$Q_0 = \Pr(G = aa) = p^2$, $Q_1 = \Pr(G = aA) = 2pq$, and $Q_2 = \Pr(G = AA) = q^2$. Let $Y_i = 1$ indicate that individual i is affected and $Y_i = 0$ is unaffected, and let $f_g = \Pr(Y = 1 \mid G = g)$ denote the genetic risk (or *penetrance*) for genotypes $g = aa, aA, AA$. Finally, let $T_{g_j g_m g_f}$ denote the transition probabilities $\Pr(G_j = g_j \mid G_m = g_m, G_f = g_f)$, given in Table 3.3. [These are composed of the *transmission* probabilities $\tau_{acd} = \Pr(A_p = a \mid G_p = \{cd\})$ (Table 3.2), the probability of a parent with genotype G_p transmitting allele A_p to an offspring, by the relationship $\Pr(G = \{ab\} \mid G_m = \{cd\}, G_f = \{ef\}) = (\tau_{acd}\tau_{bef} + \tau_{bcd}\tau_{aef})/2.$]

We consider the risk to an individual j given the disease status Y_k of a single sib k:

$$\Pr(Y_j = 1 \mid Y_k = 1) = \frac{\Pr(Y_j = 1, Y_k = 1)}{\Pr(Y_k = 1)}$$

Let us focus first on the numerator of this expression,

$$\Pr(Y_j = 1, Y_k = 1) = \sum_{g_j} \sum_{g_k} \Pr(Y_j = 1, Y_k = 1, G_j = g_j, G_k = g_k)$$

$$= \sum_{g_j} \sum_{g_k} \Pr(Y_j = 1, Y_k = 1 \mid g_j, g_k) \Pr(g_j, g_k)$$

$$= \sum_{g_j} \sum_{g_k} \Pr(Y_j = 1 \mid g_j, g_k) \Pr(Y_k = 1 \mid g_j, g_k) \Pr(g_j, g_k)$$

$$= \sum_{g_j} \sum_{g_k} \Pr(Y_j = 1 \mid g_j) \Pr(Y_k = 1 \mid g_k) \Pr(g_j, g_k)$$

$$= \sum_{g_j} \sum_{g_k} f_{g_j} f_{g_k} \Pr(g_j, g_k)$$

where, after the first line, for notational simplicity, we have written $G_j = g_j$ simply as g_j. The first step in the above derivation simply involves summing the joint probabilities of two phenotypes and the two genotypes over all possible genotype combinations. The second step decomposes this joint probability into the conditional probability of phenotypes given genotypes times the genotype probability. (These first two steps require only the laws of total and conditional probability and make no genetic assumptions.) The third step is based on the assumption that the two sibs' phenotypes are conditionally independent, given their genotypes; this is a strong assumption, tantamount to assuming that there are no other shared risk factors (other genes or environmental factors) that influence both of their phenotypes. The final step is based on the assumption that each sib's phenotype depends only on his or her own genotype, not that of his or her sib.

Now we evaluate the last term in this expression by considering the sum over all possible parental genotypes, G_m and G_f:

$$
\begin{aligned}
\Pr(G_j = g_j, G_k = g_k) &= \sum_{g_m}\sum_{g_f} \Pr(g_j, g_k \mid g_m, g_f)\Pr(g_m, g_f)\\
&= \sum_{g_m}\sum_{g_f} \Pr(g_j \mid g_m, g_f)\Pr(g_k \mid g_m, g_f)\Pr(g_m, g_f)\\
&= \sum_{g_m}\sum_{g_f} \Pr(g_j \mid g_m, g_f)\Pr(g_j \mid g_m, g_f)\Pr(g_m)\Pr(g_f)\\
&= \sum_{g_m}\sum_{g_f} T_{g_j g_m g_f} T_{g_k g_m g_f} Q_{g_m} Q_{g_f}
\end{aligned}
$$

Here the first line is again based on the laws of total and conditional probability, as used above. The second line is based on the assumption that offsprings' genotypes are conditionally independent given their parents' genotypes, which is simply Mendel's law of independent segregation. The third line is based on the assumption of random mating—that is, that parental genotypes are independent. This is a strong assumption, which is unlikely to be strictly true in practice since allele frequencies vary by ethnic group and couples tend to mate within their ethnic group. Nevertheless, this assumption is commonly made in most genetic analyses.

Finally, let us consider the denominator of our original expression, namely, the population risk

$$
\begin{aligned}
\Pr(Y_k = 1) &= \sum_g \Pr(Y_k = 1 \mid G_k = g)\Pr(G_k = g)\\
&= \sum_g f_g Q_g = f_0 p^2 + 2 f_1 pq + f_2 q^2
\end{aligned}
$$

Putting all this together, we can compute the sibling *recurrence risk* as

$$
\Pr(Y_j = 1 \mid Y_k = 1) = \frac{\sum_{g_m}\sum_{g_f}\sum_{g_j}\sum_{g_k} f_{g_j} f_{g_k} T_{g_j g_m g_f} T_{g_k g_m g_f} Q_{g_m} Q_{g_f}}{\sum_{g_j} f_{g_j} Q_{g_j}}
$$

To illustrate how easily such an algorithm might be programmed, consider the following *pseudocode:*

```
SumPY2=0 SumPY12=0
for gm=1..3
for gf=1..3
        Pmf = Q[gm]*Q[gf]
        for g1=1..3
        for g2=1..3
                Pmf12 = Pmf * T[g1,gm,gf] * T[g2,gm,gf]
                SumPY2 = SumPY2 + Pmf12 * f[g2]
                SumPY12 = SumPY12 + Pmf12 * f[g1] * f[g2]
RecRisk = SumPY12 / SumPY2
```

Table 5.4 illustrates the calculations of the population risk for a single major gene model with a particular choice of parameters. The corresponding calculations of sibling recurrence risk are more complex but can be implemented in a spreadsheet or a simple computer program. The results for this same choice of parameters are provided in Table 5.5.

Having derived this expression for the *absolute* familial risk for siblings (the recurrence risk), we now consider three alternative *relative* measures for any relationship type r:

- Risk relative to the general population: $\lambda_r = \Pr(Y_j = 1 \mid Y_k = 1)/\Pr(Y_j = 1)$. This quantity is conventionally denoted λ_s when applied to siblings, λ_m when applied to MZ twins, and λ_o when applied to offspring (Risch, 1990b);
- Familial risk ratio: $R_r = \Pr(Y_j = 1 \mid Y_k = 1)/\Pr(Y_j = 1 \mid Y_k = 0)$;
- Familial odds ratio:

$$\psi_r = \frac{\Pr(Y_j = 1 \mid Y_k = 1)/\Pr(Y_j = 0 \mid Y_k = 1)}{\Pr(Y_j = 1 \mid Y_k = 0)/\Pr(Y_j = 0 \mid Y_k = 0)}$$

This is the quantity that would be estimated by the case-control design described below.

Table 5.4 Illustrative Calculation of Population Risk for a Partially Penetrant Dominant Gene with Penetrance $f_1 = f_2 = 0.9$, a Sporadic Case Rate of $f_0 = 0.1$, and an Allele Frequency of $q = 0.01$

Genotype	$Q_g = \Pr(g)$	$f_g = \Pr(Y = 1 \mid g)$	Product
aa	$(0.99)^2 = 0.9801$	0.1	0.09801
aA	$2(0.01)(0.99) = 0.0198$	0.9	0.01782
AA	$(0.01)^2 = 0.0001$	0.9	0.00009
Total	1.0	—	0.11592

Table 5.5 Illustrative Calculation of Sibling Recurrence Risk for the Same Parameter Choices as in Table 5.4

$q = \Pr(A)$	0.01
$p = 1 - q = \Pr(a)$	0.99

		$O(G)$	
$f_0 = \Pr(Y=1 \mid G=aa)$	0.1	0.9801	0.09801
$f_1 = \Pr(Y=1 \mid G=aA)$	0.9	0.0198	0.01782
$f_2 = \Pr(Y=1 \mid G=AA)$	0.9	0.0001	0.00009
		$\Pr(Y=1)$:	0.11592

G_m	G_f	$\Pr(G_m)$	$\Pr(G_f)$	$\Pr(G_m, G_f)$
aa	aa	0.9801	0.9801	0.96059601
aa	aA	0.9801	0.0198	0.03881196
aa	AA	0.9801	0.0001	0.00019602
aA	aA	0.0198	0.0198	0.00039204
aA	AA	0.0198	0.0001	0.00000396
AA	AA	0.0001	0.0001	0.00000001

TRANSITION PROBABILITIES $\Pr(G_1, G_2 \mid G_m, G_f)$

G_m	G_f	aa / aa	aa / aA	aa / AA	aA / aA	aA / AA	AA / AA
aa	aa	1					
aa	aA	0.25	0.5		0.25		
aa	AA				1		
aA	aA	0.0625	0.25	0.125	0.25	0.25	0.0625
aA	AA				0.25	0.5	0.25
AA	AA						1

$\Pr(G_1, G_2, G_m, G_f)$

G_m	G_f	aa / aa	aa / aA	aa / AA	aA / aA	aA / AA	AA / AA
aa	aa	0.960596	0	0	0	0	0
aa	aA	0.009703	0.019406	0	0.009703	0	0
aa	AA	0	0	0	0.000196	0	0
aA	aA	2.45E-05	9.8E-05	4.9E-05	9.8E-05	9.8E-05	2.45E-05
aA	AA	0	0	0	9.9E-07	1.98E-06	9.9E-07
AA	AA	0	0	0	0	0	1E-08
$\Pr(G_1, G_2)$:		0.9703235	0.019504	4.9E-05	0.009998	1E-04	2.55E-05
$\Pr(Y_1 = 1 \mid G_1)$:		0.1	0.1	0.1	0.9	0.9	0.9
$\Pr(Y_2 = 1 \mid G_2)$:		0.1	0.9	0.9	0.9	0.9	0.9
$\Pr(Y_1 = 1, Y_2 = 1, G_1, G_2)$:		0.0097032	0.001755	4.41E-06	0.008098	8.1E-05	2.07E-05
$\Pr(Y_2 = 1, G_1, G_2)$:		0.0970324	0.009752	2.45E-05	0.008998	9E-05	2.3E-05

$\Pr(Y_1 = 1, Y_2 = 1)$	0.019663
$\Pr(Y_2 = 1)$	0.11592
$\Pr(Y_1 = 1 \mid Y_2 = 1)$	0.169626
$\Pr(Y_1 = 1 \mid Y_2 = 1) / \Pr(Y_1 = 1)$	= 1.463302

Table 5.6 Illustrative Calculation of Familial Relative Risks for Various Genetic Models

		Dominant		Recessive	
	$q =$	0.01	0.05	0.10	0.30
GRR	$\Pr(g) =$	0.0199	0.0975	0.01	0.09
2		1.01	1.04	1.00	1.03
5		1.13	1.36	1.04	1.26
10		1.57	2.00	1.20	1.74
50		6.97	4.12	4.16	3.45
100		11.8	4.75	8.24	3.99
1000		23.3	5.48	25.2	4.61
∞		25.5	5.57	30.3	4.69

Each of these quantities can be readily computed from the expressions for their component parts given above. Nevertheless, these complex formulas do not provide much insight into the quantititive relationship between the two types of risk. Table 5.6 illustrates the results of numerical evaluation of the FRR under dominant and recessive models for various combinations of allele frequency and *genetic relative risk* (*GRR*). The striking observation from this table is that the FRRs are often quite modest even when the genetic relative risk is extremely large. Peto (1980) explains this phenomenon as follows:

- The sib's disease was not necessarily hereditary.
- Even if it was, the individual at risk may not have inherited the mutant allele.
- Even if he did, he may nevertheless not get the disease.
- Conversely, if the sib is unaffected, he may still carry the susceptibility genotype, the individual at risk might have inherited it, and he might get the disease.

Thus, a small FRR does not necessarily imply that the genetic risk is small.

Similar results can be computed for other genetic models, such as a two-locus interactive model or a polygenic model. In general, familial risks will decline more rapidly with degree of relationships under multigeneic models than under single-gene models.

One might also wonder whether a familial risk can be accounted for by shared environment instead of shared genotype. In a series of papers, Khoury et al. (1988, 1993) reported the results of similar calculations based on different degrees of sharing of an unmeasured binary environmental risk factor that acts alone or in combination with a genetic factor. The conclusion of these calculations is that such a factor would have to have a very strong effect on disease risk (an *RR* of at least 10) and be highly correlated within families to induce a familial correlation of the magnitude illustrated for genetic factors in Table 5.6.

Design principles

The basic concepts of epidemiologic study design, as they relate primarily to population-based studies of unrelated individuals, were introduced in Chapter 4. Here we elaborate on some of the issues that arise specifically in designing family studies. Many of the complications in genetic epidemiology arise from the need to sample families rather than individuals. It is hard enough to find appropriate sampling frames for *individuals* from the general population in standard epidemiologic studies; finding appropriate sampling frames for *families* is even harder in most countries, including the United States. In the study of dichotomous diseases, a further complication is that multiple-case families are the most informative, and these are not efficiently identified by simple random sampling of families in the general population. For these reasons, most studies of familial aggregation of disease are based on ascertainment of *probands,* followed by identification of their family members. For efficiency, diseased probands are usually employed, but some designs also include control probands.

Population-based ascertainment of probands (both diseased and control) is highly desirable for generalizability and validity. If population-based disease and population registries are not available, then it is essential to establish the representativeness of the case (and control) series. Design principles here are no different from those in standard epidemiologic studies.

Case probands might be identified through death certificates or cancer registries over some defined geographic area and time period. One consideration that will become important when we consider analysis methods, particularly segregation analysis, is how complete the identification of cases is. Specifically, let π denote the probability that any given case in the population will be identified as a proband. We will focus on two limiting cases, *complete* ascertainment where $\pi = 1$ and *single* ascertainment where $\pi \to 0$. In both instances, only families with at least one case will be included in the sample. In complete ascertainment, multiple-case families will be represented in the sample in the same proportion as their occurrence in the population, since all such families are represented with probability 1. In contrast, in single ascertainment, multiple-case families will be overrepresented in the sample relative to the population in proportion to the number of cases in the family. Surprisingly, single ascertainment turns out to produce unbiased tests of familial aggregation, while complete ascertainment does not, unless each case in a multiple-case family is counted separately. This point will be demonstrated formally below when we discuss case-control analyses.

Control probands might be identified using any of the standard epidemiologic methods, such as sampling from population registries (e.g., voter registration lists), death certificates, neighborhood censuses, random digit dialing, or friends. One method is of particular interest in family studies, however. Spouse controls are genetically unrelated (except in the case of consanguineous marriages), but are likely to share a common adult environment and similar demographic characteristics (other than gender). Comparison of their family histories is thus matched on many of the factors we might wish to control for in testing a genetic hypothesis. (The rationale for including control families is discussed further below.)

Having identified case and perhaps control probands, one then proceeds to enumerate their families. This might be narrowly focused or quite broad, depending on the ultimate aims of the project, but in any event it should be done systematically. Thus, one might inquire only about siblings, parents, or offspring, all second-degree relatives (grandparents, aunts, uncles, grandchildren, nieces, nephews), or third-degree relatives (cousins, etc.). For whatever types of relatives to be considered, the ideal information would be number of relatives of each type at risk, their disease status (including specific diagnoses), sexes, and ages at risk (birth dates and dates of diagnosis or death). Obviously there is a trade-off between the number of relative types to be considered and the extent and quality of the information that can realistically be collected on each. Compromises might be possible: for example, one might systematically obtain all the above information on first-degree relatives and only the number of second-degree relatives at risk and the details on any cases in that group.

Reports of family histories are likely to be inaccurate, including both false positives and false negatives. There is little that can be done about false negatives without a great deal of effort. However, one might consider asking for the same information from each member of the family or do record linkage against the National Death Index and/or disease registry for the area(s) where the family members live. To facilitate these options, it might be desirable to also ask the probands for the addresses and phone numbers of family members and permission to contact them. False positives are perhaps a greater concern, because there is a tendency for families to over-report disease, particularly where the diagnosis is uncertain (e.g., "cancer" with the specific site unknown or benign disease as malignant). It is therefore important to verify the diagnosis of all reported familial cases by pathology reports, medical records, death certificates, and so on. This will also entail obtaining the necessary consent from family members. In principle, one ought to devote the same energy to this confirmation as to confirmation of the diagnosis of the original probands. The small literature on validation of family histories (Ziogas and Anton-Culver, 2003, and references therein) suggests that specificity is high for first-degree relatives (typically 80%–90%, the errors being primarily misclassification of benign tumors as malignant or misreporting the site of cancer) but much lower for second-degree relatives. Sensitivity data are more elusive, but a few reports indicate that other family members occasionally report cases missed by the proband.

It may also be desirable to obtain risk factor information, both for control of confounding and for assessment of interaction effects. Depending on the form of analysis anticipated, this might be limited to the original probands or it might extend to family members as well (recognizing that information on the latter might be quite difficult to obtain, particularly for deceased relatives). Again, compromises might be possible, perhaps using an abbreviated form for the relatives. The use of these data will be discussed below.

Analytical approaches

Case-control method. Probably the simplest analysis is to compare cases and controls as independent individuals (or matched pairs, depending on how they were selected) in terms of *family history* as an exposure variable, using standard case-control methods. Thus, for an unmatched study, one might form Table 5.7, and estimate the *OR* and test the null hypothesis $OR = 1$ using the methods described in Chapter 4 (Table 4.2 or, for a matched study, Table 4.3).

In either the matched or unmatched design, family history might be defined simply as the presence or absence of an affected relative of a particular type, or it might be extended to a multilevel scale such as

- first-degree, other relative, none;
- two or more, one, none;
- parent or sib under age 50, parent or sib over age 50, none.

Clearly, there is plenty of scope for imagination! Is there any logical basis for choosing among the alternatives? Previous literature might be a guide; for example, the breast cancer literature suggests that premenopausal cases are more likely to be genetic than postmenopausal cases. This would be an example of an interaction on an age scale, that is, that the genetic relative risk is not constant as a function of age. Suppose, however, that this is not the case. How would we expect *FRR*s to vary as a function of degree of relationship, number of relatives at risk, and their ages? Calculations similar

Table 5.7 Presentation of Data From an Unmatched Case-Control Study of Familial Aggregation

Family History	Controls	Cases	Odds Ratio
Negative	A	B	1
Positive	C	D	AD/BC

to those outlined above but extended to include multiple relatives of different types were reported by Mack et al. (1990). Before considering the numbers, let us consider the principles involved:

- The larger the family, the larger the number of familial cases expected by chance, even if the genetic relative risk is 1.
- Similarly, the older the family members, the higher their cumulative risks.
- *FRR*s are larger for first-degree relatives than for second-degree relatives, and so on.
- The more cases there are in a family, the more likely they are to be hereditary.
- If the disease is rare, the risk in someone with a negative family history is only very slightly lower than the population risk, but the risk in someone with a positive family history is much higher than the population risk.

For example, Bryant and Brasher (1994) found a stronger breast cancer FRR for sisters than for mothers, a larger difference than could be explained by differences in their expected incidence. Taken together, these observations suggest that the ideal family history index should take the expected incidence in the family into account as well as the degree of relationship. Consider sibships for the moment. Table 5.8 shows that the familial log *RR* varies roughly in proportion to the *difference* between the observed and expected number of cases in the sibship, where the expected number is computed in the usual way by summing products of age-specific person-years times standard rates over all sibs at risk. The standard rates might come from the general population or be computed internally from the cohort of all family members in the study, excluding probands. Of course, if the disease is really rare, these expected numbers might be negligible, suggesting that the number of affected members (ignoring the number at risk and their ages) might be a quite adequate index of the family history. Note, however, that the trends by number of affected sibs are not linear: in large sibships with a common disease, one or two affected may actually be fewer than expected and will therefore contribute evidence *against* a major gene segregating in such families, whereas with a high proportion affected, a point of diminishing returns is reached, with each additional case contributing less and

Table 5.8 Familial Relative Risk for Sibships Under a Dominant Model with $f_0 = 0.1$, $f_1 = f_2 = 0.9$, and $q = 0.01$

Number of Sibs at Risk	Number of Sibs Affected					
	0	1	2	3	4	5
1	0.94	1.46				
2	0.91	1.22	2.67			
3	0.89	1.07	2.13	3.89		
4	0.88	0.98	1.69	3.46	4.42	
5	0.87	0.93	1.38	2.99	4.16	4.66

less additional information, as the FRR approaches its maximum limiting value.

Standard multivariate methods of case-control analysis (e.g., matched or unmatched logistic regression) can be used to explore the modifying effects of degree of relationship, age, or other attributes of family history, as well as confounders or interactions with exposure status of the probands. This analysis would not make any use of risk factor information on the relatives (except possibly to adjust the expected numbers). Instead, the hypothesis being tested is that the effect of family history on the proband's risk is confounded or modified by his or her own risk factors.

Now let us revisit the effect of ascertainment on tests of familial aggregation. Suppose that there is no familial aggregation, that is, the phenotypes of each individual in a family are independent. Consider sibships of a fixed size s and assume that each individual had the same risk of disease p. Then the expected distribution of the number of cases r would be Binomial(s, p). Under single ascertainment, each case has probability π of being ascertained, so the probability that a family will be ascertained is πr, assuming that π is small. Likewise, control families will be ascertained from the unaffected individuals in the population, in proportion to $s - r$ times the population distribution of r. Now a case will be classified as having a positive family history if $r \geq 2$, while a control will be classified as positive if $r \geq 1$. Hence, the expected distribution of cases and controls will be as given in Table 5.9. The OR estimated from this 2×2 table is

$$OR = \frac{\sum_{r=2}^{s} r \binom{s}{r} p^r (1-p)^{s-r} \times s(1-p)^s}{\sum_{r=1}^{s-1} (s-r) \binom{s}{r} p^r (1-p)^{s-r} \times sp(1-p)^{s-1}} = 1$$

Proof of this identity requires only some straightforward algebra and is left as an exercise for the student. A similar calculation for complete ascertainment, however, does not lead to $OR = 1$ if each family is counted only once. In this case, what is required for unbiased estimation is that *every* affected family member be counted separately as a case. Under the null hypothesis, of course, their outcomes are independent, so the standard chi-square

Table 5.9 Expected Distribution of Sibships by Family History in a Case-Control Study Under Single Ascertainment of Cases

Family History	Controls	Cases
Negative	s Binom$(0 \mid s, p)$	π Binom$(1 \mid s, p)$
Positive	$\sum_{r=1}^{s-1} (s - r)$ Binom$(r \mid s, p)$	$\pi \sum_{r=2}^{s} r$ Binom$(r \mid s, p)$

test for association remains valid. However, the standard variance estimator $\mathrm{var}(\ln OR) = 1/A + 1/B + 1/C + 1/D$ will be an underestimate of the true sampling variance under the alternative hypothesis, requiring one to resort to one of the techniques for dealing with dependent data described at the end of this chapter. This problem does not arise under single ascertainment, because few if any families will be ascertained through more than one proband, so the sampled individuals are unrelated.

Cohort method. Alternatively, one might view the family members of cases and controls as two birth cohorts, one "exposed" to a case, the other not. Standard person-years methods might then be used to compare the incidence of disease between the two cohorts (Table 4.4). This analysis neatly avoids the need to reduce the entire complex family history to a single index by treating each individual in the family as a separate observation. Standard multivariate methods (e.g., Poisson or Cox regression) can be used to explore the modifying effects of age or degree of relationship to the proband. A complication with this approach that does not arise in the case-control approach is that the data on family members are dependent and require special treatment to obtain valid confidence limits and significance tests; we will return to this problem at the end of this chapter.

There is an additional subtlety in the calculation of person-years at risk due to selection for survival. The standard method treats all family members (except the proband) as having been at risk from birth to the present, their time of diagnosis, or death. However, parents of the proband must have been alive at the time of birth of the proband, and, depending on the disease, may be less likely to have had the disease before then than an unselected member of the population. This would argue for beginning their tabulation of person-years at the birth of the proband. In principle, the same argument could be applied to all ancestors of the proband. A trickier question relates to ancestors of other members of the pedigree. Consider an aunt: had she developed the disease at age 10, that event and the prior person-years would have been duly recorded as occurring in an unselected offspring of the grandparents; however, in that event, she would be unlikely to have had offspring whose events and person-years we also wish to count. This would argue in favor of excluding the person-years for all parents in the dataset accrued prior to their last offspring's birth. Fortunately, for late-onset diseases like most cancers and Alzheimer's disease, this is an academic issue, since these person-years will be multiplied by a tiny standard rate and will have negligible influence. The problem is more severe for early-onset diseases for which survival to reproductive age is unlikely, like juvenile-onset diabetes (IDDM). In this case, perhaps the simplest solution is to make an a priori decision on whether to include cousins or aunts/uncles.

A potential advantage of the cohort approach over the case-control approach is that control families are not needed if population rates are available. Instead, one simply ascertains case families and compares the cumulative incidence of disease in their family members (excluding the proband) to the expected incidence, using SIR_1, as described above. Indeed, one might wonder whether control families are ever needed in genetic epidemiology. In fact, control families are seldom used in segregation and linkage analyses. If the disease is rare, the expected yield of cases in the control families might be so small that the comparison SIR_0 would be highly unstable. In this circumstance, population rates would be expected to provide a much more stable estimate of the expected incidence in case families, since they are based on a much larger sample size. On the other hand, there are several reasons why control families might be worth including (Hopper, 2003), at least at the stage of studying familial aggregation:

- Population rates for the disease under study may not be available for the entire period under study (including the years at risk for all family members).
- Even if they are, the completeness of ascertainment of disease may be better or worse for these family members than in the population disease registry.
- The families included in the study may not be representative of the total population of affected families in terms of potential confounding factors or determinants of data quality, particularly the accuracy of the reported phenotypes.
- It may be possible to match case and control probands on age and other risk factors and on family characteristics such as sibship size, a potential confounder if cases tended to have larger or smaller families than controls.
- Nongenetic risk factors can be assessed for cases and controls that are unavailable from the population data and used to control for confounding and/or to test for interaction with familial risk.

There are two approaches to allowing for risk factors in the cohort approach. If one had such data on all relatives, then one could incorporate them in standard multivariate models to test the hypothesis that the effect of proband status on an individual's risk is confounded or modified by his or her own risk factors. This would clearly be the hypothesis of greatest interest, but obtaining the necessary data on all relatives may be nearly impossible, at least for extended families. The alternative would be to include the proband's risk factors in the analysis of the family members' outcomes. It does not make a lot of sense that one individual's exposure history would have a main effect on the risk for another family member, but it may be reasonable to ask whether it modifies that risk. For example, an individual's familial risk of breast cancer may be stronger if the affected family member (in this case the proband) was affected at an early age rather than at a late age.

Example: breast cancer. It has been known for decades that breast cancer has a tendency to run in families. Most of the relevant data on familial aggregation have come from case-control family studies. Two studies *using the same database* particularly well illustrate the contrast between the two analytical approaches described above: Sattin et al. (1985) and Claus et al. (1990) both analyzed data from the Cancer and Steriod Hormone (CASH) study, a large population-based case-control study in which cases and controls were asked about their family histories. Sattin et al. used a case-control form of analysis, while Claus et al. used a cohort form of analysis.

For both studies, cases comprised 5889 women aged 20 to 54 years with histologically confirmed primary breast cancer diagnosed between December 1, 1980, and December 31, 1982, who resided in one of eight SEER registry areas. Controls were identified by random digit dialing from the same geographic areas as the cases and were frequency matched on age. A total of 4754 controls agreed to participate. Cases and controls were interviewed in person, with the interviewer using a questionnaire that focused on reproductive, contraceptive, and family history, as well as standard breast cancer risk factors. The family history information was limited to breast cancer in mothers, sisters, daughters, and grandmothers, together with the age and vital status of each family member at risk. The number of aunts affected and at risk was also obtained but was not used in these analyses. Reported family histories were not verified; see, for example, Anton-Culver et al. (1996) and Ziogas and Anton-Culver (2003) for data on validation of breast cancer family histories and a review of similar studies.

Table 5.10 summarizes the information on family history from Sattin et al.'s case-control comparison. The effect of a first-degree relative is generally stronger than if only a second-degree relative is affected, but the effect of an affected sister or an affected mother is similar. Note also how the increased risk associated with having an affected first-degree relative is stronger

Table 5.10 Summary of Case-Control Comparison of a Family History of Breast Cancer in Cases and Controls from the Cancer and Steroid Hormone Study

Family History	Cases	Controls	OR (95% CI)
None	1804	2139	1.0 (referent)
First-degree relative only	456	231	2.3 (1.9–2.7)
Second-degree relative only	741	569	1.5 (1.4–1.8)
First- and second-degree relatives	79	42	2.2 (1.5–3.3)
Mother affected	364	196	2.1 (1.7–2.6)
Sister affected	136	74	2.1 (1.5–2.8)
Both mother and sister	35	3	13.6 (4.1–44.8)
First-degree relative under age 45	170	75	2.8 (2.1–3.7)
First-degree relative over age 45	329	190	1.9 (1.6–2.3)

Source: Sattin et al. (1985).

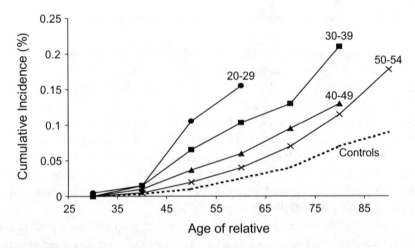

Figure 5.6 Cumulative incidence of breast cancer in first-degree relatives of breast cancer cases (solid lines) and first-degree relatives of controls (dashed line), distinguishing the age of the proband: circles 20–29, squares 30–39, triangles 40–49, crosses 50–54. (Adapted from Claus et al., 1990)

if that relative was affected before age 45, although the effect of having an affected relative did not depend strongly on the age of the proband in this analysis (3.1 for premenopausal women, 1.6 for perimenopausal women, and 3.1 for postmenopausal women with a first-degree relative affected before age 45, with a similar pattern for those with an affected relative after age 45).

Claus et al. used a person-years approach to estimating the age-specific incidence rates of breast cancer in relatives of cases and controls. The estimated rates using standard lifetable methods are shown in Figure 5.6. Note in particular the strong effect in this analysis of the age of the proband, in contrast to the lack of an effect of the proband's age in the Sattin et al. analysis.

Claus et al. also used Cox regression to incorporate covariates relating to the probands' characteristics into the analysis (no covariate information was available for the relatives themselves). The strongest predictor was the case-control status of the proband, $\hat{\beta}_1 = 2.88$, SE 0.30, reduced by −0.0474 (SE 0.0066) per year of age of the proband. Thus, the predicted relative risk for a relative of a case diagnosed at age 30 would be $\exp(2.88 - 0.0474 \times 30) =$ 4.3 (95% CI 3.3–5.6), while for a relative of a case diagnosed at age 50 it would be only 1.7 (95% CI 1.4–2.0). Having additional affected sisters or an affected mother or being a relative of a control with a history of benign breast disease further increased these risk estimates. Claus et al. later revisited these same data with a segregation analysis, as will be described in the following chapter.

A meta-analysis of 74 studies of familial risk of breast cancer (Pharoah et al., 1997) yielded estimates very similar to those given above for the CASH analysis: $RR = 2.1$ (95% CI 2.0–2.2) for first-degree relatives (2.0 for mothers, 2.3 for sisters, and 1.8 for daughters), 3.6 (CI = 2.5–5.0) for both mother and sister, and 1.5 (CI = 1.4–1.6) for second-degree relatives. It also confirmed the finding of an increased risk in women under age 50 or in those with affected family members under age 50: the relative risk to an individual under 50 with a first-degree relative affected before age 50 was 3.3 (CI 2.8–3.9) compared with 1.8 if one or the other member was under 50 or 1.7 (CI 1.5–2.0) if both were over 50.

Limited data are available on interactions of family history with other breast cancer risk factors. Andrieu et al. (1993) analyzed a case-control study of breast cancer using the case-control approach to family history in relation to the standard breast cancer risk factors and found the number of abortions to be the only significant modifier of the family history effect: $OR = 1.4$ (0.9–2.0) for women with no abortions, 1.2 (0.5–2.3) for women with one abortion, and 3.8 (1.7–8.4) for women with two or more abortions. A subsequent segregation analysis incorporation of interaction effects will be described in Chapter 6.

Other Designs

Randomization tests of familial clustering

Randomization tests were described in general terms in Chapter 4. In the context of familial aggregation, the relationships under study are assessed within families, so the relevant randomization is to permute the phenotypes among all the individuals in the dataset while keeping the family structures intact. Here family structure would include the indicators of who is related to whom, as well as the age and sex distribution that would affect the expected disease incidence under the null hypothesis. One way to accomplish the randomization would then be to stratify the subjects on age and sex and then, within each stratum, randomly permute the assignment of phenotypes across families. Alternatively, one could define the phenotype for each person as the difference between his or her observed disease status and the expected cumulative incidence, taking age and sex into account, and then permute these phenotypes across the entire dataset.

The hypothesis of familial aggregation is tested by taking as the index some summary of the *variability* in familial risks across families. For example, one might select one of the following indices:

$$Z = \begin{cases} \text{var}\,(Y_i/E_i) \\ \text{var}\,[(Y_i - E_i)/\sqrt{E_i}] \\ \sum_i \sum_j \sum_k (Y_{ij} - e_{ij})\,(Y_{ik} - e_{ik})\,\varphi_{jk} \\ \text{Avg}\,(\varphi_{jk}\,|\,Y_{ij} = 1 \text{ and } Y_{ik} = 1) \end{cases}$$

The first of these is simply the variance in the *FRRs,* where Y_i denotes the to-tal number of cases in (real or permuted) family i and E_i the corresponding expected number (both omitting probands). The difficulty with this index is that small families tend to have more variable *FRRs* than large families, so part of the variance in *FRRs* is due to variability in family size that ob-scures the variability in true *FRRs* that is of real interest. The second index overcomes this problem by dividing the $(Y-E)$s by their expected standard deviation, which should lead to a more powerful test. Neither of the first two indices exploits the types of relationships with families. The third index does this by computing a covariance between individuals within families weighted by their kinship coefficient. The final index is the average kinship coefficient over all pairs of affected relatives.

These indices are conceptually different from those described in the previous section: rather than testing for differences in *mean* familial risk between groups (case families vs. control families or population rates), the test is whether there is a larger *variance* in familial risk within a single group than would be expected by chance. This technique could also be applied to continuous phenotypes, with an appropriate definition of the index.

Although this technique can be applied to standard case-control and co-hort family studies (Chakraborty et al., 1984; Lynch et al., 1986; Schwartz et al., 1988, 1991), one of the most elegant applications of the approach has been to the Utah Mormon genealogy database (Slattery and Kerber, 1993, 1994). This database comprises over 1 million descendants of founders who were born or died on the Mormon Pioneer Trail in Utah. Each individual is linked on average to 2633 relatives (some to as many as 20,000) out to the 12th degree. The genealogy database has been linked to the Utah Cancer Registry for the years 1966–1990. Skolnick et al. (1981) used the random-ization procedure to compare the observed mean kinship coefficient for case families to that of control families matched on age of the proband. The case-control difference in kinship coefficients was found to be highly significant, compared to its randomization distribution, for prostate, breast, colorectal, and cervical/uterine cancers. Thirty-one pairs of cancer sites were found to cluster together in families, the most significant pairing being for gastroin-testinal and colon cancers (interestingly, breast/ovary cancers ranked only 21 out of the 78 combinations considered).

Twin studies

There are two basic subtypes of twin studies: twin cohort studies and twin concordance studies. In the twin cohort design, a cohort of twin births is established from birth certificate registries and followed to assess disease outcomes. In the twin concordance design, a set of twin individuals with the disease of interest is identified from disease registries, by advertisements, or by other methods, and the disease status of their cotwin is determined. Twins can also be used to investigate continuous phenotypes. In this case, random samples of twin pairs may be quite suitable, and the analysis is generally a special case of the variance components methods described above (for details, see Khoury et al., 1993, pp. 212–214). In the remainder of this section, we will focus on the analysis of binary disease traits.

For example, Hrubek et al. (1984) identified Swedish twin pairs born between 1891 and 1930 and sent them a questionnaire in 1951 or 1961 (depending on their date of birth). Those pairs for whom both were alive and disease free at that time and both of whom returned the questionnaire then formed the cohort for prospective follow-up. Their cancer outcomes were identified by linkage to the Swedish cancer registry. For the analysis described below, 475 breast cancers were identified in the cohort of 11,581 female pairs, including 25 concordant pairs.

In contrast, Mack et al. (2000) identified 2729 breast cancer cases among twins throughout North America by advertising in newspapers. Of these twins, 437 reported having a cotwin who also had breast cancer. This series was intended primarily as a source of matched pairs for conventional case-control studies, for which representativeness is not a crucial issue since any selection bias would affect both members of the pair equally. A particularly appealing aspect of using twins for case-control studies is that each can report not only on his or her own history but also on the cotwin's, allowing comparisons of both absolute and relative exposures (Hamilton and Mack, 2000). However, for analysis of concordance rates or genetic parameters derived from them (as described below), such a series is potentially biased in relation to such factors as zygosity, concordance, vital status, age, gender, and geographic proximity (Mack et al., 2000).

The parameters that are of primary interest in twin analysis for dichotomous traits are the concordance rates in MZ and DZ twins. Under the assumption that MZ and DZ twins share environmental factors equally, the comparison of these two rates can be used to derive an estimate of *heritability*. It goes without saying that the assumption of equal sharing is highly questionable; one commonly used refinement is to restrict the DZ pairs to same-sex pairs. There are several subtleties, however. First, the definition of the concordance rate depends on the question being asked and on the way the twins were ascertained. Second, heritability is defined in terms of a continuous trait and requires adaptation for binary traits. And third, some allowance for censoring is needed.

Three definitions of concordance are in widespread use:

- *Casewise concordance rate:* $2C/(2C + D)$, where C is the number of concordant affected twin pairs and D is the number of discordant pairs, is an estimator of the probability that one twin is affected given that the other is affected.
- *Pairwise concordance rate:* $C/(C + D)$ is an estimator of the proportion of twinships in the population who are concordant when twinships have been identified by complete ascertainment; in the case of single ascertainment, C should be divided by 2.
- *Probandwise concordance rate:* $(2C_2 + C_1)/(2C_2 + C_1 + D)$ where C_2 and C_1 are the numbers of concordant two-proband and one-proband twin pairs, respectively, and D is the number of discordant pairs. This is an estimator of the risk of disease to an individual with an affected cotwin.

The choice of which measure to use depends on the questions being asked. In a genetic counseling situation, for example, one might want to know the risk to a currently unaffected twin given that the cotwin is already affected; here, the casewise concordance rate is appropriate. On the other hand, if one wishes to know whether both twins are affected given that *at least one* twin is affected, the pairwise or probandwise concordance rates are appropriate, depending on the sampling scheme.

The concordance rate is related to the ratio of the cumulative probabilities A and B in the bivariate distribution shown in Figure 5.7B. To estimate heritability, the most widely used concept is the *liability model* introduced by Falconer (1967; Falconer and MacKay, 1994). This is very similar to the frailty model discussed below, except that (*1*) each member of a twinship is assumed to have his or her own liability, the pair of liabilities being assumed to be bivariate normally distributed, and (*2*) an individual is affected

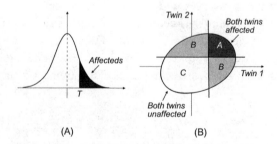

(A)   (B)

Figure 5.7 (A) Postulated normal distribution of liabilities: individuals with liability greater than the threshold T are affected. (B) Bivariate distribution of liabilities: pairs for which both members' liabilities are greater than the threshold are concordant (region A), those in which one is greater than T are discordant (region B), and the remainder are unaffected (region C).

if his or her liability exceeds some threshold that depends on the population rate of the disease (possibly age-dependent). It is also closely related to the polygenic model introduced in the next chapter.

Liability, in turn, can be decomposed into genetic and environmental components (as in the familial correlation models described above), and the correlation between the two liabilities is then the parameter of interest. In particular, heritability is defined in terms of the proportion of the total variance in liability that is due to genotype and environmentality is the corresponding proportion due to shared environment. These parameters can be estimated by comparing concordance rates between MZ and DZ twins and the population rate. Estimation of the underlying bivariate normal correlation r from data on the relative frequencies of these three sectors, A, B, and C, is known as the *tetrachoric* correlation, for which standard tables are available (Smith, 1970). The values of the correlation (r) are algebraically approximated to within 5% by

$$\tan\left[\frac{\pi}{4}(1-r)(1+r^5)\right] = \log q_R / \log q_P$$

where q_R is the incidence in the relatives of affected individuals and q_P is the incidence in the population.

Table 5.11 provides a summary of the standard analysis of breast cancer in the Swedish twin cohort. The overall risk in the cohort was 0.019, so it is evident that both MZ and DZ twins have substantially elevated familial risks. The estimate of heritability was $\hat{h}^2 = 2(\hat{r}_{MZ} - \hat{r}_{DZ}) = 14.0\% \pm 14.0\%$ and that of environmentality was $\hat{e}^2 = 2\hat{r}_{DZ} - \hat{r}_{MZ} = 26.0\% \pm 7.4\%$, suggesting that shared environment may be more important than shared genotype.

The methods described above do not properly allow for the fact that some twins may not have fully expressed their risk, due to premature death from competing causes or truncation of follow-up, or due to age or calendar year effects. For diseases with variable age at onset, survival analysis techniques are more appropriate, and the frailty models described at the end of this chapter are the natural solution. Thomas et al. (1990) illustrated the application of this method to the Swedish breast cancer data and compared it to standard concordance methods. They found a frailty variance of

Table 5.11 Proband Concordance Rates and Correlation in Liability for Breast Cancer Among Swedish Twins

Zygosity	Concordant Pairs	Discordant Pairs	Proband Concordance Rate	Correlation in Liability
MZ	10	140	0.125	0.38
DZ	15	285	0.095	0.31

$\eta = 1.37$ ($p = 0.015$), corresponding to 95% of the population having an *RR* between 0.19 and 5.0 compared with the general population risk. The frailty variance was nearly double for MZ compared to DZ twins.

The multivariate nature of these models also allows easy incorporation of risk factors and interactions. Addition of year of birth, cigarette smoking, and weight to the model did not substantially alter the frailty variance, but there was a significant interaction with year of birth, indicating a stronger familial risk at younger ages.

There have been a large number of other twin studies of breast cancer (Forsti et al., 2001; Holm, 1981; Holm et al., 1980; Hubinette et al., 2001; Kaijser et al., 2001; Segal, 2000; Verkasalo et al., 1999; Whiteman et al., 2000). One that received considerable attention (Lichtenstein et al., 2000) studied 44,788 twin pairs from the combined Swedish, Danish, and Finnish twin registries and found significant concordance for stomach, colorectal, lung, breast, and prostate cancers. Their estimate of heritability for breast cancer was 27% (95% CI 4%–41%), on the basis of which they concluded that shared environment likely plays a more important role. In another report, Peto and Mack (2000) pointed out that the incidence rate of breast cancer in MZ cotwins, following diagnosis in the first twin, was high and virtually constant, mirroring a similar pattern that is seen for the risk of cancer in the contralateral breast of the same individual, or in nontwin siblings (at a lower rate), but very different from the rapidly rising rate of cancer in the general population. On this basis, they argued for a new theory of carcinogenesis in which the age at which individuals move from a relatively low risk to a high constant risk varies between individuals (thus accounting for the rising rate with age) and is genetically determined. An alternative view was put forward in an accompanying editorial (Easton, 2000), suggesting that breast cancer was caused by a combination of a few major genes, like *BRCA1*, and a larger number of lower-risk polymorphisms, perhaps related to estrogen metabolism. The constancy of the absolute risk of second cancers was then simply a reflection of a declining relative risk with age.

In a further analysis of these twin data, Hamilton and Mack (2003) found no association between breast cancer status and age at menarche among disease discordant twins, but a strong association ($OR = 5.4$, 95% CI 2.0–4.5) with age at onset among concordant MZ twins. They interpret this finding as evidence that, among women with the strongest genetic susceptibility, breast cancer is not related to cumulative exposure to hormones, but rather to an unusual sensitivity to hormones at the time of puberty. In commenting on these findings, Hartge (2003) points out that no such interaction has been seen with *BRCA1* or *BRCA2* and FH, but that concordant MZ twins are more likely to carry potent combinations of common low-penetrance genes, some of which may be more directly related to hormone metabolism than *BRCA1/2*.

Various extensions of the twin design include comparisons of twin adoption studies and twin family studies. The twin adoption study design involves the ascertainment of twins who have been reared apart. Thus, each member of the pair has two sets of parents, their biological parents (shared) and their adoptive parents (separate). In one variant of the design, phenotype data are obtained only on the twins, but by comparing twins reared together and twins reared apart, it is possible to estimate the effect of both genotype and shared environment without having to assume that MZ and DZ twins have equal sharing of environmental factors. (However, instead one must assume that twins reared apart and twins reared together have the same baseline risk of disease.) The addition of phenotype data on both biological and adoptive parents provides an even more powerful design, allowing estimation of path models of considerable complexity.

Finally, twins could be the starting point for a variety of interesting family studies. Some possible designs include the following:

- Concordant pairs are highly likely to be gene carriers and thus a particularly efficient means of ascertaining hereditary families for segregation and linkage analysis.
- Twins and their spouses provide a novel variant on the standard case-control design, in which one might compare the case to the unaffected cotwin or either twin to his or her spouse.
- The unaffected member of a discordant MZ pair can be taken as the case for a case-control study when a measured genotype is under study and the case is no longer available. In particular, if a phenotypic assay is needed that can be distorted by the disease process, the unaffected cotwin could provide a more accurate measure of the phenotype than the case. For example, see Los et al. (2001) for a discussion of the use of twins for studying intermediate phenotypes for asthma, and Cozen et al. (in press) for an application to Hodgkin's lymphoma.
- DZ twins can be compared with non-twin siblings. While the two types of pairs have the same degree of genetic sharing, twins also share a common uterine environment and have a greater similarity of childhood environmental factors.
- Shared environmental factors can be compared between concordant and discordant twin pairs, treating the pair as the unit of observation. Factors that are more common among concordant pairs would be interpreted as risk factors. Differences in relative risks between MZ and DZ pairs would be evidence of an interaction effect.

Adoption studies

The study of twins reared apart is an elegant design for separating genetic and environmental influences, in part because it offers natural comparisons of both genetic influences (MZ vs. DZ twins) and environmental influences (those raised together vs. those raised apart). However, adopted twins are difficult to identify and sample sizes tend to be small, particularly for rare disease traits. An alternative is therefore to use adoptees without limiting the design to twins.

Consider first a continuous trait such as blood pressure, and let us focus on a single relationship, say parent–child (since not all adoptees need have both biological and adopted siblings) and random samples. In principle, there are four possible comparisons one might make: (*1*) between parents and their biological offspring they reared (sharing both genetic and environmental influences); (*2*) between parents and their biological offspring raised apart (sharing genetic but not environmental influences); (*3*) between parents and their adopted children (sharing environmental but not genetic influences); and (*4*) between adoptive parents and the other children of the biological parents of their adoptee (sharing neither). In practice, the last of these correlations should estimate zero, and hence the observed estimate does not add any useful information. Using variance components methods (or the equivalent path analysis representation), we could write the expected covariances (denoting biological parents by p_b, adoptive parents by p_a, natural offspring by o, and adopted children by a) as follows:

$$\text{cov}\left(Y_{p_b}, Y_o\right) = \frac{1}{2}\sigma_A^2 + \sigma_E^2$$

$$\text{cov}\left(Y_{p_b}, Y_a\right) = \frac{1}{2}\sigma_A^2$$

$$\text{cov}\left(Y_{p_a}, Y_a\right) = \sigma_E^2$$

$$\text{cov}\left(Y_{p_a}, Y_o\right) = 0$$

This assumes that the extent of environmental correlation is the same between parents and their natural children as with their adoptive children and also that adopted children have the same genetic correlation with their biological parents as nonadopted children. The latter may seem obvious, but there are important selection biases in who is placed for adoption. For this reason, adoption studies are frequently limited to the adoptees, without comparing them to other children raised by their biological parents (in either the source or destination families).

A good example is the Montreal Adoption Study (Mongeau et al., 1986), a cross-sectional survey of cardiovascular risk factors in 756 adopted French-Canadian children and 445 natural children living in the same households and their 1176 parents. Highly significant correlations in blood pressure were found between parents and their biological children but not with their adopted children. Maximum likelihood estimates of heritability, derived from joint analysis of parent–child and sib–sib correlations of the different types, yielded an estimate of 61% for systolic and 58% for diastolic blood pressure. Annest et al. (1979a, 1979b, 1983) provide detailed analyses of the familial aggregation of various risk factors.

For binary disease traits, the limiting factor is likely to be the number of *affected* adoptees, suggesting that some form of ascertainment design will be needed. There are a number of ways this could be done. Again, focusing on parent–child relationships, one could draw a sample of affected adoptees as cases and a matched control group of unaffected adoptees, a case-control sample of biological parents, or a case-control sample of adoptive parents. The schizophrenia study described in Chapter 1 is an example of the former, although earlier studies had used disease in either the biological parent (Higgins, 1976) or the adoptive parent (Wender et al., 1974) as the basis for ascertainment. Ingraham and Kety (2000) provide an excellent discussion of the advantages and disadvantages of the alternative designs.

Random samples are, however, sometimes used with disease traits. For example, Sorensen et al. (1988) studied 960 families that included adopted children born between 1924 and 1926 in Denmark and studied the adoptees' risk of dying of specific causes as a function of their biological and adoptive parents' outcomes for the same cause. Specifically, they compared the risk of death at ages 15–58 in adoptees with the risk in a parent (biological or adopted) who died of that cause before age 50 compared with those whose parents were still alive at age 50. For cancer, the relative risk was 1.2 (95% CI 0.2–9.0) for a biological parent who died of cancer but 5.2 (1.2–22) for adoptive parents, suggesting that environmental factors predominate. In contrast, for infections, the corresponding *RR*s were 5.8 (2.5–13) versus unity, and for cardiovascular and cerebrovascular causes they were 4.5 (1.2–15) versus 3.0 (0.7–13), suggesting that genetic factors were more important for these causes.

Analyses of multivariate survival data are not straightforward, and these data could yield more information. One approach would be to take the adoptees as the unit of analysis in a Cox regression, using two fixed covariates, one for their biological parents' outcomes and one for their adoptive parents' outcomes, each coded as $\sum_j (Y_j - E_j)$, where Y_j is an indicator for parent j having died of the specific cause and E_j is the cumulative incidence up to that parent's age at death or censoring, as discussed elsewhere in this chapter. This would have the advantage that the individuals in the analysis are independent and thus no allowance for residual familiality needs to be taken into account, but it would limit the analysis to a single individual in each family. An appealing alternative would be to view each family (comprising both biological and adoptive relatives) as a stratum and form Cox risk sets within the family, taking each death from the cause of interest as a case and comparing them to all other family members who survived to the same age. The comparison would be made for two time-dependent covariates, the number of biological relatives and the number of adoptive relatives who had succumbed to the disease of interest by that age. Thus, comparisons could be made in either direction, early death of a parent as a risk factor for the death of an offspring at a later age, or vice versa. In this way, all of the information would be fully exploited, but because risk sets are formed within families, no further allowance for residual familiality is needed. However, when families are ascertained through affected individuals over a fixed time window, additional complications arise, as discussed by Langholz et al. (1999b). Other techniques for dealing with dependent data are discussed in the following section.

Approaches to Dependent Data

We noted earlier that the cohort-style analysis assumes that the outcomes of each family member are independent. This assumption is clearly violated if the null hypothesis being tested is false: if two family members are both at increased risk because they are related to the same case proband, then their outcomes must also be dependent on each other. This does not produce a bias in the estimated *FRR,* but it does tend to inflate the effective sample size, leading to liberal significance tests and confidence limits that are too narrow. On the other hand, if the null hypothesis is true, then it also follows that family members' outcomes should be independent of each other and hence the test of the null hypothesis is valid. It is not the most powerful test of familial aggregation (nor is the case-control test described above) because neither test exploits the information contained in the correlations among the outcomes among nonproband family members.

Figure 5.8 represents the conceptual basis of the standard case-control and cohort analyses of familial aggregation. The case-control approach treats family history as a risk factor for predicting the disease status of the case and control subjects (denoted Y_1), thereby reducing their complex history information to a single variable. The cohort approach treats the probands' disease status as a risk factor for predicting the family members' outcomes ($Y_2, \ldots, Y_5$) but ignores the potential dependencies among the family members. What is really needed is a unified analysis that exploits

Figure 5.8 Schematic representation of relationships among family members in case-control and cohort data and the need for methods of dependent data analysis.

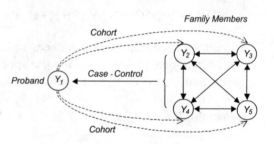

all the relationships in the families, conditional on how the probands were originally selected. There is a growing statistical literature on methods of analysis of dependent data. Here we briefly introduce four basic methods for dealing with this problem.

Genetic models

The method this book will explore in greatest detail is *genetic modeling*, in which we postulate an explicit model for the unobserved genotypes (major genes and/or polygenes) and fit the model using maximum likelihood. This approach will be treated in Chapters 6 and 7. In essence, we will postulate one or more unobserved (*latent*) variables—major genes and/or polygenes—and form a likelihood by summing or integrating over all possible values of the unobserved quantities. For example, in segregation analysis, we might propose a major gene G and maximize a likelihood of the form

$$\mathcal{L}(\mathbf{f}, q) \equiv \Pr(\mathbf{Y} \mid \mathbf{f}, q) = \sum_{\mathbf{G}} \Pr(\mathbf{Y} \mid \mathbf{G}; \mathbf{f}) \; \Pr(\mathbf{G} \mid q)$$

One is then interested in the estimates of the penetrances $\mathbf{f}$ and the population mutant allele frequency q, and especially in testing particular hypotheses about penetrance models (e.g., a global null hypothesis of no genetic effect $H_0 : f_0 = f_1 = f_2$ vs. a dominant hypothesis $H_1 : f_1 = f_2$ vs. the general unrestricted alternative hypothesis).

Regressive models

A second approach is known as *regressive models* (Bonney, 1986). Here one includes as covariates in a multivariate model for each individual the phenotypes of all individuals in the family who appear before him or her in the dataset. This relies on the basic law of conditional probability that

$$\begin{aligned}
\Pr(\mathbf{Y}) &= \Pr(Y_1, \ldots, Y_k) \\
&= \Pr(Y_1) \Pr(Y_2, \ldots, Y_k \mid Y_1) \\
&= \Pr(Y_1) \Pr(Y_2 \mid Y_1) \Pr(Y_3, \ldots, Y_k \mid Y_1, Y_2) \\
&\cdots \\
&= \Pr(Y_1) \Pr(Y_2 \mid Y_1) \Pr(Y_3 \mid Y_1, Y_2) \ldots \Pr(Y_k \mid Y_1, \ldots, Y_{k-1})
\end{aligned}$$

The basic modeling decision that needs to be made is how to specify the various conditional probabilities, but it is appealing to take them all to be of the same basic form. Thus, for example, in a logistic model, one might write

$$\operatorname{logit} \Pr(Y_i = 1 \mid Y_p, Y_1, \ldots, Y_{i-1}) = \alpha + \beta Y_p + \gamma \sum_{j < i} (Y_j - E_j) \qquad (5.3)$$

where Y_i is the disease status of the individual whose risk we are currently computing, Y_p is the disease status of the proband, Y_j are the disease status of the other family members, and E_j are their corresponding expected numbers, computed as described above. Any subjects whose disease status is unknown would simply be omitted from the summation, including their expected values. (Including the Es in this way is preferable to Bonney's original suggestion of coding the Ys as 1 for affected, -1 for unaffected, and 0 for missing, because the expected value of Y would not be 0 unless the prevalence were $1/2$. Bonney also suggested setting up a separate set of coefficients for missingness indicators, but this seems wasteful of degrees of freedom.) Covariates can be added in a natural way simply by adding each individual's own covariate to his or her own logistic probability.

Bonney (1986) proposed a number of variants of this basic approach for use in family data, allowing for different types of relationships. Thus, if one orders the individuals so that parents precede their offspring and sibs are ordered by age, then one might allow for different regression coefficients for the effects of one spouse on the other, for parents on offspring, and for older sibs on younger sibs. Among sibs, one might regress each sib on the mean or sum of the effects of his or her older sibs or perhaps just on the immediately preceding sib. Thus, letting Y' denote the residuals $Y - E(Y)$, one could fit the model by arranging the data in the form shown in Table 5.12 and using any standard linear or logistic regression program.

Frailty models

The third approach, known as *frailty models*, is similar to the first in that it postulates an unobserved risk factor (the *frailty*) that is shared by members of a family. The difference from a real genetic model is that all members of a family unit are assumed to share a common value of this frailty rather than to transmit alleles from parents to offspring. As a consequence, this analysis

Table 5.12 Arrangement of Data from a Nuclear Family for Input to a Linear or Logistic Regression Program to Fit the Regressive Model, Where $Y' = Y - E(Y)$

Dependent Variable	β	Covariates		
		γ_{Sp}	γ_{PO}	γ_{Sib}
Y_f	Z_f	0	0	0
Y_m	Z_m	Y_f'	0	0
Y_1	Z_1	0	$Y_f' + Y_m'$	0
Y_2	Z_2	0	$Y_f' + Y_m'$	Y_1'
Y_3	Z_3	0	$Y_f' + Y_m'$	$Y_1' + Y_2'$
$\ldots$	$\ldots$	$\ldots$	$\ldots$	$\ldots$
Y_s	Z_s	0	$Y_f' + Y_m'$	$\sum_{j=1}^{s-1} Y_j'$

is much simpler, but it should be thought of as only a descriptive model for estimating the variability in risk between families. It is also a special case of the liability models for twin data discussed earlier. In brief, a proportional hazards model is assumed for the age-specific disease rate $\lambda_{ij}(t)$ for member j of family i of the form

$$\lambda_{ij}(t) = \lambda_0(t) X_i\, e^{\mathbf{Z}'_{ij}\beta}$$

where the unobserved frailty X_i for family i is assumed to have a gamma distribution with unit mean and variance η that is the parameter of interest, and $\mathbf{Z}_{ij}$ is a vector of covariates for individual j in family i. (For simplicity, we will omit covariate effects in the remainder of this section.) The model is fitted using a marginal likelihood obtained by integrating the usual survival likelihood over all possible values of the unknown frailties, leading to another proportional hazards model in which the frailties are replaced by their expected values, which can be shown to be

$$\mathrm{E}(X_i) = \frac{1 + \eta Y_i}{1 + \eta E_i}$$

where Y_i is the total number of cases in the family and E_i is the corresponding expected number. Individual risk factors can easily be incorporated into this analysis using standard survival regression techniques (e.g., adding a factor of the form $e^{\beta Z_{ij}}$). For more details, see Clayton (1991) and Hougaard and Thomas (2002).

Proof: The standard parameterization of the gamma distribution with parameters α and η

$$\Pr(X) = \exp(-X/\eta) X^{\alpha-1}/\eta^\alpha \Gamma(\alpha)$$

has mean $\alpha\eta$ and variance $\alpha\eta^2$. To obtain a distribution with unit mean and variance η, we therefore set $\alpha = \eta^{-1}$ to obtain

$$\Pr(X) = \exp(-X/\eta) X^{\eta^{-1}-1}/\eta^{\eta^{-1}} \Gamma(\eta^{-1})$$

This is a convenient distribution to use because it is of the same form— in terms of its dependence on X—as the Poisson distribution used for the likelihood (assuming that $Y_i \sim \mathrm{Poisson}(E_i X)$),

$$\Pr(Y_i \mid X, E_i) = \exp(-E_i X)(E_i X)^{Y_i}/Y_i!$$

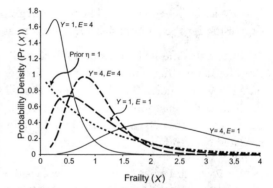

Figure 5.9 Shapes of gamma distributions: dotted line, prior with $\eta = 1$; dashed lines, posterior with $Y=1, E=1$ and $Y=4, E=4$ (equivalent to priors with $\eta = 2$ and 5, respectively; solid lines, posterior with $Y=1, E=4$ and $Y=4, E=1$).

Thus, the posterior distribution of $X_i \mid Y_i, E_i$ can be obtained by Bayes' formula as

$$\Pr(X \mid Y, E) = \frac{\Pr(Y \mid X, E)\Pr(X)}{\int \Pr(Y \mid X, E)\Pr(X)\, dX}$$

$$\propto \exp(-EX)X^Y \times \exp(-X/\eta)X^{\eta^{-1}-1}$$

$$= \exp[-(E+\eta^{-1})X]X^{(Y+\eta^{-1})-1}$$

where in the second line we have retained only the factors that depend on X. Thus, X has a gamma distribution with parameters $Y+\eta^{-1}$ and $(E+\eta^{-1})^{-1}$. Its mean is given by $E(X_i) = (1 + \eta Y_i)/(1 + \eta E_i)$, as given above (Fig. 5.9).

Now what about the unknown frailty variance parameter η? This is estimated from the *marginal* likelihood, obtained by integrating out the unobserved frailties. Although an analytic expression for this likelihood is available (see below), maximization of the likelihood with respect to η generally requires numerical methods.

Proof: The likelihood can be written as follows:

$$\mathcal{L}(\eta) = \prod_i \Pr(Y_i \mid E_i; \eta) = \prod_i \int \Pr(Y_i \mid E_i X)\Pr(X \mid \eta)\, dX$$

$$\propto \prod_i \int \exp[-(E_i + \eta^{-1})X]X^{(Y_i+\eta^{-1})-1}/\eta^{\eta^{-1}}\Gamma(\eta^{-1})\, dX$$

$$= \frac{\prod_{i=1}^{N}\left[\left(\frac{\eta}{1+\eta E_i}\right)^{\eta^{-1}+Y_i}\Gamma(\eta^{-1}+Y_i)\right]}{[\eta^{\eta^{-1}}\Gamma(\eta^{-1})]^N}$$

The last line can be derived by recognizing that the integrand in the numerator is simply the numerator of another gamma distribution with parameters

$Y + \eta^{-1}$ and $(E + \eta^{-1})^{-1}$, and hence it integrates to the denominator in the expression for the gamma distribution given above.

Fitting this model by maximum likelihood can be difficult, so an attractive alternative that will be developed further in Chapters 6 and 7 relies on MCMC methods. The basic ideas of MCMC methods were described in Chapter 4. Clayton (1991) has described a Gibbs sampling approach to frailty models that essentially involves the following sequence of operations, repeated over and over again:

- For each family i, sample a frailty conditional on Y_i, E_i and the current estimate of η. As shown above, this simply entails sampling a random gamma deviate with parameters $Y_i + \eta^{-1}$ and $(E_i + \eta^{-1})^{-1}$.
- Update $\lambda_0(t)$ and any measured individual covariates Z_{ij} treating these new frailties X_i as known covariates, using a standard Cox regression model.
- Update η by sampling from $\prod_i \Pr(X_i \mid \eta)$, again treating the X_i as known.

This algorithm is quite easy to implement and can be generalized in various ways, including to models with person-specific frailties that are correlated within families. The polygenic model, to be discussed in Chapter 6, can be considered an example of such a correlated frailty model.

Generalized estimating equations

GEE methods, introduced in the previous chapter, are appealing for the analysis of dependent data because they require specification of only the first few moments (e.g., means, variances, covariances) of the observed data, without having to specify the entire distribution. Thus, inferences on the parameters of these *marginal models* are much more robust to model misspecification because there are fewer assumptions involved. GEE methods have been used for analyses of familial aggregation in two ways. First, one might be interested in testing hypotheses about covariate effects on the means model while allowing for the dependency between family members' phenotypes; in such analyses, the residual familiality is treated as a nuisance parameter and GEE-1 methods are used. Second, one might be primarily interested in estimating or testing hypotheses about the familial dependencies themselves, in which case GEE-2 methods are needed.

As an example of the first approach, let us revisit the cohort approach to testing for familial aggregation while now trying to allow for the dependency between the probands' relatives. Suppose that we adopt a marginal model of the form

$$\text{logit}(\mu_{ij}) = \beta_0 + \beta Y_{ip} + \mathbf{Z}_{ij}'\boldsymbol{\gamma}$$

where $\mu_{ij} = \Pr(Y_{ij} = 1 \mid Y_{ip}, \mathbf{Z}_{ij})$, Y_{ip} denotes the case-control status of the proband in family i, and $\mathbf{Z}_{ij}$ denotes a vector of person-specific covariates. The parameter β now tests the same hypothesis tested by the cohort design, that is, the dependence of each family member's risk of disease on whether he or she is a relative of a case or a relative of a control. The difference is that when the robust variance estimate is used, asymptotically valid confidence limits on $\hat{\beta}$ and valid tests of $H_0 : \beta = 0$ can be obtained that correctly allow for the dependency between family members. However, this dependency is simply *allowed* for as a nuisance; it does not contribute to the estimation of β per se. For this purpose, one might simply adopt as a working covariance matrix $\mathbf{W}_i$, an independence structure $\sigma^2 \mathbf{I}$, or an exchangeable structure $\sigma^2 \mathbf{I} + \tau^2 \mathbf{1}$, where the variance components are estimated in a separate step from the residuals from the fitted model at each iteration, as described by Liang et al. (1992). This approach was first introduced by Liang et al. (1986) with an application to chronic obstructive pulmonary disease. Such an analysis is implemented in standard statistical programs such as procedure GENMOD in the S.A.S. package.

In the second approach, one would specify a particular model for the form of the dependency between relatives. For example, one might fit a model of the form

$$E(C_{ijk}) = \alpha_0 + \alpha_1 \varphi_{ijk} \tag{5.4}$$

where φ_{ijk} is the coefficient of relationship between relatives j and k of family i. For this purpose, one might be particularly interested in testing the hypothesis $\alpha_1 = 0$. Applications of this general approach to censored survival time phenotypes have been described by Prentice and Hsu (1997).

Conclusions

Studies of familial aggregation are normally the first step in investigating a possible genetic etiology for a disease or trait since one that does not run in families is unlikely to have a strong genetic component. As the name implies, such studies require the collection of family data. However, the actual sampling plan might comprise only a set of unrelated individuals (probands, such as cases and controls), who are then asked about their family histories without formally enrolling their family members as study subjects. In this approach, the outcomes of the probands could be analyzed in relation to their family histories as predictor variables (a case-control approach) or the reported outcomes of the family members could be treated as a vector of response variables to be analyzed in relation to the disease status of the proband (a cohort approach). In the latter case, some allowance is needed for the dependence of family members' outcomes on each other. The analyses of breast cancer in the CASH study by Sattin et al. (1985) and Claus et al. (1990) provide examples of these two approaches, both showing a roughly 2-fold relative risk, declining with age. More complex sampling plans, such as those based on twins or adoptees, can also be used.

In addition to testing the null hypothesis of no familial aggregation, these studies have the potential to provide estimates of the relative magnitude of the contribution of genes (heritability) and unmeasured environmental factors (environmentality) using variance components models (for a continuous trait) or liability models (for a binary trait). The analysis of a cohort of Scandinavian twins (Lichtenstein et al., 2000), for example, appeared to show a stronger effect of environment than of genetics on breast cancer risk. However, such analyses usually require untestable assumptions about the distribution of the unobservable shared environmental influences (e.g., the assumption in a twin study that MZ and DZ twins have similar degrees of a common environment). Testing hypotheses about the specific mode of inheritance (major genes, polygenes, environment, or combinations thereof) and estimating the parameters of a genetic model is the job of segregation analysis, as discussed in the following chapter.

6

Segregation Analysis

Segregation analysis refers to the process of fitting genetic models to data on phenotypes of family members. For this purpose, no molecular data are used, the aim being to test hypotheses about whether one or more major genes and/or polygenes can account for the observed pattern of familial aggregation, the mode of inheritance, and to estimate the parameters of the best-fitting genetic model. As in the previous chapter on familial aggregation, the technique can be applied to various types of traits, including continuous and dichotomous traits and censored survival times. However, the basic techniques are essentially the same, involving only appropriate specification of the penetrance function $\Pr(Y \mid G)$ and the ascertainment model.

The presentation of analysis methods here is divided into three parts: (*1*) classical methods for sibships, allowing us to develop the basic ideas in the simplest form; (*2*) pedigree likelihoods, the standard method for *complex segregation analysis;* and (*3*) a some recent methodological advances. But before describing these methods, we briefly consider study design principles.

Design Issues

Ascertainment of families

As discussed in Chapter 5, families may be ascertained in a number of ways, depending on the nature of the trait under study. In almost any study, however, families are usually identified through a single individual, called the *proband,* and the family structure around that person is then discovered, since (at least in North American society) there are few resources that would be suitable for sampling entire families. For continuous traits (and common dichotomous ones), it is not unusual for the probands to be simply random members of the population (at least with respect to their trait), in which case no special ascertainment correction is needed. However, for rare disease traits, probands are usually selected from registries of affected individuals. Similarly, for continuous traits with highly skewed distributions, thought to be due to the presence of a rare major gene, it may also be more efficient to select as probands individuals with extreme values of the trait. In either case, some correction for the method of ascertainment will be needed in the analysis to allow for the fact that families with cases are over-represented in the sample relative to the source population to which we wish to generalize.

In the case of a binary trait we distinguish a range of ascertainment models, based on the probability π that a random case in the population will be selected as a proband. In the situation where $\pi = 1$, known as *complete ascertainment,* all families with cases are included. In the opposite situation where $\pi \to 0$, known as *single ascertainment,* the probability that a family is selected is proportional to the number of cases in the family. Thus, multiple-case families will be considerably over-represented, and it is unlikely that any families will be independently ascertained through more than one proband. In intermediate situations, known as *multiple ascertainment,* there are likely to be multiple probands in some families. The implications of these different situations for the analysis will be discussed below.

In the case of a continuous trait, the most commonly used ascertainment model is *threshold ascertainment,* which assumes that probands are representative of all members of the population with phenotypes greater than some minimum value (the *threshold;* see Fig. 5.7). Ascertainment correction is simplest in this situation, so if this is the intent, it is desirable that the study design reflect it, that is, that probands be selected at random from a pool of all cases above some predefined threshold. The reality is often quite different, with probands simply being patients from a clinic that specializes in treating individuals with extreme values of the trait. The analyst may then be forced to define the threshold after the fact as the smallest proband phenotype in the sample, but one should recognize that within this group, higher values may be over-represented. Another possible analytical strategy might be to assume that the probability of ascertainment is proportional to the trait value (or some function thereof), but this may be mathematically intractable and unrealistic.

For a dichotomous or survival trait, it is common to perform segregation analysis on families ascertained through a previous case-control study aimed at testing familial aggregation. (The CASH study [Claus et al., 1990] is a good example.) In this situation, the families are actually a mixture of case families (for whom single ascertainment may be a reasonable model) and control families (for whom random ascertainment ought to be reasonable). However, the yield of multiple-case families from the controls may be so low that it is hardly worthwhile to include them, particularly if further data collection (e.g., extended family histories) is planned. Piggybacking segregation (and linkage) analyses on an existing case-control study can be a very efficient strategy, but one might reasonably restrict the genetic part of the study to the case families.

Sequential sampling

When the probands have been identified, it is then necessary to assemble a pedigree for each of them, including their phenotypes. This is normally done by working outward from the proband, confirming information by interviewing other family members and obtaining medical records or other documentation. This must be done very carefully to avoid introducing bias. For example, one must guard against selectively including individuals with positive phenotypes and omitting those one doesn't hear about. The starting point is usually an interview and/or a questionnaire with the proband, inquiring in a structured manner about all first- and perhaps second-degree relatives. As discussed in Chapter 5, it is important to obtain medical confirmation about all reported cases if possible, but one should not simply omit unconfirmed cases either, since that strategy could be even more biased than including unconfirmed cases. Case-control studies seldom inquire beyond second-degree relatives because of the difficulty of doing so systematically. One could, of course, stop there and do segregation analysis on only first-degree relatives; indeed, the classical methods we shall discuss first are restricted to sibships.

However, there is a considerable increase in power if one is able to assemble large pedigrees (particularly for linkage analysis, which we will discuss in Chapter 7). To avoid bias in segregation analysis, such large families must be built systematically, but one does not want to waste effort investigating families that are unlikely to be informative. To fulfill these conflicting requirements, a clever strategy known as *sequential sampling of pedigrees* was developed by Cannings and Thompson (1977). They enumerated the following principles:

- The initial identification of the family must follow a systematic ascertainment scheme that one can characterize in the analysis.
- At each stage of the pedigree-building process, ascertainment of phenotype information about the individuals identified so far must be done in an unbiased manner.
- In deciding whether to extend a pedigree in a particular direction, it is legitimate to use the following information: (*1*) the phenotype information accumulated systematically so far (to judge the likelihood that a mutation is segregating in that branch of the family) and (*2*) knowledge of the family structure in the extension being considered (to judge the potential yield of further work); however, one must not be influenced by any anecdotal information one might have learned about the presence of disease in that branch.

• Once a branch has been extended, all the phenotype data obtained must be included in the analysis; one must not selectively omit branches that turn out to be negative.

Through a subtle mathematical argument, Cannings and Thompson show that if one proceeds in this manner, then one need only correct the analysis for the original ascertainment event.

Consider the pedigree shown in Figure 6.1. If initially all one had was the nuclear family shown in panel A, then one would be entitled to decide to

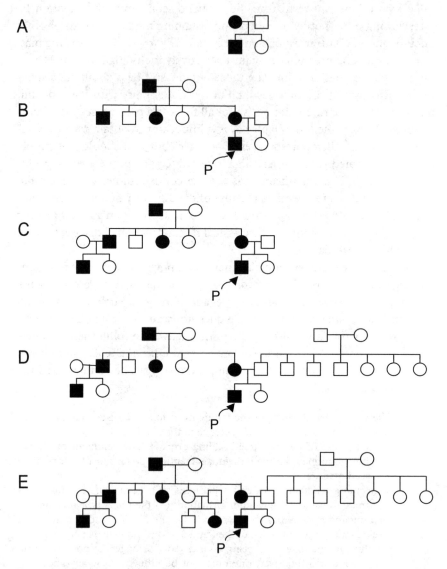

Figure 6.1 Hypothetical example of sequential sampling of a pedigree.

pursue the maternal branch first, since the mother was affected and hence was more likely to be the source of any mutant allele. Suppose that this resulted in the expanded pedigree shown in panel B. By the same reasoning, one could choose to investigate the offspring of the affected maternal uncle to produce the pedigree shown in panel C. Now suppose that one decided to pursue the paternal branch on the grounds that one already knew the father had many siblings. Even though it turned out that none of them was affected (panel D), it would then be necessary to include them all in the analysis. But suppose that in the course of talking with family members, one happened to learn that the unaffected maternal aunt had had an affected offspring (panel E). One would not be entitled to include this information in the analysis because it was anecdotally obtained, not based solely on the information already available.

Classical Methods for Sibships

Sibships represent the simplest structure on which it is possible to do segregation analysis. For this purpose, we ignore the phenotypes of the parents. In the classical method, we do not try to estimate penetrances and allele frequencies separately. Instead, we wish to estimate a quantity known as the *segregation ratio p,* defined as the probability that an offspring of a particular mating type of interest is affected. Suppose that a gene is fully penetrant and there are no phenocopies. Then if the gene is dominant, the segregation ratio for offspring of an $aA \times aa$ mating (affected × nonaffected) will be 1/2. Similarly, if the gene is recessive, the segregation ratio for offspring of an $aA \times aA$ mating (carrier × carrier) will be 1/4. To complete the story, if sibships are ascertained through affected probands, then most parental matings in the sample will be of these types. Thus, by testing whether the segregation ratio is 1/2 or 1/4 in the appropriate mating type, one can indirectly test whether a dominant or recessive major gene is involved.

Suppose that the observed data consist of the distribution N_{rs} of sibships of size s with r affected members and we wish to compute the probability of observing such data. Since each sibship is an independent unit, the overall likelihood is simply the product of the probabilities for each type of sibship separately:

$$\mathcal{L}(p) = \prod_r \prod_s \Pr(r \mid s, p)^{N_{rs}} \tag{6.1}$$

If one had a random sample of matings of the desired type, the probability of observing r affected individuals among s at risk would simply be the binomial probability

$$P_{rs} = \Pr(r \mid s, p) = \binom{s}{r} p^r (1-p)^{s-r} \tag{6.2}$$

under the assumption that the offspring's phenotypes were conditionally independent given the parental mating type. One could then test the null hypothesis by comparing the observed distribution against the expected numbers, $E_{rs} = N_{\cdot s} P_{rs}$, using a simple chi-square test $\sum_{rs}(N_{rs} - E_{rs})^2/E_{rs}$. For a fixed sibship size, this would have a chi-square distribution on s degrees of freedom. For a mixture of sibship sizes, the degrees of freedom would be the sum of s over all observed sibship sizes, likely leading to sparse data and a test with low power. A more powerful test would be a 1 df chi-square test of trend in proportions (Armitage, 1971), given by

$$\chi^2 = \frac{\left[\sum_{rs} r(N_{rs} - p_0 N_s)\right]^2}{\sum_{rs} r^2 p_0 N_s} = \frac{(R - Sp_0)^2}{Sp_0(1 - p_0)}$$

where $R = \sum_{rs} r N_{rs}$ is the total number of cases and $S = \sum_{rs} s N_{rs}$ is the total number at risk.

To motivate the development of the general framework for complex segregation analysis, it is helpful to recast the above tests in terms of maximum likelihood. The loglikelihood from Eqs. (6.1) and (6.2) is $\ell(p) = R \ln(p) + (S - R) \ln(1 - p)$. The score-estimating equation is thus $U(p) = R/p - (S - R)/(1 - p)$, leading to the MLE $\hat{p} = R/S$. The Fisher information is $S/p(1 - p)$, leading to the score test given by the Armitage trend test above. The variance of $\hat{p}$ is given by the inverse of the Fisher information, the usual binomial variance estimator $\mathrm{var}(\hat{p}) = \hat{p}(1 - \hat{p})/S$.

Worked example. Suppose that we have ascertained $N = 100$ sibships of size $s = 5$ (so $S = 500$), and we have observed the distribution of affecteds r shown in Table 6.1, with $R = 200$ affecteds in total. The overall chi-square test is $\chi^2_5 = 22.08$ for $p_0 = 1/2$ (dominant) and 77.75 for $p_0 = 1/4$ (recessive), both highly significant. The 1 df trend test results are $\chi^2_1 = 20.00$ and 16.00, respectively, also highly significant. The segregation ratio is simply the proportion of the total number at risk who are affected, $\hat{p} = R/S = 200/500 = 0.40$ with $\mathrm{var}(\hat{p}) = 0.4 \times 0.6/500 = 0.00048$. Approximate 95% confidence limits are $\hat{p} \pm 1.96\sqrt{\mathrm{var}(\hat{p})} = (0.357, 0.443)$. All these analyses suggest that neither the dominant nor the recessive models provide a good fit to the data and that the best estimate of the segregation ratio is intermediate between the two alternatives.

Table 6.1 Example of the Classical Method of Segregation Analysis for Sibships of Size $s = 5$

r	N_r	rN_r	Expected (E_r)	
			$p = 1/2$	$p = 1/4$
0	8	0	3.1	23.7
1	26	26	15.6	39.6
2	34	68	31.3	26.4
3	23	69	31.3	8.8
4	8	32	15.6	1.5
5	1	5	3.1	0.1
Total	100	200	100	100

Ascertainment correction

The difficulty with this approach is that we do not have a random sample of matings, but rather a random sample of probands. We must therefore compute instead the *conditional* probability distribution of r given that the sibships were ascertained in the first place.

Consider sibships of a fixed size s. Suppose first that we ascertain all such sibships with at least one case (complete ascertainment, $\pi = 1$, as defined above). Thus, we wish to compute the conditional distribution

$$\Pr(r \mid s, r \geq 1) = \frac{\Pr(r \mid s)}{\Pr(r \geq 1 \mid s)}$$

$$= \frac{\binom{s}{r} p^r (1 - p)^{s-r}}{\sum_{r=1}^{s} \binom{s}{r} p^r (1 - p)^{s-r}} \qquad (6.3)$$

$$= \frac{\binom{s}{r} p^r (1 - p)^{s-r}}{1 - (1 - p)^s}$$

Now suppose instead that the ascertainment probability π is very small (single ascertainment). Then

$$\Pr(\text{family with } r \text{ cases is ascertained})$$

$$= 1 - \Pr(\text{family with } r \text{ cases is not ascertained})$$

$$= 1 - \prod_{k=1}^{r} \Pr(\text{case } k \text{ is not ascertained})$$

$$= 1 - \prod_{k=1}^{r} (1 - \pi)$$

$$= 1 - (1 - \pi)^r$$

As π approaches 0, Pr(family with r cases is ascertained) $= 1 - (1 - \pi r + \pi^2 r(r-1)/2 + \cdots) \approx \pi r$. Then the probability of ascertaining a family is approximately proportional to the number of affecteds in the family, πr, the denominator in Eq. (6.3) becoming $\sum_r \pi r \Pr(r \mid s, p) = \pi p$. Thus, the conditional probability becomes

$$
\Pr(r \mid s, r \geq 1) = \frac{\pi r \binom{s}{r} p^r (1-p)^{s-r}}{\pi p s}
$$

$$
= \binom{s-1}{r-1} p^{r-1} (1-p)^{s-r}
$$

which is simply a binomial probability for the remaining members of the sibship, excluding the proband.

Worked example (continued). Consider the same population distribution as before, P_r being 1000 times the numbers given in the previous table, now under single ascertainment. Families are represented in proportion to the total number of cases ($C_r = r P_r$), and there are no families in the sample without cases. Suppose that we ascertain a sample of 200 such families (i.e., $\pi = 0.001$). Their expected distribution is given in Table 6.2. Excluding the probands (200), there are a total of $F = 322$ familial cases out of 800 sibs at risk, leading to $\hat{p} = 0.403$ with 95% CL $= (0.369, 0.436)$. The expected distributions are computed by multiplying $N = 200$ by the binomial probabilities for $r - 1$ given $s - 1 = 4$ and $p = 0.5$ or 0.25. The overall chi squares are now $\chi_4^2 = 32.52$ for $p_0 = 1/2$ (dominant) and 119.57 for $p_0 = 1/4$ (recessive). The test for the trend produces $\chi_1^2 = 30.42$ and 99.23, respectively.

Now consider the same distribution as in the original random sample, but excluding the eight sibships with no affecteds (complete ascertainment). The expected distribution of the remaining 92 sibships is given in Table 6.3.

Table 6.2 Expected Distribution Under Single Ascertainment

r	P_r $\pi = .001$	C_r $r P_r$	N_r $\pi r P_r$	F_r $(r-1)N_r$	Expected (E_r) $p = 1/2$	Expected (E_r) $p = 1/4$
0	8,000	0	0	0	0.0	0.0
1	26,000	26,000	26	0	12.5	63.3
2	34,000	68,000	68	68	50.0	84.4
3	23,000	69,000	69	138	75.0	42.2
4	8,000	32,000	32	96	50.0	9.4
5	1,000	5,000	5	20	12.5	0.8
Total	100,000	200,000	200.0	322	200.0	200.0

Table 6.3 Expected Distribution Under
Complete Ascertainment

		Expected (E_r)	
r	N_r	$p = 1/2$	$p = 1/4$
1	26	14.8	47.7
2	34	29.7	31.8
3	23	29.7	10.6
4	8	14.8	1.8
5	1	3.0	0.1

There are still a total of 200 cases, now out of $92 \times 5 = 460$ sibs at risk. The naive estimate $200/460 = 0.435$ is an overestimate because of the truncated ascertainment. There is no simple way to estimate $\hat{p}$ from these data, but iterative search leads to $\hat{p} = 0.401$ with 95% CL $(0.351, 0.452)$. We can, however, test the null hypotheses easily. The expecteds are computed by multiplying $N = 92$ by the binomial probabilities for r given $s = 5$ and $p = 0.5$ or 0.25, but eliminating the case $r = 0$ and adjusting the probabilities accordingly. The overall chi squares are now $\chi_4^2 = 14.98$ for $p_0 = 1/2$ and 53.12 for $p_0 = 1/4$. The score tests are $\chi_1^2 = 14.06$ and 44.50, respectively.

Multiple ascertainment. In the general case of multiple ascertainment, $0 < \pi < 1$, similar reasoning leads to an expression for the conditional probability of the observed data of the form

$$\Pr(r \mid s, r \geq 1) = \frac{\Pr(r \mid s) \times \Pr(A \mid r, s)}{\Pr(A \mid s)}$$

$$= \frac{\binom{s}{r} p^r (1-p)^{s-r} \times [1 - (1-\pi)^r]}{1 - (1 - \pi p)^s} \tag{6.4}$$

In principle, one could use this expression to estimate both p and π, but if π is known, one would obtain more precise estimates of p by constraining it to that value.

Complex segregation analysis. The segregation ratio is, of course, a mixture of penetrances and transition probabilities for each *mating type (MT)*:

$$p_m = \Pr(Y = 1 \mid MT = m) = \sum_g \Pr(Y = 1 \mid G = g)\ \Pr(G = g \mid MT = m)$$

For example, for testing a dominant model, we would focus on the $aA \times aa$ mating type, for which $p = (1/2)f_0 + (1/2)f_1$. For testing a recessive model, we would focus on the $aA \times aA$ mating type, for which $p = (1/4)f_0 + (1/2)f_1 + (1/4)f_2$. For fully penetrant genes with no phenocopies, substitution of $f_0 = 0$, $f_1 = 0$ (recessive) or 1 (dominant), and $f_2 = 1$ produces $p = 1/2$ in the dominant case or $p = 1/4$ in the recessive case. More generally, we might want to estimate these penetrances by substituting this expression for p into the appropriate conditional probability above. However, as soon as we admit the possibility that the disease is not fully penetrant or that there are phenocopies, we must also allow for the possibility that we are wrong about the genotypes of the parents of probands. The segregation ratio thus becomes an average of segregation ratios over all possible genotypes of the parents

$$p = \sum_m p_m \Pr(MT = m \mid q)$$

if the parent's phenotypes are unknown; if they are known, one would simply include the expression $\Pr(Y_m \mid G_m) \Pr(Y_f \mid G_f)$ in the summand. We describe how to do this in greater detail using maximum likelihood in the following section.

Likelihood Methods for Pedigree Analysis

General model

This section presents a general likelihood approach to testing genetic hypotheses and estimating parameters in genetic models for arbitrary pedigree structures. Readers are referred to Chapter 4 for a review of the general principles of likelihood inference. The likelihood for a pedigree is the probability of observing the phenotypes, $\mathbf{Y}$, given the model parameters $\Theta = (\mathbf{f}, q)$ [where $\mathbf{f} = (f_0, f_1, f_2)$] and the method of ascertainment A, that is, $\Pr(\mathbf{Y} \mid \Theta, A)$. Setting aside the ascertainment issue for the moment, we recognize that the outcomes are dependent due to shared genetic and possibly other influences. Chapter 5 introduced regressive models that allow for this by modeling the dependency of each person's phenotypes on the phenotypes of those appearing previously in the dataset. We now take a different approach, modeling the dependencies among the underlying genotypes, as introduced at the end of Chapter 5. In some instances it may be desirable to allow for both types of dependency, but for now we assume that the dependency between phenotypes can be completely accounted for by our model for shared genotypes. Thus, we assume that *conditional on genotypes, individuals' phenotypes are independent:*

$$\Pr(\mathbf{Y} \mid \mathbf{G}) = \Pr(Y_1 = y_1 \mid G_1 = g_1) \times \cdots \times \Pr(Y_n = y_n \mid G_n = g_n) \quad (6.5)$$

However, since we do not observe the genotypes, the marginal probability of the phenotypes must be computed by summing over all possible combinations of genotypes:

$$\mathcal{L}(\Theta) = \Pr(\mathbf{Y} \mid \Theta) = \sum_{\mathbf{g}} \Pr(\mathbf{Y}, \mathbf{G} = \mathbf{g}) = \sum_{\mathbf{g}} \Pr(\mathbf{Y} \mid \mathbf{G} = \mathbf{g}; f) \Pr(\mathbf{G} = \mathbf{g} \mid q)$$

$$(6.6)$$

The first factor in the summation is simply Eq. (6.5). The second is obtained in the same way as in regressive models described in Chapter 5 as

$$\Pr(\mathbf{G}) = \Pr(G_1) \Pr(G_2 \mid G_1) \Pr(G_3 \mid G_1, G_2) \cdots \Pr(G_n \mid G_1, \ldots, G_{n-1})$$

$$(6.7)$$

Some simplifications are possible, however, because under Mendelian laws, one's genotype depends only on the genotypes of one's parents, f_i and m_i, or the population allele frequency q if one is a founder or a marry-in. Thus, Eq. (6.7) can be rewritten as

$$\Pr(\mathbf{G}) = \prod_{i=1}^{N} \begin{cases} \Pr\left(G_i = g_i \mid G_{m_i} = g_{m_i}, G_{f_i} = g_{f_i}\right) & \text{nonfounders} \\ \Pr(G_i = g_i \mid q) & \text{founders} \end{cases} \quad (6.8)$$

where the probability on the right is either the transition probabilities shown in Table 1.4 or the Hardy-Weinberg probabilities $((1-q)^2, 2q(1-q), q^2)$. Putting this all together, one obtains

$$\mathcal{L}(\Theta) = \sum_{\mathbf{g}} \prod_{i} \Pr(Y_i \mid g_i) \times \begin{cases} \prod \Pr\left(g_i \mid g_{m_i}, g_{f_i}\right) & \text{nonfounders} \\ \prod \Pr(g_i \mid q) & \text{founders} \end{cases} \quad (6.9)$$

The fundamental difficulty in computing genetic likelihoods is that the sum over $\mathbf{g}$ can in principle entail a very large number of terms—3^N for a single diallelic major gene or 10^N in the simplest linkage analysis problem. For a 13-member pedigree, for example, there would be over a million terms to evaluate, although many of these would be inconsistent with the observed data and/or Mendelian laws and thus would have zero probability. Brute force enumeration of all possible genotypes is therefore not usually feasible. Instead, a recursive algorithm known as *peeling* (Elston and Stewart, 1971) is used (described below).

To complete the specification of the likelihood, one must condition Eq. (6.9) on the ascertainment process. The appropriate conditional likelihood is

$$\mathcal{L}_A(\Theta) = \Pr(\mathbf{Y} \mid \Theta, A, \pi) = \frac{\mathcal{L}(\Theta)\,\Pr(A \mid \mathbf{Y}; \pi)}{\Pr(A \mid \Theta, \pi)} \qquad (6.10)$$

where A denotes the event that the family was ascertained and

$$\Pr(A \mid \Theta, \pi) = \sum_{\mathbf{y}} \Pr(A \mid \mathbf{Y} = \mathbf{y}; \pi)\,\Pr(\mathbf{Y} = \mathbf{y} \mid \Theta)$$

is the probability of ascertainment, which is computed along the lines described above. By following the rules of sequential sampling of pedigrees, it becomes necessary to condition only on the initial ascertainment event, not on the entire pedigree. Although these ideas are straightforward in principle when applied to sibships, they become much more complicated in practice when applied to extended pedigrees, in part because the families that are identified independently through separate probands could link up later into larger pedigrees. For further discussion, see Burton et al. (2000), Dawson and Elston (1984), Elston (1995), Hodge and Vieland (1996), Vieland and Hodge (1995, 1996), and Vieland and Logue (2002).

Polygenic and mixed models

So far, we have considered only major gene models. In a polygenic model, each person's genotype is the sum over a large number of genes, each making a small independent contribution to the phenotype. By the Central Limit Theorem, this sum, denoted Z, is normally distributed and, without loss of generality, can be taken to have zero mean and unit variance, $Z \sim \mathcal{N}(0, 1)$. To calculate $\Pr(Z \mid Z_m, Z_f)$, we let $Z = Z_{ft} + Z_{mt}$, where Z_{ft} represents the polygene inherited from the father and Z_{mt} the polygene inherited from the mother (Fig. 6.2). Z_f can, in turn, be decomposed into the sum of Z_{ft} and

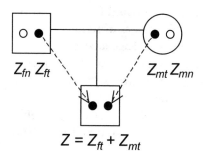

Figure 6.2 Polygenic model.

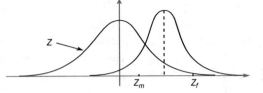

Figure 6.3 Distribution of genotypes for a polygenic model.

Z_{fn}, the nontransmitted portion of the father's polygene, with both components having the same $\mathcal{N}(0, 1/2)$ distribution, and likewise for the mother's polygene. The distribution of these polygenes is shown in Figure 6.3. Since half of the polygenes come from each parent, it follows that an offspring's polygene will be normally distributed with mean $\bar{Z} = (Z_m + Z_f)/2$ and variance $1/2$. The mean $\bar{Z}$ is commonly referred to as the *breeding value,* a term derived from animal and plant breeding experiments.

A likelihood can be formed exactly as in Eq. (6.9), except that the sum over **g** is replaced by a multiple integral over **z**,

$$\mathcal{L}(\Theta) = \int\!\!\int \cdots \int \prod_{i=1}^{N} \Pr(Y_i \mid Z_i = z_i) \Pr\left(z_i \mid z_{m_i}, z_{f_i}\right) d\mathbf{z} \qquad (6.11)$$

where the last factor is $\mathcal{N}(0, 1)$ for a founder or $N[\bar{z}, 1/2]$ for a nonfounder. Thus, the term $\Pr(\mathbf{Z})$ can be expressed as a multivariate normal density with zero mean and covariance matrix $\mathbf{C}$, for example, for a nuclear family with two offspring,

$$\mathbf{C} = \begin{pmatrix} 1 & 0 & 1/2 & 1/2 \\ 0 & 1 & 1/2 & 1/2 \\ 1/2 & 1/2 & 1 & 1/2 \\ 1/2 & 1/2 & 1/2 & 1 \end{pmatrix} \qquad (6.12)$$

where the first two rows and columns relate to the parents and the second two to the offspring. It remains to specify the penetrance function $\Pr(Y \mid Z; \mathbf{f})$. For a continuous trait, the linear model with normally distributed residuals is convenient because the integral above can be evaluated in closed form as another multivariate normal density. Suppose that we write $Y_i = \alpha + \beta Z_i + \epsilon_i$, where $\epsilon \sim \mathcal{N}(0, \sigma^2)$; then the vector **Y** turns out to have density $MVN(\mu\mathbf{1}, \beta^2\mathbf{C} + \sigma^2\mathbf{I})$. (This is exactly equivalent to assuming that the polygene has variance β^2 and the phenotype is $Y_i = \alpha + Z_i + \epsilon_i$, a formulation commonly seen in the variance components models literature.) Likewise, for a binary trait, a loglinear model $\Pr(Y = 1 \mid Z) = \exp(\alpha + \beta Z)$ allows for a closed-form expression of the integral for a rare disease as

$Pr(\mathbf{Y}) = \exp(\alpha \mathbf{Y}'\mathbf{1} + \beta^2 \mathbf{Y}'\mathbf{CY})$. For general penetrance models, the Elston-Stewart algorithm can be used to expedite the calculations. We will discuss the specification of penetrance functions in greater detail shortly.

The mixed model (Morton and MacLean, 1974) involves both major genes and polygenes, thus requiring both a multiple summation over $\mathbf{g}$ and a multiple integral over $\mathbf{z}$. Unfortunately, this model is intractable by the Elston-Stewart algorithm without invoking some approximations that are beyond the scope of this book (Hasstedt, 1982, 1991). The regressive model provides a particularly convenient approximation to the mixed model as a combination of major gene and residual phenotypic dependencies. All that is done is to add the phenotypes of all individuals appearing previously in the pedigree to the penetrances in Eq. (6.9). For example, if the phenotype is continuous, one might use a linear regression model of the form (Bonney, 1986)

$$Y_i = f_{g_i} + \beta_f Y'_{f_i} + \beta_m Y'_{m_i} + \gamma Y'_{s_i} + \delta \sum_{j \in O} Y'_j + \epsilon_i \qquad (6.13)$$

where Y' denotes deviations of the phenotypes from their means (zero if missing), s_i a spouse if (s)he appears earlier in the dataset, O the set of older sibs, and ϵ_i an independent $\mathcal{N}(0, \sigma^2)$ error. This is the *Class D* model of Bonney (1986), implemented in the REGC procedure of the S.A.G.E. package.

Penetrance models

Continuous phenotypes. In a pure major gene model, the penetrance function for a continuous phenotype is usually treated as being normally distributed, with means and variances that depend on the genotype, that is, $Y \sim \mathcal{N}(\mu_g, \sigma_g^2)$, although some transformations of the phenotype may be necessary in some circumstances. Initially one might test whether the three variances are equal before proceeding to test for differences in means and dominance effects (two means being equal). In a polygenic model, one would assume a linear regression model of the form $Y \sim \mathcal{N}(\alpha + \beta Z, \sigma^2)$. The regressive model for major gene and residual phenotypic dependencies was discussed above.

Binary phenotypes. The penetrance function for a dichotomous phenotype simply requires three Bernoulli probabilities for $Pr(Y = 1 \mid G = g) = f_g$. If, however, one wishes to add additional covariate or regressive effects to the model, one might use a logistic regression model

$$\text{logit } \Pr(Y = 1 \mid G = g, Z) = f_g + \beta' Z$$

where Z denotes individual covariates and/or others' phenotypes. See Chapter 4 for further discussion of the use of the logistic model to describe the joint effects of several variables, including interaction effects. Several options are available for specifying the penetrance function in a polygenic model. The traditional model is a threshold model along the lines of the liability models (Fig. 5.7), where $\Pr(Y = 1 \mid Z) = 1$ if $Z > T$, 0 otherwise. Alternatively, one might postulate a continuous dependence of risk on Z, but approximations are needed for the integrals in Eq. (6.11) to be tractable.

Censored age-at-onset phenotypes. For late-onset diseases, one must allow for the fact that unaffected family members may not have expressed their risk by their time of death or by the end of the observation period. Furthermore, most late-onset diseases have rates that depend strongly on age (and possibly on calendar year or other factors). Let us represent the phenotype Y as a pair of variables (D, T) where D represents disease status $(1 = \text{affected}, 0 = \text{unaffected})$ and T represents the age at onset (diagnosis, death) if affected or the age last known to be disease free if unaffected (age at death from a competing cause, loss to follow-up, or current age). The traditional approach to censored age-at-onset phenotypes was based on the assumption that ages were a normally distributed continuous phenotype: if affected, the normal density at age t is used as the penetrance; if unaffected, the cumulative probability for all ages after t is used instead. The modern approach is to model the age-specific incidence rates $\lambda(t)$ (Eq. 4.1) instead: the penetrance is then $\lambda(t)^D S(t)$, where $S(t) = \exp(-\int_0^t \lambda(u)\, du)$ is the probability of surviving to age t. One possibility for modeling the incidence rates is the proportional hazards model

$$\lambda(t \mid G = g) = \lambda_0(t) \exp(\beta_g)$$

which can easily be extended to allow for additional covariates (environmental risk factors, interactions, regressive effects, etc.).

However, this model implicitly assumes that the disease is inevitable for everybody if they were not censored first, unless the rates decline to zero as $t \to \infty$ such that $\int_0^\infty \lambda(u)\, du$ remains finite. An alternative model incorporated into the procedure REGTL in S.A.G.E. (Sellers et al., 1990) allows either the lifetime risk and/or its age distribution to depend on genotype and other risk factors. Specifically, a logistic risk model is used to specify

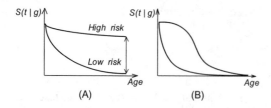

Figure 6.4 Some alternative possibilities for the lifetime risk and age distribution as a function of genotype.

the lifetime risk and a logistic density function to model the age at onset among those who are susceptible:

$$\Pr(D = 1, T = t \mid G = g) = \Pr(D = 1 \mid G = g) \Pr(T = t \mid D = 1, G = g)$$

$$= \left(\frac{e^{\gamma_g}}{1 + e^{\gamma_g}} \right) \frac{\alpha e^{\beta_g + \alpha t}}{(1 + e^{\beta_g + \alpha t})^2} \qquad (6.14)$$

Thus, for example, Figure 6.4A illustrates the case where the lifetime risk differs by genotype but the shape of the age distribution does not, whereas Figure 6.4B illustrates the case where the lifetime risk is the same but the shape of the age distribution differs.

Incorporating covariates and interactions. In addition to the genetic factors being modeled by segregation analysis, the phenotype under study may depend on a variety of host or environmental factors. This must be allowed for, if only to improve the power for testing genetic hypotheses, but also because these covariates may also aggregate in families, masquerading as a genetic effect. Perhaps the simplest way to address this problem is to do a preliminary regression analysis of these factors and then take the residuals from this analysis as the phenotype for genetic analysis. This is something of an approximation, since the familial dependencies are usually ignored in doing the preliminary regression modeling; however, use of simple regressive models or just adding a *family history* covariate to the model will go a long way toward addressing this problem. More seriously, this strategy is effective only for analysis of continuous traits. For binary or survival time traits, residuals from a logistic or proportional hazards model are no longer binary and cannot be analyzed using the penetrance models that would be appropriate for the original phenotypes. Finally, the residual approach adjusts only for the main effects of the covariates, not for any interactions with the genetic effects.

For all these reasons, it is preferable to incorporate the covariates directly into the penetrance functions, as described above for the different types of phenotypes. For example, in a segregation analysis of lung cancer,

Sellers et al. (1990) extended the logistic models for age at onset (the second factor in Eq. [6.14]) by adding pack-years of smoking as a covariate, while allowing genotype to affect either age at onset (β_g) or lifetime risk (γ_g), but not both, thus implicitly assuming a multiplicative model for the joint effects of smoking and genotype. In a subsequent reanalysis, Gauderman et al. (1997b) tested this assumption by allowing each genotype to have a different slope coefficient for pack-years in a proportional hazards model and found no significant departure from multiplicativity.

A problem that frequently arises in incorporating covariates into a segregation analysis is missing data. It can be very difficult to obtain complete data on all members of a pedigree, particularly for deceased members. Missing covariate data is generally a more serious problem in genetic analysis than in epidemiology (where individuals with missing data are frequently simply omitted from the analysis), because omitting such people entirely would destroy the pedigree structure, and exclusion of entire pedigrees with any missing data is likely to leave one with too little data. One approach is to omit only the penetrance contributions from the likelihood for subjects who are missing any relevant data. This is valid under the assumption that missingness is unrelated to the true values of the missing data and unrelated to their genotype (at least conditional on any other factors included in the model). However, this strategy could lead to omitting valuable phenotype information for individuals for whom only some covariates are missing, so some imputation of missing values is desirable. One approach is to replace them with a mean or, better, with an expected value given any other relevant information that is available (e.g., birth year, age, phenotype, other family members' covariates). Later in this chapter, we describe a better approach based on the principle of multiple imputation (see "Gibbs Sampling").

The Elston-Stewart peeling algorithm

Fortunately, it is not really necessary to sum (or integrate) over all possible genotypes to evaluate likelihood (Eq. 6.9), because it is possible to carry out the calculations sequentially in such a way that the amount of computing rises only linearly with pedigree size rather than exponentially.

First, consider the likelihood for a single nuclear family, which we can write as $\mathcal{L}(\Theta) = \sum_g \Pr(\mathbf{Y}, \mathbf{G} = \mathbf{g})$. This would appear to require a summation over all possible combinations of genotypes $\mathbf{g}$, a calculation of 3^{s+2} terms for a family with s siblings, but the calculations can be simplified by exploiting the conditional independence of the siblings given the parents' genotypes. Thus, letting subscripts p and o indicate the genotype and phenotype vectors of parents and offspring, respectively,

$$\mathcal{L}(\Theta) = \sum_{\mathbf{g}_p} \sum_{\mathbf{g}_o} \Pr(\mathbf{Y}_p, \mathbf{G}_p = \mathbf{g}_p) \Pr(\mathbf{Y}_o, \mathbf{G}_o = \mathbf{g}_o \mid \mathbf{G}_p = \mathbf{g}_p)$$

$$= \sum_{\mathbf{g}_p} \Pr(\mathbf{Y}_p, \mathbf{g}_p) \left(\prod_{o=1}^{s} \sum_{g_o} \Pr(Y_o, g_o \mid \mathbf{g}_p) \right)$$

This follows from the distributive law, since $\sum_x \sum_y \Pr(x) \Pr(y) = (\sum_x \Pr(x))(\sum_y \Pr(y))$. This way, the calculation requires only $3s$ terms for each of the nine possible parental genotypes. In fact, 10 of the 27 terms for each offspring are zero, so the total number of calculations required is only $17s$. For example, for $s = 4$, this reduces the calculations from $3^6 = 729$ terms to only $17 \times 4 = 68$ terms.

For extended pedigrees, the Elston-Stewart algorithm involves an ordering of the pedigree into nuclear families, the results of each calculation being *peeled* onto the individual who links that family to the rest of the pedigree for use in later calculations. We begin by describing the calculations for a *simple* pedigree, in which only one member of a mating has parents in the pedigree. In this case, it is easiest to describe if we begin at the bottom and work upward. (Although genes are transmitted *down* a pedigree, it is generally easier to do the calculations working upward, as this allows us to use the distributive law of multiplication over addition in a manner similar to that described above.)

To illustrate the calculations for extended pedigrees, consider the hypothetical pedigree shown in Figure 6.5, divided into three nuclear families, A, B, and C, with persons 4 and 5 being the linking individuals. We begin the calculations with nuclear family A and wish to compute the likelihood of the phenotypes of the spouse and offspring in the family, given all the

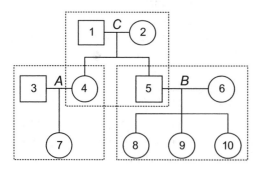

Figure 6.5 Hypothetical pedigree used to illustrate peeling calculations for simple pedigrees.

possible genotypes of the linking individual 4:

$$A(g_4) \equiv \Pr(Y_3, Y_7 \mid G_4 = g_4)$$

$$= \sum_{g_3} \sum_{g_7} \Pr(Y_3, Y_7, G_3 = g_3, G_7 = g_7 \mid G_4 = g_4)$$

$$= \sum_{g_3} \sum_{g_7} \Pr(Y_3 \mid g_3) \Pr(Y_7 \mid g_7) \Pr(g_7 \mid g_3, g_4) \Pr(g_3)$$

(assuming random mating, so that g_3 and g_4 are independent.)

In a similar way, we compute the likelihood of the phenotypes in family B, given the possible genotypes for the linking individual 5. Since there are several offspring in this family, this might appear to require a multiple summation over all possible genotypes. However, since the offspring's genotypes are independent, given their parents, this can be done simply by multiplying three single summations:

$$B(g_5) \equiv \Pr(Y_6, Y_8, Y_9, Y_{10} \mid g_5)$$

$$= \sum_{g_6} \sum_{g_8} \sum_{g_9} \sum_{g_{10}} \Pr(Y_6 \mid g_6) \Pr(Y_8 \mid g_8) \Pr(Y_9 \mid g_9) \Pr(Y_{10} \mid g_{10})$$

$$\times \Pr(g_8 \mid g_5, g_6) \Pr(g_9 \mid g_5, g_6) \Pr(g_{10} \mid g_5, g_6) \Pr(g_6) \qquad (6.15)$$

$$= \sum_{g_6} \Pr(Y_6 \mid g_6) \Pr(g_6) \prod_{i=8}^{10} \left(\sum_{g_i} \Pr(Y_i \mid g_i) \Pr(g_i \mid g_5, g_6) \right)$$

Finally, we compute the likelihood for all phenotypes in the pedigree, given the genotypes of mating 1–2, using the peeled likelihoods for individuals 4 and 5:

$$C(g_1, g_2) \equiv \Pr(Y_3, \ldots, Y_{10} \mid g_1, g_2)$$

$$= \left(\sum_{g_4} A(g_4) \Pr(Y_4 \mid g_4) \Pr(g_4 \mid g_1, g_2) \right)$$

$$\times \left(\sum_{g_5} B(g_5) \Pr(Y_5 \mid g_5) \Pr(g_5 \mid g_1, g_2) \right)$$

A final sum over g_1 and g_2 concludes the calculation of the likelihood

$$\Pr(Y_1, \ldots, Y_{10}) = \sum_{g_1} \sum_{g_2} \Pr(Y_1 \mid g_1) \Pr(Y_2 \mid g_2) C(g_1, g_2) \Pr(g_1) \Pr(g_2)$$

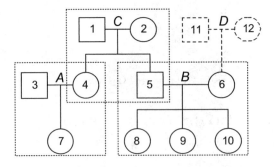

Figure 6.6 Adding family D to the pedigree creates a complex pedigree.

Suppose now that individual 6 also has parents (call them individuals 11 and 12 to create family D), so that we have a *complex* pedigree, but still with no inbreeding loops (Fig. 6.6). Then, when evaluating Eq. (6.15), we must now replace $Pr(g_6)$ by the joint probability of g_6 and his parents' phenotypes:

$$D(g_6) \equiv Pr(Y_{11}, Y_{12}, g_6)$$
$$= \sum_{g_{11}} \sum_{g_{12}} Pr(Y_{11} \mid g_{11}) Pr(Y_{12} \mid g_{12}) Pr(g_6 \mid g_{11}, g_{12}) Pr(g_{11}) Pr(g_{12})$$

Thus, in complex pedigrees, peeling may have to be done both upward and downward. The order in which the nuclear families are processed is called the *peeling sequence*. For any given pedigree, there could be several possible peeling sequences, the choice between them being a matter of convenience. In this example, one could proceed in the sequence D–B–C–A or A–C–B–D and get exactly the same answer.

For both simple and complex pedigrees, each linking individual (e.g., person 4) divides the pedigree into two pieces that are conditionally independent given the genotype of that linking person. Thompson (1986) defines the *lower neighborhood* of a linking individual to be all those subjects connected to the linker through spouse(s) and offspring and the upper neighborhood to be all subjects connected to the linker through his or her parents. For example, in the complex pedigree, the lower neighborhood of person 5 includes subjects 6, 8, 9, 10, 11, and 12, and his upper neighborhood includes subjects 1, 2, 3, 4, and 7. In a simple or complex pedigree, the lower and upper neighborhoods of a linking subject are conditionally independent given the genotype of the linker.

If there are inbreeding loops, the peeling calculations become substantially more difficult. Suppose, for example, that individuals 2 and 11 were siblings, with parents 13 and 14 (Fig. 6.7). The problem is that now no single subject defines an upper and a lower neighborhood that are independent. Considering subject 5, for example, we see that his grandparents (13 and 14) are members of both his upper neighborhood (through parent 2)

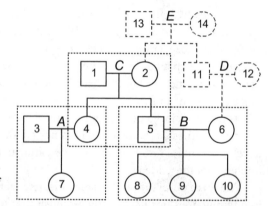

Figure 6.7 Adding family E to the pedigree creates an inbreeding loop consisting of members 2, 11, 5, and 6.

and his lower neighborhood (through spouse 6). The solution is to define a *cutset* of two or more individuals that break the pedigree into two independent pieces. In the example pedigree, subjects 2 and 5 form a cutset, since conditional on their genotypes, the phenotypes of subjects above 2 and below 5 are independent of the remaining subjects' phenotypes. Once a cutset is defined, likelihood computation proceeds as it does without loops. However, the equations can be cumbersome since they require computation of the distribution of phenotypes conditional on the joint genotypes of all members of a cutset. In highly inbred pedigrees, cutsets may include several individuals, rendering likelihood calculations computationally infeasible. Most computer packages, including S.A.G.E., do not allow inbred pedigrees. An approximate solution is to break loops by ignoring certain relationships, for example ignoring subjects 13 and 14, or treating one or the other of their offspring as founders. Clearly, this is wasteful of potentially valuable information. Another solution is to use the Monte Carlo method of Gibbs sampling, which is described in more detail later in this chapter.

We have described the peeling algorithm in some detail for a major gene model. The same principles apply in a polygenic model, with the summations over g replaced by integrals over z. This is not as difficult as it may seem if the penetrances are normal densities, since the integral of a product of normal densities is also normal. Thus, it suffices to compute the mean and variance of the resulting normal at each step of the peeling process. Details can be found in Khoury et al. (1993, §8.4.2).

Hypothesis testing

A basic principle of scientific inference is that a good fit of a model to a set of data never proves the truth of the model. Science progresses only by *rejecting* null hypotheses. The same is true in genetics.

Specifically, before one can conclude that a major gene is involved in a particular disease, one must (*1*) reject the null hypothesis that there is no familial aggregation, (*2*) reject the null hypothesis that the apparent aggregation is explainable by a polygene or other forms of residual familial dependency, and (*3*) fail to reject the null hypothesis of Mendelian inheritance in favor of a more general model for transmission of some discrete *type* other than a major gene. Likelihood ratio tests provide a statistical basis for testing hypothesis among a family of nested alternatives. In this section, we develop a general family of hypotheses, known as the *ousiotype model*, which implements these ideas.

The mere observation that some discrete factor appears to be segregating in a family does not necessarily establish that that factor is a gene. Certain discrete environmental factors, for example, might also appear to be transmitted through families in a fashion that could mimic a major gene. Only a major gene, however, would be required to follow the laws of Mendelian inheritance (the transition probabilities and Hardy-Weinberg equilibrium), although other factors might not depart significantly from these probabilities. For example, McGuffin and Huckle (1990) showed that a segregation analysis of the phenotype of going to medical school appeared to follow a Mendelian major gene model, although it seems more likely that this trait would be determined by cultural transmission than by a single major gene. To provide a plausible alternative to a major gene that would include Mendelian inheritance as a special case, Cannings et al. (1978) introduced the concept of an *ousiotype*, or *type* for short. We postulate that types occur in three forms, denoted tt, tT, and TT, with probabilities p_0, p_1, and p_2, respectively. Type T is "transmitted" independently from each parent to offspring with probabilities τ_0, τ_1, or τ_2, depending on the parental type. Thus, the transition matrix above is replaced by the ousiotype matrix shown in Table 6.4.

Table 6.4 Transmission Probabilities Under the Ousiotype Model

Father's Ousiotype	Mother's Ousiotype	Offspring's Ousiotype		
		tt	tT	TT
tt	tt	$(1 - \tau_0)^2$	$2\tau_0(1 - \tau_0)$	τ_0^2
tt	tT	$(1 - \tau_0)(1 - \tau_1)$	$\tau_0(1 - \tau_1) + (1 - \tau_0)\tau_1$	$\tau_0\tau_1$
tt	TT	$(1 - \tau_0)(1 - \tau_2)$	$\tau_0(1 - \tau_2) + (1 - \tau_0)\tau_2$	$\tau_0\tau_2$
tT	tt	$(1 - \tau_1)(1 - \tau_0)$	$\tau_1(1 - \tau_0) + (1 - \tau_1)\tau_0$	$\tau_1\tau_0$
tT	tT	$(1 - \tau_1)^2$	$2\tau_1(1 - \tau_1)$	τ_1^2
tT	TT	$(1 - \tau_1)(1 - \tau_2)$	$\tau_1(1 - \tau_2) + (1 - \tau_1)\tau_2$	$\tau_1\tau_2$
TT	tt	$(1 - \tau_2)(1 - \tau_0)$	$\tau_2(1 - \tau_0) + (1 - \tau_2)\tau_0$	$\tau_2\tau_0$
TT	tT	$(1 - \tau_2)(1 - \tau_1)$	$\tau_2(1 - \tau_1) + (1 - \tau_2)\tau_1$	$\tau_2\tau_1$
TT	TT	$(1 - \tau_2)^2$	$2\tau_2(1 - \tau_2)$	τ_2^2

Several submodels of the major ousiotype model are distinguished:

- No transmission—$H_0 : p_1 = p_2 = 0$; τ's irrelevant because there is only a single type.
- *Environmental* transmission—$H_1 : \tau_0 = \tau_1 = \tau_2$. [This is something of a misnomer, as it has nothing to do with environmental factors per se. Instead, it assumes that there exist three discrete types in the population but that the parental types are independent of the offspring types. As a special case of this model, if $p_0 = (1 - \tau)^2$, $p_1 = 2\tau(1 - \tau)$, $p_2 = \tau^2$, then these prevalences of the three types will remain constant between generations.]
- Mendelian transmission—$H_2 : \tau_0 = 0$, $\tau_1 = 1/2$, $\tau_2 = 1$ and $p_1 = 2p_0(1 - p_0)$, $p_2 = (1 - p_0)^2$ (i.e., the types obey the transmission probabilities given in Table 1.3 and are in Hardy-Weinberg equilibrium).
- General model—$H_3 : \tau$'s and p's are unconstrained.

To implement the strategy described above, we test H_0 against H_2 to test the hypothesis of no genetic transmission, H_1 against H_3 to test the hypothesis of environmental transmission, and H_2 against H_3 to test the hypothesis of Mendelian inheritance. In addition to using these major ousiotype models, one should reject a pure polygenic model against the mixed model. Given the difficulties with the general mixed model mentioned above, the easiest way to do this is to add a regressive component to the Mendelian and general models above. The pure Mendelian and pure regressive models are then each tested against the mixed model. Certain other packages, such as PAP and Pointer, support various approximations to the mixed model that can also be used in this way.

Before we leave this topic, it is worthwhile to emphasize the tenuousness of most inferences about genetic mechanisms from pure segregation analysis. Based on various examples, like the study of the propensity to attend medical school mentioned above, there is some skepticism among geneticists about the utility of segregation analysis and a reluctance to conclude that a major gene has been demonstrated until it has at least been supported by linkage analysis. Two factors in particular contribute to this concern. The first is the statistical power of the various tests described above. On the one hand, low power for the comparison of the no-transmission model against the Mendelian alternative could lead to failure to detect a gene; on the other hand, low power for the comparison of the Mendelian model against the general alternative could lead to spurious conclusions about the existence of a major gene. Violation of some of the assumptions of the model, such as skewness in the distribution of a continuous phenotype assumed to be normally distributed, can also produce spurious evidence for a major gene. MacLean et al. (1975), Go et al. (1978), Burns et al. (1984), and Boehnke et al. (1988) provide further discussion of power.

The other major factor is the possibility of genetic heterogeneity—multiple factors, genetic or environmental, that represent distinct pathways to the disease. A classic example is retinitis pigmentosa, which has dominant, recessive, and X-linked genetic as well as environmental forms (Bleeker-Wagemakers et al., 1992; Humphries et al., 1992). Straightforward application of segregation analysis to such a condition could fail to detect a major gene or provide meaningless estimates of penetrance and allele frequencies. If important $G \times G$ or $G \times E$ interactions are ignored in the analysis, the results are also likely to be misleading. In the breast cancer example discussed below, we now know that there are at least two major genes involved (*BRCA1* and *BRCA2*), but both act in a dominant fashion with broadly similar penetrances, so the estimated allele frequency should be roughly the sum of the allele frequencies for the two genes and the penetrances would be roughly a weighted average of the two gene-specific penetrances, assuming no interactions between them. Some approaches have been proposed for fitting multilocus models or models that assume that the population comprises a mixture of families with different etiologies (Greenberg, 1989; Moll et al., 1984), but little is known about their power. Khoury et al. (1993, pp. 279–283) provide an excellent review of this literature and a discussion of these problems of interpretation.

Alternative Methods

Gibbs sampling

The computational difficulties with the peeling algorithm have led various investigators to search for alternative methods of computing genetic likelihoods. One of the most promising approaches involves the use of Monte Carlo methods to sample from the set of possible genotypes with the right probability rather than have to enumerate all possibilities systematically. A particular variant of this approach is the technique of *Gibbs sampling*, which constructs a Markov chain on the genotype set (hence the term *Markov chain Monte Carlo;* see Chapters 4 and 5 for additional background). When applied for segregation analysis, the basic approach is as follows:

1. Initialize the process with any legal assignment of genotypes to all members of the pedigree. (For example, $G = dD$ for everyone is a legal assignment, provided that $f_g \neq 0$ for all three genotypes.)
2. At each cycle:
   a. Consider each member of the pedigree in turn and select a new genotype for that person from its posterior distribution, conditional on his or her phenotype and the current assignment of genotypes for his or her immediate relatives (denoted $\mathbf{g}_{-i}$, based on the current model parameters)

$$\Pr(G_i = g_i \mid \mathbf{g}_{-i}, Y_i) \propto \Pr(Y_i \mid g_i) \Pr\left(g_i \mid g_{m_i}, g_{f_i}\right) \prod_k \Pr\left(g_{o_k} \mid g_i, g_{s_i}\right)$$

     b. For a fully Bayesian analysis, sample new values of model parameters, treating the genotypes as known. For example, the full conditional distribution of the allele frequency is $q \sim \text{Beta}(N, 2F)$, where N is the number of D alleles currently assigned to the F founders. Likewise, the penetrances are $f_g \sim \text{Beta}(Y_g, R_g)$, where Y_g is the number of affecteds with genotype g and R_g is the total number at risk.

3. Repeat this process until it stabilizes; thereafter, accumulate distributions of genotypes, model parameters, likelihood contributions, and so on.

Under suitable conditions, this process can be shown to generate the joint marginal distribution of all the unknowns (genotypes and model parameters), given the observed data. If flat priors are used for the parameters, their posterior distribution can be taken as an estimate of the likelihood itself. Alternatively, one can constrain the model parameters to a particular null value and use this method to compute the likelihood ratio as a function of model parameters. Specifically

$$LR(\Theta : \Theta_0) \approx \frac{1}{N} \sum_{\mathbf{G}_n | \mathbf{Y}, \Theta_0} \frac{\Pr(\mathbf{Y}, \mathbf{G} \mid \Theta)}{\Pr(\mathbf{Y}, \mathbf{G} \mid \Theta_0)}$$

where $\mathbf{G}_n$, $n = 1, \ldots, N$ are sampled from their full conditional distribution, given $\mathbf{Y}$ and Θ_0 (see Eq. [4.9] for the derivation). Details of both approaches, together with a discussion of some of the limitations of the technique in genetics, are provided in Thomas and Gauderman (1996) and Gauderman and Thomas (1994). This approach appears to offer a solution to some of the presently intractable problems in likelihood methods, such as inbred pedigrees, the mixed major gene/polygene model, and linkage with multiple polymorphic markers. However, problems arise in the case of complete penetrance (e.g., with marker data), where this process is not guaranteed to generate the full distribution of all possible genotypes, even if run infinitely long (see Chapter 7). These problems remain an active research area.

Missing data. Gibbs sampling also provides a natural way to address the problem of missing covariate data, under the assumption that the data are *missing at random (MAR)*, meaning that the probability of missingness does not depend on the true value or other unknown variables (although it can depend on measured variables) (Little and Rubin, 1989). One simply treats each missing datum as one more unknown in the system and, at each cycle of the Gibbs sampler, samples a random covariate value for each missing value, conditional on any other available information for the subject, including his or her phenotype, other covariates, his or her currently assigned genotype, and perhaps information on other family members. This approach was used by Gauderman et al. (1997b) in a reanalysis of the Sellers et al. (1990) lung cancer data, allowing many more subjects to be included in this analysis.

The advantage of this approach over standard *multiple imputation* methods (Rubin, 1987) is that the assignment of missing values can depend on the unknown genotypes.

Generalized Estimating Equations

Another way to overcome the computational problems is to use GEE methods, as outlined briefly in Chapters 4 and 5. When these methods are applied to segregation analysis, the basic idea is to model the means and the covariances between individuals' phenotypes as a function of the penetrances and allele frequency. An extension of the estimating equations for the means (GEE-1, described in Chapter 5) to include the covariances (GEE-2) is used to adjust the model parameters to fit the observed data. Lee et al. (1993) have shown that the means and covariances do not provide enough information to estimate both the penetrances and allele frequency simultaneously, and they suggest a profile likelihood approach to this problem. More recent work has explored the use of higher moments of the joint distribution of phenotypes to resolve this identifiability problem (Lee and Stram, 1996). The compelling advantage of GEE methods, aside from their apparent computational simplicity, is that estimates of model parameters require only the first few moments of the distribution, not the full distribution, and thus can be expected to be more robust than likelihood methods to misspecification of model assumptions.

Applications to Breast Cancer

The most widely quoted estimates of genetic parameters (age-specific penetrances and allele frequencies) for breast cancer—before the cloning of *BRCA1* and *BRCA2*—were from a reanalysis of the CASH data described in Chapter 5. In a second paper, Claus et al. (1991) described the fit of two segregation analysis models to the data on mothers and sisters of white cases and controls. Second-degree relatives and nonwhites were excluded (as in their previous analyses) because of under-reporting of the disease for these groups. Daughters were also excluded, as they were very young (the probands being under age 55 themselves), and thus only four of them were affected (two from cases and two from controls). Parametric analyses were carried out using the program Pointer (Lalouel and Morton, 1981), and maximum likelihood analyses using a step-function specification of the age- and genotype-specific incidence rates were conducted using MAXLIK (Kaplan and Elston, 1972). Table 6.5 summarizes the likelihood obtained with a variety of alternative genetic models. Thus, the purely sporadic model

Table 6.5 Alternative Genetic Models Fitted to the Cancer and Steroid Hormone Study Data

Model	q	h^2	$\chi^2 (df)$
Sporadic	—	—	0.00 —
Polygenic	—	0.25	205.51 (1)
Pure major gene			
Recessive	0.1612	—	230.36 (2)
Additive	0.0023	—	295.85 (2)
Dominant	0.0023	—	296.40 (2)
Mixed (dominant)	0.0023	0.00	296.40 (4)

Source: Adapted from Claus et al. (1991).

is rejected against all the alternative models, but any of the major gene models fit substantially better than a purely polygenic model. The mixed model, incorporating both major genes and polygenes, converges to the pure major gene model, with the dominance parameter diverging to its limit of 1.0 (corresponding to a dominant model). This general alternative model provides a 3 df chi-square test of the polygenic model, $296.40 - 205.51 = 90.89$, showing that the major gene model fits significantly better ($p < 10^{18}$).

Figure 6.8 shows the estimated penetrance function from the step-function method. The cumulative incidences $F_g(t) = 1 - S_g(t) = \exp(-\int_0^t \lambda_g(u)\,du)$ shown in the left panel were provided in Table 2 of Claus et al. (1991), and the incidence rate ratios $r(t) = \lambda_1(t)/\lambda_0(t)$ were provided in their Table 3. From the tabulated $F_g(t)$, the incidence rates can be calculated from $\lambda_g(t) = \ln[S(t_{k+1})/S(t_k)]/(t_{k+1} - t_k)$. Similar fits were obtained by assuming that the distribution of ages at diagnosis $f_g(t) = \lambda_g(t)S_g(t)$ was normal, with a mean at age 55 in carriers and 69 in noncarriers and a

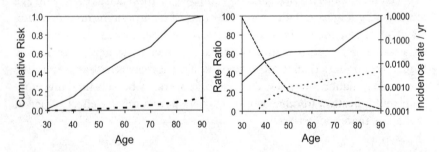

Figure 6.8 Penetrance estimates from the segregation analysis of the CASH data using a step function for the age-specific incidence rates. Left: cumulative incidence in carriers (solid line) and noncarriers (dotted line). Right: age-specific incidence rates in carriers (solid line) and noncarriers (dotted line), both on a log scale (right axis) and rate ratios (dashed line) on the linear scale (left axis). (Adapted from Claus et al., 1991, Table 2.)

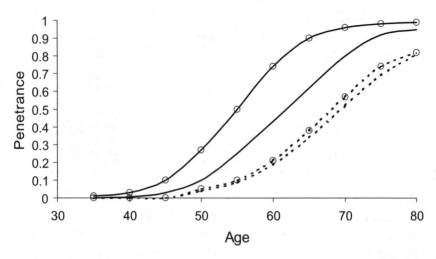

Figure 6.9 Penetrance estimates in carriers from a French family study (Andrieu and Demenais, 1997) incorporating age at menarche as a main effect and a modifier. Solid lines: women under age 15 at menarche; dotted lines: women aged 15 years or more at menarche. Lines without symbols come from a multiplicative model for the effect of menarche and genotype; lines with symbols incorporate an interaction effect.

common standard deviation of 15 years. The latter model yielded an estimate of $q = 0.0033$, which has been widely used in most subsequent linkage analyses, together with the penetrance estimates shown above.

Andrieu and Demenais (1997) conducted segregation analyses of the French family data discussed in Chapter 5, with the aim of further exploring interaction effects. Using the REGRESS program, which implements the Class D regressive logistic models of Bonney (1986), they found interactions between the major gene, age, and reproductive factors such as parity and age at menarche. Figure 6.9 illustrates the effect of incorporating an interaction effect of age at menarche on the estimates of penetrance in carriers. In either analysis, women with a young age at menarche have dramatically higher penetrances than those with older ages at menarche—as seen in the general population—but the difference appears to be substantially more than multiplicative; in other words, carriers have a greater effect of age at menarche than noncarriers.

Conclusions

Segregation analysis is the basic technique used to test whether a familial aggregation of a trait or disease appears to be due to major genes, polygenes, a shared environment, or some combination thereof. This is done by comparing the statistical fits of alternative genetic models, which usually involves summing over a set of unobservable genes or other factors that are transmitted within families. These models are generally fitted by the technique of maximum likelihood, using the Elston-Stewart peeling algorithm to expedite the calculations. For valid inference, the likelihood function must allow for the way in which the families were ascertained. In addition to tests of various null hypotheses, the method yields maximum likelihood estimates and confidence limits on the parameters of the alternative models, such as the penetrance function and allele frequencies for major gene(s) and the heritability of a polygenic component.

Based on segregation analyses of the CASH data, Claus et al. (1991) concluded that a dominant major gene fitted much better than pure environmental, pure polygenic, or recessive major gene models. Their estimates of the lifetime risk of breast cancer in gene carriers approached 100%, with an estimated population frequency of the mutant allele of 0.3%. The next chapter will pursue this story as researchers sought to localize the gene. As we shall see, two major genes (*BRCA1* and *BRCA2*) have already been identified, and subsequent segregation analyses in families not segregating mutations in either of these genes suggest the existence of one or more additional major genes, possibly acting in a recessive manner (Antoniou et al., 2002; Cui et al., 2001).

7

Linkage Analysis

Linkage analysis is the process of determining the approximate chromosomal location of a gene by looking for evidence of *cosegregation* with other genes whose locations are already known (i.e., *marker* genes). Cosegregation is a tendency for two or more genes to be inherited together, and hence for individuals with similar phenotypes to share alleles at the marker locus. Gene mapping is a huge topic, for which only a general introduction can be given here. Those interested in more detail can read one of the excellent textbooks by Ott (1999), Haines and Pericak-Vance (1998), or Pawlowitzki et al. (1997). Terwilliger and Ott (1994) provide a useful how-to manual of the mechanics of conducting a linkage analysis, based mainly on the LINKAGE package.

Before considering methods of linkage analysis per se, we review some fundamental concepts about the biological processes of meiosis and recombination introduced in Chapter 2 and their mathematical implications. Recall that during meiosis, linkage is possible only if two loci are situated on the same chromosome. In fact, the degree of linkage is a function of how close the loci are to each other, with widely spaced loci on the same chromosome behaving as if they were unlinked, thereby making it possible to estimate the location of an unknown gene relative to one or more known markers.

The most informative meioses are those from *doubly heterozygous* parents with *known phase*, meaning that the parent is heterozygous at both loci and we can tell with certainty which alleles at the two loci are paired with each other (e.g., by inference from the parents' genotypes). The total number of recombinants out of all such informative meioses has a binomial distribution with parameter θ. Standard methods can then be used to estimate $\hat{\theta}$, its confidence limits, and to test the null hypothesis ($\theta = 1/2$) (e.g., the McNemar chi-square test).

In practice, many meioses are not fully informative, so more complex methods are needed to exploit all available data. This chapter describes the two most widely used methods of linkage analysis—relative pair methods and lod score (likelihood) methods. Relative pair methods compare the identity by descent of markers among relatives. No assumptions about penetrance or allele frequencies are needed (hence, they are frequently called *nonparametric*). When analyzing dichotomous disease traits, researchers generally use pairs of affected siblings (*affected sib pairs*), testing the hypothesis that such pairs are more likely to share marker alleles IBD in the neighborhood of the disease locus than are random pairs of sibs. The sib pair method for quantitative traits is also presented here, its hypothesis being that there is greater similarity in phenotypes between sib pairs that share alleles IBD than between those that do not.

A more powerful test, known as the *lod score* method, is based on maximum likelihood, which can be applied either to nuclear families or to extended pedigrees. Indeed, for linkage analysis, pedigrees with many cases are the most informative. Obviously, it would be difficult to identify many heavily loaded families using a population-based sampling scheme, particularly for a rare disease, so such families cannot ordinarily be used to estimate all the parameters of a genetic model. Instead, the disease model parameters are usually fixed on the basis of prior segregation analysis of population-based data, although I will describe methods for joint segregation and linkage analysis that may be applicable even to data that are not population-based. I introduce these ideas with *two-point linkage* between a single disease gene and a single marker gene, and later describe more powerful *multipoint linkage analysis* methods, in which the disease locus is identified through the location of *flanking markers* (Kruglyak and Lander, 1995; Kruglyak et al., 1996). Procedures for whole-genome scanning for linkage and testing for heterogeneity are discussed, concluding with a brief discussion of some approaches to determining power or sample size.

Recombination and Map Functions

Genes are transmitted from parents to offspring through the process of *meiosis* (see Chapter 2). In the process of separation, the two chromosomes *cross over* at various points, and some of the material from one chromosome gets attached to the other chromosome. If the entire chromosome could be observed, we would be able to see these crossovers directly, but as markers are typically available only at discrete intervals, all we can tell is whether two consecutive markers derive from the same parental chromosome. When they derive from different parental chromosomes, the event is called a *recombination*.

Although crossover events themselves cannot be directly observed, the results of recombination are observable by tracing which grandparent the alleles at the two loci originally came from, using the techniques of linkage analysis discussed below. Two loci, A and B, separated by a single crossover event will thus appear as a recombinant. If these loci are separated by two crossover events, they will appear as a nonrecombinant since the transmitted alleles will have originated from the same chromosome. Such an event is indistinguishable from zero crossovers unless one observes a third locus, C, between A and B with recombinants both between A and C and between C and B. Thus, in general, all we can say is that a recombination relates to an odd number of crossovers and a nonrecombination to an even number. If the recombination fraction is small, the probability of two or more events is very small indeed, so a recombinant is likely to relate to a single crossover and a nonrecombinant to zero crossovers. As the crossover rate becomes large, multiple crossovers will become common so that eventually the probability of an even number of events is about the same as the probability of an odd number; hence the limiting value of the recombination fraction becomes 1/2.

During meiosis each chromosome segregates independently, so that a pair of genes on two different chromosomes are as likely to have one combination of alleles in a particular gamete as any other combination. For example, suppose that at one locus a parent has alleles a, A and at another locus the parent has alleles b, B (Fig. 7.1). Then if the two loci are on different chromosomes, the four possible gametes ab, aB, Ab, and AB are equally likely to occur (Fig. 7.1A), since linkage can occur only if two loci are on the same chromosome.

Now suppose that the two loci were on the same chromosome and further suppose that one member of the chromosome pair had alleles ab and the other AB. (Thus, we write the genotype as $ab \mid AB$, the vertical bar indicating which alleles were on the same chromosome, i.e., their *phase*.) If all chromosomes were transmitted intact during meiosis (Fig. 7.1B), then we would observe only two transmitted *haplotypes*, ab and AB; hence, by looking at transmission of markers, we would be able to tell which chromosome the gene we were looking for was on, but we would have no way of determining exactly where on the chromosome it was located (short of directly sequencing the entire chromosome).

Fortunately for the gene hunter, whole chromosomes are not transmitted intact; instead, the two members of the pair are scrambled through the process of crossing-over and recombination. This happens at multiple random points along the chromosome so that widely spaced loci segregate essentially at random, just as if they were on completely separate chromosomes. On the other hand, recombination is very unlikely to occur between two loci that are immediately adjacent to each other, so that the scenario described in the

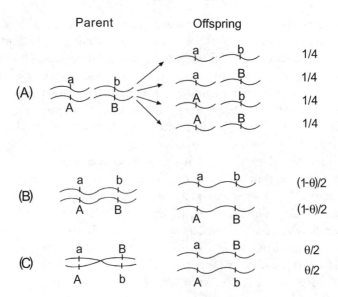

Figure 7.1 Schematic representation of pairs of loci A and B from one parent to an offspring. (A) Two loci on different chromosomes segregate independently, each possibility having probability $1/4$. (B) Two loci on the same chromosome segregating without recombination, with probability $1 - \theta$ or (C) with recombination, with probability θ.

previous paragraph would likely apply. At intermediate distances, recombination is likely to occur, so that all four possible haplotypes will be seen, but not with equal frequency. The probability of recombination increases with the physical distance between the two loci, from zero for adjacent loci to a limiting value of $1/2$ (Fig. 7.2), at least in the absence of *interference* or nonrandom assortment (Ott, 1999). It is this gradient in recombination probabilities that allows linkage analysis to determine the probable location

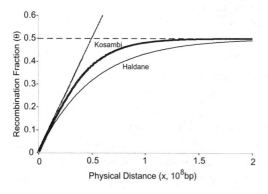

Figure 7.2 Map function showing the relationship between physical distance (x) in base pairs (bp) and recombination fraction (θ) in Morgans (M). Note the linearity at short distances and the asymptote of $\theta = 1/2$ at long distances.

of a gene. Thus, either a nonrecombinant haplotype ab or AB might be transmitted (Fig. 7.1B), each with probability $(1 - \theta)/2$, or a recombinant haplotype aB or Ab (Fig. 7.1C), each with probability $\theta/2$.

Suppose that crossovers occurred purely randomly, in the sense that the number of events between two loci followed a Poisson distribution, with the expected number of crossovers x proportional to the physical distance between them. Thus, the probability of c crossovers is $e^{-x}x^c/c!$. Since we can only tell whether an even or odd number of crossovers have occurred (as nonrecombinant or recombinant events, respectively), the probability of a recombination θ would be

$$\begin{aligned} \theta &= \Pr(c = 1 \mid x) + \Pr(c = 3 \mid x) + \Pr(c = 5 \mid x) + \cdots \\ &= e^{-x}(x + x^3/3! + x^5/5! + \cdots) \\ &= e^{-x}\sinh(x) \\ &= (1 - e^{-2x})/2 \end{aligned}$$

where $\sinh(x) = (e^x - e^{-x})/2$. The inverse function is

$$x = -\ln(1 - 2\theta)/2$$

This is known as the *Haldane* (1919) *map function,* expressing the relationship between map distances and recombination fractions. Map distances express the location of markers relative to an established panel of other markers whose order and locations have already been established (at least approximately). These distances x are expressed in units of Morgans (M), where 1 M represents the distance over which the expected number of crossovers is 1. Since this is such a large distance, the more commonly used unit is 1/100 of this, or a centiMorgan (cM), representing a 1% probability of crossover. Hence, for example, a map distance of $x = 0.29$ (29 cM) corresponds to a recombination fraction of $\theta = 0.22$. Recombination fractions, being a probability, are dimensionless quantities, usually expressed in percent, although the terms *cM* and *percent* are often used interchangeably. Physical distance is measured in base pairs (bp) of DNA, with 1 cM corresponding on average to about 1 million bp, although this proportionality factor varies across the genome, by gender, and by other factors.

In fact, crossovers do not really occur randomly. Given that a crossover has occurred at one location, the probability of another crossover nearby is somewhat lower than the overall rate, a phenomenon known as interference. Based on various mathematical theories about interference, a variety of other map functions have been derived. Perhaps the most commonly used map function is that of Kosambi (1944):

$$\theta = \tanh(2x)/2 = \frac{1}{2}\frac{e^{4x}-1}{e^{4x}+1}$$

$$x = \tanh^{-1}(2x)/2 = \frac{1}{4}\ln\left(\frac{1+2\theta}{1-2\theta}\right)$$

For a more complete discussion of map functions, see Ott (1999, §1.5 and 6.4). At very short intervals (a few kb or less), the linear relationship between physical and genetic distance can be distorted by the phenomenon of *gene conversion*—the transfer of short sequences from one chromosome to another, not necessarily at the same location, leaving the donor sequence intact (Strachan and Reed, 1999, pp. 220–222)—leading on average to a local increase in the apparent recombination rate. Assuming a geometric distribution of track lengths, Frisse et al. (2001) derive an expression for the expectation of the relationship of the form $\theta \propto r[x + 2(g/r)L(1 - e^{-x/L})]$, where, as before, x denotes physical distance in bp, θ the recombination rate in Morgans, and r, g and L are parameters giving the average rate of recombination per bp, the rate of gene conversion events per bp, and the mean track length in bp, respectively. For the purpose of linkage analysis, the level of resolution at which this phenomenon comes into play is too small to be important in family-based studies of recombination rates, but could be relevant for fine-scale mapping studies using linkage disequilibrium methods discussed in Chapter 10.

Although in principle knowledge of the correct map function should allow one to take a recombination fraction estimate and determine the precise physical location of the gene being sought, in practice the estimates of θ are too imprecise and the true map function too uncertain for this to be of much help in localizing genes. In addition to the phenomenon of interference, for example, the recombination rate is nonuniform across the genome (Kong et al., 2001). Thus, one normally proceeds by searching for more markers in the region until one reaches the point where further recombinants are unlikely to be found. At this point, other *fine mapping* techniques, as discussed at the end of this chapter and in Chapter 10, are used to narrow down the location to a point where direct sequencing becomes feasible.

Direct Counting Methods

Suppose for the moment that one could observe recombinants directly. How would we draw an inference about their statistical distribution? Let us denote the probability of recombination between a pair of loci by θ. Suppose that

Table 7.1 Transmission of Haplotypes Through the Process of Recombination

Parental Genotype	Transmitted Haplotype			
	dm	dM	Dm	DM
$dm \mid dm$	1	0	0	0
$dm \mid dM$	1/2	1/2	0	0
$dM \mid dM$	0	1	0	0
$dm \mid Dm$	1/2	0	1/2	0
$dm \mid DM$	$(1-\theta)/2$	$\theta/2$	$\theta/2$	$(1-\theta)/2$
$dM \mid Dm$	$\theta/2$	$(1-\theta)/2$	$(1-\theta)/2$	$\theta/2$
$dM \mid DM$	0	1/2	0	1/2
$Dm \mid Dm$	0	0	1	0
$Dm \mid DM$	0	0	1/2	1/2
$DM \mid DM$	0	0	0	1

one locus is an unknown disease susceptibility locus with alleles d and D and the other is a known marker locus with alleles m and M. Only *doubly heterozygous* parents (genotypes $dm \mid DM$ or $dM \mid Dm$) are informative about linkage. (Consider instead a parent with genotype $dm \mid dm$: he or she would transmit the same haplotype, dm, whether a recombination occurred or not, so one could not tell whether the specific d and m alleles had come from the same member or different members of the chromosome pair.) Depending on the parent's phase, the probability of each of the four possible haplotypes being transmitted to the offspring is given in Table 7.1. The only entries that involve θ are those for transmissions from double heterozygotes.

In principle, we therefore look for parent-offspring pairs (meioses) in which a parent is doubly heterozygous and count the number of occasions for which the transmitted haplotype is a recombinant or a nonrecombinant. Letting r and s denote the number of these two events and letting $n = r + s$ be the total number of informative meioses, the probability of the observed data is simply $\text{Binom}(r \mid n, \theta)$:

$$\Pr(r \mid n) = \binom{n}{r} \theta^r (1-\theta)^{n-r}$$

Thus, we would estimate θ in the obvious way as $\hat{\theta} = r/n$ and $\text{var}(\hat{\theta}) = rs/n^3$. The usual McNemar chi-square test

$$\chi_1^2 = \frac{(|r-s| - 1/2)^2}{n}$$

would be used to test the significance of the null hypothesis $H_0 : \theta = 1/2$.

In practice, unless the disease gene is fully penetrant with no pheno-copies, we cannot unambiguously determine the genotypes of the individuals at the disease locus, and even if we could, we might not always be able to

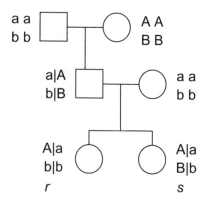

Figure 7.3 Hypothetical pedigree illustrating codominant inheritance of two markers.

figure out the phase. Thus linkage analysis generally uses the relative pair or lod score methods described later. Nevertheless, it is instructive to explore further the principles of direct counting to set the stage for the practical methods that follow.

Consider first two codominant loci with complete penetrance so that we can unambiguously determine the genotypes of each individual. A hypothetical pedigree is shown in Figure 7.3. Here we have no way of determining the phase of the grandparents or the mother, but since all three are homozygous at each locus, it does not matter. Since the A and B alleles for the father could only have come from his mother (paternal grandmother), we can be certain of the phase of his genotype, and in the same way, we can unambiguously determine the phase of his offspring. Because the mother is homozygous, her meioses are uninformative. Of the two paternal meioses, the first must have been a recombinant and the second a nonrecombinant. We would therefore score this pedigree as $r = 1, s = 1$. By scoring other pedigrees in the same way, we could obtain the total numbers r and s and test for linkage as described above.

Suppose that in this manner we were able to count 100 meioses and observed $r = 35$ recombinants. We would then estimate $\hat{\theta} = 35/100 = 0.35$ with a standard error of $\sqrt{35 \times 65/100^3} = 0.048$. The chi-square test would be 9.89, corresponding to a one-tailed p-value of 0.0008. (A one-tailed test is used because values of $\theta > 0.5$ are of no interest.)

Now suppose that one of the two loci is a disease susceptibility locus with only two possible phenotypes, affected or not. Then we cannot distinguish two of the possible genotypes, depending on dominance. Suppose, however, that the gene is autosomal dominant with complete penetrance, and suppose further that the mutant allele is rare so that genotype DD is extremely rare. Now consider the hypothetical pedigree shown in Figure 7.4, where the affected individuals (the shaded symbols) are assumed to be genotype dD

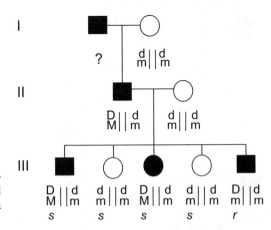

Figure 7.4 Hypothetical pedigree illustrating autosomal dominant inheritance with complete penetrance.

and the unaffected individuals dd. Again, we have no way to determine the phase of the grandfather, but since the grandmother is doubly homozygous, it is evident that the father must have phase $DM \mid dm$. Similarly, since the mother is also doubly homozygous, it is evident that the first four offspring are all nonrecombinant and the last is recombinant (from the father). We would therefore score this pedigree as $r = 1, s = 4$.

If we did not know the genotype of the grandmother, we would be in a quandary. Is the father's genotype $DM \mid dm$ or $Dm \mid dM$? If it is the latter, we would have to score the pedigree as $r = 4, s = 1$. Under the null hypothesis, both possibilities would be equally likely, so we might be tempted to average the two scores to produce $r = 2.5, s = 2.5$, leading to $\hat{\theta} = 0.5$. Thus, such a pedigree would therefore appear to be uninformative. As we shall see, this is not the right thing to do, as there is indeed some linkage information in such a pedigree, but less than if the grandparents were typed.

A similar situation arises when the gene is recessive or not fully penetrant, so that the trait genotypes cannot be unequivocally determined. Consider the hypothetical pedigree shown in Figure 7.5 and suppose that the gene is autosomal recessive and fully penetrant, with a rare mutant allele. Thus all affected individuals have genotype DD and the parents must be carriers $D \mid d$. Given the markers of the grandparents, we can determine the phase for both parents with certainty ($D1 \mid d2$ and $D3 \mid d4$, respectively). The first affected offspring must therefore be a double nonrecombinant, but what of the other three unaffected offspring? We cannot tell whether or not they are carriers. If the second offspring were genotype $D1 \mid d4$, she would also be a double nonrecombinant, but if she were $d1 \mid D4$ she would be a double recombinant, and if she were $d1 \mid d4$ she would have one of each type. By direct scoring, such individuals could not be counted and the pedigree would

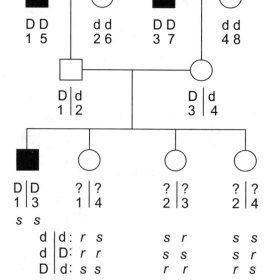

Figure 7.5 Hypothetical family illustrating autosomal recessive inheritance with complete penetrance.

be scored as $r = 0, s = 2$. We shall revisit these ambiguous situations in the section "lod Score Methods" and see how additional information can be gleaned from them.

Relative Pair Methods

Relative pair methods consider all possible pairs of relatives in a particular type of relationship and determine whether pairs with similar phenotypes tend to share marker alleles more than would be expected by chance, given the nature of their relationship. These methods offer quite simple significance tests for the null hypothesis but no estimate of the recombination fraction. They are thus particularly useful for rapid screening of a large number of marker loci to look for evidence of linkage, but they are less useful for fine mapping. Because the test of the null hypothesis does not require any assumptions about penetrance, these methods are often called *nonparametric* or *model free* and are generally believed to be more robust to the choice of a specific test than is the lod score approach. On the other hand, the methods are likely to be less powerful than lod score methods if the assumptions of the latter are correctly specified. As noted by Whittemore (1996), the choice of the *optimal* test depends on knowledge of the disease model, so she advocates using the term nonparametric rather than model free to describe this class of tests.

The particular methods are distinguished by the way they handle similarity in phenotypes, the way they handle similarity in marker alleles, and what types of relationships are considered. For continuous phenotypes, all individuals are potentially informative and similarity within pairs is usually assessed by the squared difference in phenotypes. For dichotomous disease phenotypes, affected pairs are much more informative than affected-unaffected or unaffected-unaffected pairs (assuming the mutant allele is rare), so usually only affected pairs are used. (This will be demonstrated later in the section "Power and Sample Size"; see Table 7.11.)

Similarity in alleles at any locus can be determined on an IBS or an IBD basis. These concepts were introduced in Chapter 5 in the context of genetic relationships between individuals and gene identity at a disease locus. We now apply these principles to an observable marker gene rather than to the unobserved disease gene.

Identity by state and by descent

Consider the simple nuclear families shown in Figure 7.6 illustrating a four-allele marker system. (For present purposes, we can ignore the disease phenotypes since at this point we are only interested in similarity of marker alleles.) Since each member of a pair has two marker alleles, a pair of individuals can share either zero, one, or two alleles. In panel A, the two siblings have no alleles in common, so IBS = IBD = 0. In panel B, the two sibs share the *a* allele from the father, the allele from the mother being different for each sib; hence IBS = IBD = 1. In panel C, the sibs share two alleles and there is no ambiguity about their sources, so IBS = IBD = 2.

Figure 7.7 illustrates more complicated situations. In panel A, the sibs share the *b* allele by state, but it is evident that these two copies may not

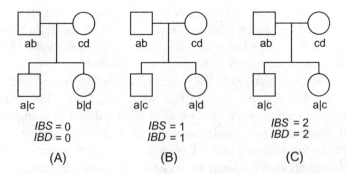

Figure 7.6 Hypothetical pedigrees illustrating unambiguous assignments of IBD sharing.

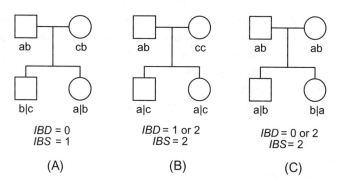

Figure 7.7 Hypothetical pedigrees illustrating the difference between IBD and IBS allele sharing.

have come from the same parent, since both parents carry the *b* allele. In this instance, the brother's *b* allele must have come from his father (since his *c* allele could only have come from his mother); similarly, the sister's *b* allele must have come from her mother. The two *b* alleles did not come from the same source and are therefore not identical by descent. Thus, we say that they share zero alleles IBD.

If a parent is homozygous, we cannot determine identity by descent (if all that is available is that one marker; we will discuss the use of multiple marker loci later). Consider the nuclear family shown in Figure 7.7B. It is obvious that the *a* alleles shared by the two sibs must both have come from the father and the two *c* alleles must both have come from the mother, but the IBD requirement is stronger—they must also have the same grandparental source. Since the mother has two *c* alleles, one sib's allele might have come originally from the maternal grandfather and the other's from the maternal grandmother. Since we cannot tell which is which, we do not know whether to score this pair as sharing one or two alleles IBD, although we can say with certainty that they share two alleles IBS. In panel C the two sibs each have one *a* and one *b* allele, but because both parents also have both *a* and *b* alleles, it is not clear whether either sib has ordered genotype *a | b* or *b | a*. Thus, they could share either zero or two alleles IBD.

The advantage of knowing IBD relationships is that the probabilities under $H_0 : \theta = 1/2$ that any two relatives share one or two alleles are simple constants, depending only on their type of relationship. For example, a parent and offspring share exactly one allele IBD, since the parent transmits one allele to the offspring and the offspring's other allele must come from the other parent, even if it happens to be the same allele (by state). Monozygotic twins must, of course, share both alleles IBD. Sibs can share zero, one, or two alleles IBD, with probabilities 1/4, 1/2, and 1/4, respectively.

Table 7.2 Probabilities of Sharing Alleles Identical by Descent (IBD) for Different Types of Relationships

Type of Relative Pair	Probability of Sharing IBD Alleles		
	π_0	π_1	π_2
Monozygotic twins	0	0	1
Full sibs	1/4	1/2	1/4
Parent-offspring	0	1	0
First cousins	3/4	1/4	0
Double first cousins	13/16	1/8	1/16
Grandparent-grandchild, half-sibs, avuncular	1/2	1/2	0

The probabilities π_a of sharing a alleles IBD under the null hypothesis of no linkage for various types of relationships are given in Table 7.2 (see the derivation of these probabilities in Eq. [5.1]).

In contrast, the null probability of sharing alleles IBS is more complicated, as they depend on the population allele frequencies. Suppose that there are only two alleles, a and b, with allele frequencies $\mathbf{p} = (p_a, p_b)$. Then intuitively, if $p_a > p_b$, it is more likely that a pair of sibs would share one or more copies of the a allele than that they would share one or more copies of the b allele. If the parents are untyped, the null probability distribution for the number of alleles shared IBS depends on which allele(s) is (are) shared and is calculated by summing over all possible combinations of parental genotypes. Letting $\mathbf{M}_p$ denote the parental and $\mathbf{M}_o$ the offspring marker genotypes,

$$\Pr(\text{IBS} = n) = \sum_{\mathbf{M}_p} \Pr(\mathbf{M}_p \mid \mathbf{p}) \ \Pr(\text{IBS} = n \mid \mathbf{M}_p)$$

$$= \sum_{\mathbf{M}_p} \Pr(\mathbf{M}_p \mid \mathbf{p}) \sum_{\mathbf{M}_o} \Pr(\mathbf{M}_o \mid \mathbf{M}_p) \ I(\text{IBS} = n \mid \mathbf{M}_o)$$

Table 7.3 illustrates the calculations. The totals by the number of alleles shared IBS are obtained by considering all the possible probabilities for each number of shared alleles. Thus, for $p_a = 0.25$, the probability of sharing one allele IBS is $0.059 + 0.246 = 0.305$, and the probability of sharing two alleles IBS is $0.024 + 0.431 + 0.223 = 0.678$. Here the probability of sharing the a allele IBS is computed as

$$\frac{1}{2}\left(2p_a^3 p_b\right) + \frac{1}{2}\left(2p_a^3 p_b\right) + \frac{1}{4}\left(4p_a^2 p_b^2\right) = 0.0234 + 0.035 = 0.058$$

Even in the case of $p_a = 0.5$, the distribution of the number of alleles shared IBS is not the same as the distribution by IBD. Rather, one will find

Table 7.3 Calculation of the Probabilities of Sharing Alleles Identical by State (IBS), Summing Over the Possible Combinations of Parental Genotypes

Father's Genotype	Mother's Genotype	Joint Probability	Probability of Sharing Alleles IBS					
			—	a	aa	b	bb	ab
aa	aa	p_a^4	0	0	1	0	0	0
aa	ab	$2p_a^3 p_b$	0	1/2	1/4	0	0	1/4
aa	bb	$p_a^2 p_b^2$	0	0	0	0	0	1
ab	aa	$2p_a^3 p_b$	0	1/2	1/4	0	0	1/4
ab	ab	$4p_a^2 p_b^2$	1/8	1/4	1/16	1/4	1/16	1/4
ab	bb	$2p_a p_b^3$	0	0	0	1/2	1/4	1/4
bb	aa	$p_a^2 p_b^2$	0	0	0	0	0	1
bb	ab	$2p_a p_b^3$	0	0	0	1/2	1/4	1/4
bb	bb	p_b^4	0	0	0	0	1	0
Totals	$p_a = 0.50$		0.031	0.188	0.141	0.188	0.141	0.313
	$p_a = 0.25$		0.018	0.059	0.024	0.246	0.431	0.223
	$p_a = 0.10$		0.004	0.010	0.003	0.154	0.731	0.098
	$p_a = 0.01$		0.000	0.000	0.000	0.020	0.970	0.010

Totals by number of alleles shared IBS*		0	1	2
	$p_a = 0.50$	0.031	0.375	0.594
	$p_a = 0.25$	0.018	0.305	0.678
	$p_a = 0.10$	0.004	0.164	0.832
	$p_a = 0.01$	0.000	0.020	0.980

*$0 = \{-\}, 1 = \{a, b\}, 2 = \{aa, ab, bb\}$ in the panels above.

more sharing IBS than IBD. The difficulty is that the true marker allele frequencies **p** may not be known, and misspecification of this quantity will lead to biased estimates of the expected allele sharing under the null hypothesis and an inflation of the Type I error rate (Borecki, 1999; Freimer et al., 1993; Korczak et al., 1995; Mandal, 2000). Ideally, estimates of **p** would come from sample data for the population in which the study is being conducted. Data typically available from high-throughput genotyping laboratories may approximate this but could also reflect a mixture of populations they happened to have previously typed. For that matter, if the study sample itself is heterogeneous, then no single estimate will adequately describe this variation and false positive linkages could also result. Hence the investigator should endeavor to stratify the sample by race or ethnicity and use subgroup-specific estimators where possible. If no external estimates of marker allele frequencies are available, the investigator could use the empirical estimates from the founders in the dataset at hand (Boehnke, 1991), but these too could be biased if the marker is in linkage disequilibrium with the causal locus, since the associated allele would be over-represented in a sample of families ascertained through affected pairs.

While these calculations are relatively straightforward for sib pairs, they can in principle be extended to more distant relatives or to larger sets of relatives, as will be discussed further below. This would allow linkage analysis to be conducted in situations where the IBD status cannot be determined, such as when some of the linking members of the pedigree are not available for genotyping.

Recent developments in multipoint analysis (Kruglyak and Lander, 1995; Kruglyak et al., 1996), discussed below, allow these probabilities to be computed as a continuous function $\pi_n(x)$ of the location x along a chromosome in relation to multiple markers, using all the data in a modest-sized extended pedigree. Here we introduce the general approach for the simplest case of a single marker and a sib pair with parental genotypes unavailable, deferring the general treatment of multipoint linkage in general pedigrees until later. The remainder of this section is somewhat technical and can be skipped by the less mathematically inclined.

First, we compute the probability Q_a^A that IBD $= a = 0, 1, 2$ at the marker locus A itself, given the available marker information. For example, in panel C of Figure 7.7, we saw that $Q_0^A = 1/2$, $Q_1^A = 0$, and $Q_2^A = 1/2$. When parents are not available, the calculation of these probabilities is similar to that described above for IBS sharing, summing over all possible parental genotypes and segregation indicators, thereby involving the marker allele frequencies. Then we combine these quantities with the conditional probabilities T_{ab} of IBD at locus B given IBD at locus A to obtain the desired probability $\pi_b(\theta)$ of IBD at any locus B given the available marker information at A, as a continuous function of recombination distance θ between the two loci.

To compute the IBD probabilities at the marker locus, we proceed as follows. Let $Z^A = 0, 1, 2$ denote the pair's IBD status at locus A and let $\mathbf{M}_p^A, \mathbf{M}_o^A$ denote the observed offsprings' and unobserved parents' genotypes at locus A.

$$Q_a^A = \Pr\left(Z_A = a \mid \mathbf{M}_o^A\right) = \frac{\Pr(\mathbf{M}_o^A \mid Z^A = a)\,\Pr(Z^A = a)}{\sum_a \Pr(\mathbf{M}_o \mid Z^A = a)\,\Pr(Z^A = a)} \tag{7.1}$$

where

$$\Pr\left(\mathbf{M}_o^A \mid Z^A = a\right) = \sum_{\mathbf{m}} \Pr(\mathbf{M}_p^A = \mathbf{m} \mid \mathbf{p}^A)\,\Pr(\mathbf{M}_o^A \mid \mathbf{M}_p^A = \mathbf{m}, Z^A = a)$$

$$= \sum_{\mathbf{m}} \Pr(\mathbf{M}_p^A = \mathbf{m} \mid \mathbf{p}^A) \sum_{\mathbf{s}} I(Z^A = a \mid \mathbf{S}^A = \mathbf{s})$$

$$\times I\left(\mathbf{M}_o \mid \mathbf{M}_p^A = \mathbf{m}, \mathbf{S}^A = \mathbf{s}\right)$$

Now to compute the transition probabilities from one locus to the next, let $\mathbf{s} = (s_1, s_2, s_3, s_4)$ denote the segregation indicators for the two alleles each for a pair of siblings at locus A and let $\mathbf{t} = (t_1, t_2, t_3, t_4)$ denote the corresponding segregation indicators at locus B. Then we could write the number of recombinants as $r_{\mathbf{st}} = \sum_{k=1}^{4} |s_k - t_k|$. Likewise, the IBD status at the two loci would be given by $Z^A = 2 - |s_1 - s_3| - |s_2 - s_4|$ and $Z^B = 2 - |t_1 - t_3| - |t_2 - t_4|$. Then the joint probability of the IBD status at the two loci can be computed by summing over all possible pairs of segregation indicators:

$$T_{ab} = \Pr(Z^B = b \mid Z^A = a)$$

$$= \frac{\sum_{\mathbf{s}} \sum_{\mathbf{t}} I(Z^A = a \mid \mathbf{s}) \, I(Z^B = b \mid \mathbf{t}) \, \theta^{r_{\mathbf{st}}} (1 - \theta)^{4 - r_{\mathbf{st}}}}{\Pr(Z^A = a)} \qquad (7.2)$$

where $\Pr(Z) = (1/4, 1/2, 1/4)$. Although this would appear to require a total of $2^4 \times 2^4 = 256$ terms, one can easily see that there are symmetric relations among them, so only 16 terms are really needed. The end result is shown in Table 7.4 and Figure 7.8.

Finally, the IBD probability at locus B, given the available information at marker locus A, would be computed as

$$\pi_b^B = \Pr(Z^B = b \mid \mathbf{M}^A) = \sum_a \Pr(Z^B = b \mid Z^A = a)$$

$$\times \Pr(Z^A = a \mid \mathbf{M}^A) = \sum_a T_{ab} \, Q_a^A$$

Letting $\mathbf{Q}_A = (Q_0^A, Q_1^A, Q_2^A)$, $\mathbf{T}_{AB} = (T_{ab})_{a=0..2, b=0..2}$, and $\boldsymbol{\pi}(\theta) = (\pi_0^B, \pi_1^B, \pi_0^B)$, we can represent this calculation in matrix notation as $\boldsymbol{\pi}(A) = \mathbf{Q}_A \mathbf{T}_{AB}$. These probabilities can then be used in any of the sib pair linkage methods described below whenever the IBD status cannot be determined with certainty.

Affected sib pair methods

Sib pair methods test the hypothesis that pairs who have similar phenotypes (and are therefore more likely to share one or both alleles at the disease

Table 7.4 Conditional Probabilities T_{ab} of Identical by Descent (IBD) at One Locus Given IBD at Another Locus at a Recombination Fraction of θ

	$\mathrm{IBD}_B = 0$	$\mathrm{IBD}_B = 1$	$\mathrm{IBD}_B = 2$
$\mathrm{IBD}_A = 0$	$(1 - 2\theta + 2\theta^2)^2$	$4\theta(1 - \theta)(1 - 2\theta + 2\theta^2)$	$4\theta^2(1 - \theta)^2$
$\mathrm{IBD}_A = 1$	$2\theta(1 - \theta)(1 - 2\theta + 2\theta^2)$	$(1 - 2\theta + 2\theta^2)^2 + 4\theta^2(1 - \theta)^2$	$2\theta(1 - \theta)(1 - 2\theta + 2\theta^2)$
$\mathrm{IBD}_A = 2$	$4\theta^2(1 - \theta)^2$	$4\theta(1 - \theta)(1 - 2\theta + 2\theta^2)$	$(1 - 2\theta + 2\theta^2)^2$

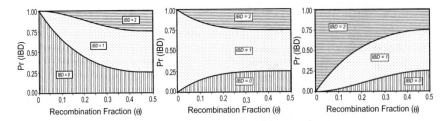

Figure 7.8 Conditional probabilities $T_{b|a}(\theta)$ of IBD at one locus given IBD at another locus at a recombination fraction of θ. Left panel, $\text{IBD}_a = 0$; center panel, $\text{IBD}_a = 1$; right panel, $\text{IBD}_a = 2$.

locus) also tend to share similar marker alleles. If a disease is rare, then an affected individual is much more likely to carry one or more mutant alleles than a random member of the population, while an unaffected individual is only slightly less likely to carry a mutant allele than a random member of the population. Thus affected individuals are much more informative than unaffected individuals. For this reason, the most widely used relative pair method for dichotomous disease traits is based only on affected pairs. In this case, we recast the hypothesis as follows: pairs of affected sibs are more likely to share marker alleles IBD than random pairs of sibs.

As noted above, a random pair of siblings would be expected to share two alleles IBD with probability $\pi_2 = 1/4$, to share one allele IBD with probability $\pi_1 = 1/2$, and to share neither allele IBD with probability $\pi_0 = 1/4$. This would be true, regardless of their disease status, if the marker under study were unlinked to any disease locus. If two sibs are both affected by the disease and the disease is linked to a particular marker, then one would expect to see more sharing of marker alleles IBD than expected by chance. One therefore tabulates the number of affected sib pairs by their IBD status and compares that distribution to the expected distribution, as shown in Table 7.5. (Here N is the number of affected sib pairs, not the number of individuals or the number of alleles.) In accumulating the table of observed IBD sharing, ambiguous pairs should not be excluded but should be counted fractionally. For example, the pair shown in Figure 7.7C

Table 7.5 Distribution of Affected Sib Pairs by Marker Allele Sharing

	Number of Alleles Shared IBD			
	0	1	2	Total
Observed	A	B	C	N
Expected	$N/4$	$N/2$	$N/4$	N

IBD, identical by descent.

would be counted as $1/2$ in IBD $= 0$ and $1/2$ in IBD $= 2$. While a 2 *df* chi-square test, $[4(A - N/4)^2 + 2(B - N/2)^2 + 4(C - N/4)^2]/N$, could be used to test the significance of the difference between observed and expected distributions, a more powerful test is provided by a 1 *df* chi-square test for trend in proportions:

$$X^2 = (A - C)^2/(A + C) \sim \chi^2_{1,\alpha}$$

using a two-tailed test. An alternative formulation (Blackwelder and Elston, 1985) uses a *t*-test to compare the mean proportion of alleles shared IBD, $\bar{\pi} = \pi_1/2 + \pi_2$, which is estimated as $\hat{\bar{\pi}} = (B + 2C)/2N$ to the null value of $1/2$ using its empirical standard error $SE(\hat{\bar{\pi}}) = \sqrt{(AB + 4AC + BC)/4N^3}$. This should be tested against a *t* distribution with $N - 1$ degrees of freedom to obtain the correct test size, and it appears to have slightly better power than the chi-square test. This is known in the linkage analysis literature as the *means test* because it tests $H_0 : \bar{\pi} = 1/2$.

For example, consider the hypothetical data shown in Table 7.6. An overall test for any differences between observed and expected is

$$\frac{(20 - 25)^2}{25} + \frac{(45 - 50)^2}{50} + \frac{(35 - 25)^2}{25} = 5.50 \sim \chi^2_2$$

leading to $p > 0.05$. Focusing instead on the shift in the distribution from zero to two alleles, the trend test yields $\chi^2_1 = (35 - 20)^2/(35 + 20) = 4.09$ with a one-tailed $p = 0.022$, while the means test variant yields $t = \sqrt{4.27} = 2.065$ with $p = 0.018$. Either of these tests tends to be more powerful for testing linkage than the 2 *df* test for an additive or rare dominant gene. For a recessive gene, however, the expected proportion of pairs with IBD $= 1$ departs from $1/2$ as θ becomes small, so a more powerful test for tight linkage is $(3C - 2B - A)^2/(9C + 4B + A)$. However, the advantage of the means test is that it does not require knowledge of the disease model: it will have the correct test size (asymptotically) whatever the disease model and is the locally most powerful test for weak linkage for any disease model.

Table 7.6 Example of Affected Sib Pair Test

| | Number of Alleles Shared IBD | | | |
	0	1	2	Total
Observed	20	45	35	100
Expected	25	50	25	100

IBD, identical by descent.

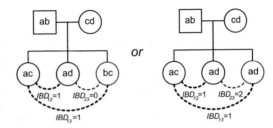

Figure 7.9 Some possible configurations of IBD status in sibships of size three.

Sibships with three or more affected individuals will contribute more than one pair to this analysis: three affected will contribute three pairs; four affected will contribute six pairs; and so on. Consider a sibship of size three (Fig. 7.9). The IBD status of any pair of sibs is independent of that of any other; hence, we say they are *pairwise independent*. But given the IBD status of two pairs, we can usually predict the IBD status of the third pair, as shown in Table 7.7. In every case but the fourth, we see that the IBD status of the third pair is uniquely determined by that of the other two pairs, but in the fourth case, two alternative configurations are possible. Thus, the third pair is not independent of the other two, yet it still contributes some additional information; hence we say that they are not *jointly independent*. In general, the information content of a sibship of size S is greater than S but less than the total number of pairs $S(S-1)/2$. Numerous papers have been written on the subject of how to weight sibships as a function of their size (see Hodge, 1984; Ott, 1999, pp. 276–277, for further discussion). The GEE methods described below provide a natural way of addressing this problem by using the robust variance estimator.

Alternatively, one could proceed as follows. First, note that if we rearrange the entries in Table 7.7, there are only four distinguishable configurations: the first and third lines both have two pairs with IBD = 0 and one with IBD = 2; and likewise, the fourth line is equivalent to the second and fifth lines. Letting $N_{002}, N_{011}, N_{112}, N_{222}$ denote the observed number of trios with the indicated IBD configurations, we can see that the corresponding

Table 7.7 Identical by Descent (IBD) Status Prediction in Sibships with Three Affected Individuals

IBD_{12}	IBD_{13}	IBD_{23}	Example
0	0	2	ac, bd, bd
0	1	1	ac, bd, ad
0	2	0	ac, bd, ac
1	1	0 or 2	ac, ad, bc or ac, ad, ad
1	2	1	ac, ad, ac
2	2	2	ac, ac, ac

probabilities are

$$\Pi_{002} = E(N_{002}) = \pi_0^2 + 2\pi_0\pi_2$$

$$\Pi_{011} = E(N_{011}) = 2\pi_0\pi_1 + \frac{\pi_1^2\pi_0}{\pi_0 + \pi_2}$$

$$\Pi_{112} = E(N_{112}) = 2\pi_1\pi_2 + \frac{\pi_1^2\pi_2}{\pi_0 + \pi_2}$$

$$\Pi_{222} = E(N_{222}) = \pi_2^2$$

Under $H_0 : \pi_0 = 1/4, \pi_1 = 1/2, \pi_2 = 1/4$, we obtain $\Pi_{002} = 3/16, \Pi_{011} = 3/8$, $\Pi_{112} = 3/8$, and $\Pi_{222} = 1/16$. The proper analog of the 2 df chi-square test would thus be

$$\frac{(N_{002} - 3N/16)^2}{3N/16} + \frac{(N_{011} - 3N/8)^2}{3N/8} + \frac{(N_{112} - 3N/8)^2}{3N/8} + \frac{(N_{222} - N/16)^2}{N/16}$$

To obtain a trend test, we set $\pi_1 = 1/2$ and $\pi_0 = 1/2 - \pi_2$ to obtain

$$\Pi_{002} = \frac{1}{4} - \pi_2^2$$

$$\Pi_{011} = \frac{3}{4} - \frac{3\pi_2}{2}$$

$$\Pi_{112} = \frac{3\pi_2}{2}$$

$$\Pi_{222} = \pi_2^2$$

The likelihood is then

$$\mathcal{L}(\pi_2) = \Pi_{002}^{N_{002}} \times \Pi_{011}^{N_{011}} \times \Pi_{112}^{N_{112}} \times \Pi_{222}^{N_{222}}$$

which could be used to form any of the three likelihood-based tests described in Chapter 4. In particular, the score test becomes

$$X^2 = \frac{[-(8/3)N_{002} - 4N_{011} + 4N_{112} + 8N_{222}]^2}{(64/9)N_{002} + 16N_{011} + 16N_{112} + 64N_{222}}$$

Similar reasoning applies to sibships with four or more affected. For four affected, there are eight distinguishable configurations, shown in Table 7.8, together with the corresponding weights in the 1 df chi-square trend test $[\sum_c (N_c - E_c) W_c]^2 / \sum_c E_c W_c^2$. For a sample of sibships with varying numbers of affected members, one would simply accumulate each sibship's contribution to the numerator and denominator separately, using the appropriate expecteds and weights.

Table 7.8 Possible Configurations of Identical by Descent (IBD) Status Among Sibships of Size 4, Together with Their Expected Frequencies E_c and Weights W_c for the Chi-Square Trend Test

Number of Pairs by IBD Status			Example of Marker Genotypes				Expected Frequency	Weight
0	1	2	Sib 1	Sib 2	Sib 3	Sib 4	E_c	W_c
0	0	6	ac	ac	ac	ac	1/64	+12
0	3	3	ac	ac	ac	ad	8/64	+8
3	0	3	ac	ac	ac	bd	4/64	0
0	4	2	ac	ac	ad	ad	6/64	+8
1	4	1	ac	ac	ad	bc	12/64	0
2	3	1	ac	ac	ad	bd	24/64	−8/3
4	0	2	ac	ac	bd	bd	3/64	−4
2	4	0	ac	ad	bc	bd	6/64	−8

Although the affected pairs are the most informative for linkage (as discussed further in the section "Power and Sample Size" below), the unaffected members of a sibship can also be useful. First, if parents are unavailable or not fully informative, the availability of additional siblings can help the determination of the IBD status. Also, the comparison of $\bar{\pi}$ for the affected pairs against a theoretical null value of $1/2$ can be biased if the IBD status cannot be determined with certainty and estimates of marker allele frequency have to be used to estimate it. In this case, comparison of affected to discordant pairs can provide a useful control and in some circumstances may also yield a more powerful test (Guo and Elston, 2000). To guard against the possibility of heterogeneity in allele frequencies across sibships, a within-sibship test should be used. Kerber et al. (2002) suggest a test of the form $t = (\bar{\pi}_i^A - \bar{\pi}_i^D)/SE(\bar{\pi}_i^A - \bar{\pi}_i^D)$, where π_i^A and $\bar{\pi}_i^D$ are the mean IBD in affected and discordant pairs within sibship i, respectively. For sibships with only affected individuals available for typing, $\bar{\pi}_i^D$ could be set to $1/2$.

Affected relative pair methods

In principle, the affected sib pair method can be generalized to any form of relative pairs. All that would be needed is to stratify Table 7.5 by type of relative, replacing the expecteds using the proportions given in Table 7.2, add up the numbers observed and expected across relative types, and use the means test as described above.

In practice, however, IBD relationships can be difficult to determine for more distant relatives and IBS methods are more commonly used. If the population marker allele frequencies were known, one might simply form a contingency table for each type of relationship in the same way as above, deriving expected distributions of allele sharing following the general procedures outlined in the two-allele, sib-pair case in Table 7.3. In general, however, the allele frequencies are not known and must be estimated from the data, so the significance test should reflect the sampling variability in these estimates. Also, reducing the table to the number of alleles shared wastes information; instead, the calculations use the specific alleles shared by each pair. Even more powerful tests can be formed using larger sets of affected relatives rather than just pairs (Whittemore and Halpern, 1994). The method is somewhat complex, requiring computer programs; see Weeks and Lange (1988) and the references in Ott (1999, pp. 277–278) for further details.

Sib pair methods for quantitative traits

For quantitative traits, the hypothesis might be formulated as follows: sib pairs (or other relative pairs) that share alleles IBD tend to have greater similarity in their phenotypes than pairs that do not; pairs that share two alleles IBD tend to have even greater similarity. Operationally, the means of testing this hypothesis is to regress the squared differences in phenotypes on the number of shared alleles. The basic method is given by Haseman and Elston (1972).

In this approach, as in the affected sib pair methods discussed earlier, it is not always possible to infer IBD sharing with certainty. The Haseman-Elston method addresses this problem by regressing the squared phenotype differences $D_i = (Y_{i1} - Y_{i2})^2$ on the *expected* proportion of alleles shared IBD, $\bar{\pi} = \pi_1/2 + \pi_2$, where π_n is the probability of sharing n alleles IBD based on the available marker information (Fig. 7.10). To allow for dominance, the regression model was extended to $E(D_i) = \beta\bar{\pi}_i + \gamma(\pi_{i1} - 1/2)$. Haseman and Elston showed that $E(\beta) = 2\sigma_A^2(1 - 2\theta)^2$ and $E(\gamma) = \sigma_D^2(1 - 2\theta)^4$, where σ_A^2 and σ_D^2 are the additive and dominance components of variance defined in Chapter 5.

Recently, it has been recognized that the squared trait difference does not capture all the linkage information in the sample (Wright, 1997), and a modified version of the test has been introduced that also exploits the squared

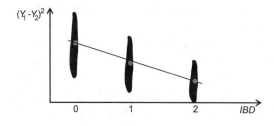

Figure 7.10 Haseman-Elston method for IBD sharing inference.

sum of trait values (Elston et al., 2000). Letting $S_i = (Y_{i1} + Y_{i2} - 2\mu)^2$ be the square of the sum of mean corrected phenotypes, and letting $C_i = (Y_{i1} - \mu)(Y_{i2} - \mu)$ be the contribution of pair i to the covariance of the traits, it is easy to show that $4C_i \equiv S_i - D_i$. Thus, any pair of these measures captures all the relevant information about their covariance structure. Now suppose that sibs' traits have a bivariate Normal distribution with mean $\mu\mathbf{1}$ and covariance matrix $\mathbf{C}$, with marginal variance σ^2 and a correlation ρ that depends on the IBD status as

$$\mathrm{E}(\rho) = \left[(\sigma^2 - \sigma_E^2) - \frac{\beta}{2}\left(\bar{\pi} - \frac{1}{2}\right) + \frac{\gamma}{2}\left(\pi_1 - \frac{1}{2}\right) \right] \Big/ \sigma^2$$

Wright (1997) and Drigalenko (1998) pointed out that D and S contribute independent information for estimating ρ. Thus, the full likelihood can be written as

$$f(\mathbf{y} \mid \mu, \sigma^2, \rho) = \frac{1}{2\pi\sqrt{|\mathbf{C}|}} \exp[-(\mathbf{Y} - \mu\mathbf{1})^T \mathbf{C}^{-1}(\mathbf{Y} - \mu\mathbf{1})/2]$$

$$= \frac{1}{2\pi\sigma^2\sqrt{1-\rho^2}} \exp\left[-\frac{D}{4\sigma^2(1-\rho)} + \frac{S}{4\sigma^2(1+\rho)} \right]$$

$$= \mathcal{N}(D \mid 0, 2\sigma^2(1-\rho)) \times \mathcal{N}(S \mid 0, 2\sigma^2(1+\rho))$$

Both components have the same dependence on ρ, but with opposite signs. Elston et al. (2000) regress C_i on $\bar{\pi}_i$ and π_{1i}. The advantage of this approach is that it can include multiple loci (as well as both additive and dominance components of each) on the right-hand side of the equation. Sham et al. (2002) instead regress π_i on D_i and S_i. This approach allows separate estimation of the effects of S and D. Palmer et al. (2000) have pointed out, however, that the use of the mean-corrected cross-products can lead to worse power than the original Haseman-Elston test with samples that are not representative of the general population. In this case, they found that the greatest power was obtained when μ was fixed at some value intermediate between the population and the ascertained sample mean. Further work on estimation of μ in ascertained samples is needed. Schaid et al. (2003) provide an excellent discussion of regression models for linkage, including their use for incorporating covariates, testing gene–environment and gene–gene interactions, and linkage heterogeneity. T. Cuenco et al. (2003) review several variants of these statistics and conclude that several alternatives that take a somewhat different weighting of S_i and D_i provide the best power. These include a statistic introduced by Sham and Purcell (2001) based on a regression of $A_i = S_i/(1+\rho)^2 - D_i/(1+\rho)^2$ on $\bar{\pi}_i$ and a variant of a score statistic introduced by Tang and Siegmund (2001) of the form

$$\frac{\sum_i A_i(\bar{\pi}_i - 1/2)}{\sqrt{1/n\left(\sum_i A_i^2\right)\sum_i(\bar{\pi} - 1/2)^2}}$$

To improve power, one could also restrict the sample to a set of sib pairs, such as "extreme-discordant sib pairs," in which one member is in top 10% of the phenotype distribution and the other in the bottom 10% (Risch and Zhang, 1995) or a combination of extreme-discordant and extreme-concordant pairs (Risch and Zhang, 1996). Conventionally, these are then analyzed treating the phenotype as dichotomous using the techniques discussed earlier for affected and discordant pairs. Szatkiewicz et al. (2003) compare the power of a broad range of statistics and conclude that treating the phenotype as continuous leads to better power and allows less-extreme pairs (which would be more frequent) to be included.

Generalized estimating equation methods

The GEE approach described in Chapters 4–6 provides a general framework that unifies all the above approaches. Essentially, one derives a model for the expected covariances between the phenotypes of each pair of relatives (of any type) as a function of their sharing of marker alleles. Because only the means and covariances are used rather than the full parametric distribution, the approach retains the robustness of relative pair methods while correctly allowing for the dependency among the multiple pairs of relatives. It also provides a natural way to incorporate covariates in either the means or covariances.

As described in earlier chapters, genetic analyses using GEE methods rely on models for the covariances in family members' phenotypes to estimate parameters of interest. For example, in Eq. (5.4), these covariances were expressed in terms of variance components and the coefficients of relationship between different relative types, while in Chapter 6, they were expressed in terms of the segregation parameters $(\mathbf{f}, q)$. In the context of linkage analysis, one might naturally express them in terms of a regression model incorporating the marker data, specifically the estimated IBD probabilities $\pi_{ijk}(x)$ at locus x between members j and k of family i, given their observed marker data.

Thomas et al. (1999) described a GEE-2 approach involving regression models for both the means and covariances of the form

$$E(Y_{ij}) = \mu_{ij} = \boldsymbol{\beta}'\mathbf{X}_{ij} + \cdots$$

$$E(C_{ijk}) = E[(Y_{ij} - \mu_{ij})(Y_{ik} - \mu_{ik})] = \alpha_0 + \alpha_1\varphi_{ijk} + \alpha_2\pi_{ijk}(x) + \cdots$$

where the parameter α_2 tests the hypothesis that these covariances depend on the IBD probabilities at location x, while allowing for residual familial aggregation (due to other genes or a shared environment) via the regression on the coefficients of relationship φ_{ijk}. Here "..." means that additional covariates or interaction effects could be added. For example, associations with environmental exposures or candidate genes could be included in the means model. Shared environmental effects could be allowed for in the covariance model by including covariates of the form $(X_{ij} - X_{ik})^2$ or $(X_{ij} - \bar{X}_i)(X_{ik} - \bar{X}_i)$. $G \times E$ interactions could be tested by including products of such covariates with π_{ijk} and $G \times G$ interactions by including products of π's at different loci. This basic approach was first developed by Amos (1994) in a variance-components context and implemented in the SOLAR package by Almasy and Blangero (1998).

So far, this method has been fully developed only for quantitative traits (Almasy and Blangero, 1998; Amos, 1994). However, Prentice and Hsu (1997) have developed GEE methods for censored survival data that may allow a generalization to linkage analysis. Rather than restrict such an analysis to affected pairs, one would use all pairs, taking as the phenotype the deviation between observed and expected incidence for each subject. Zhao et al. (1998b, 1998c, 1999) have described a unified GEE approach to linkage analysis.

Lod Score Methods

Two-point linkage

We now reformulate the direct counting methods described above in terms of maximum likelihood and show how to address some of the situations that arise when recombinants cannot be unequivocally determined. We begin with a discussion of some of the simple examples described earlier and then describe the likelihood calculations in generality.

Suppose first that all meioses can be classified as recombinants or non-recombinants. Then, as described earlier, the likelihood function is simply the binomial distribution

$$\mathcal{L}(\theta) = \binom{n}{r} \theta^r (1 - \theta)^{n-r}$$

Maximization of this function leads to the familiar estimator

$$\ln \mathcal{L}(\theta) = r \ln(\theta) + (n - r) \ln(1 - \theta)$$

$$U(\theta) = \frac{\partial \ln \mathcal{L}(\theta)}{\partial \theta} = \frac{r}{\theta} - \frac{n - r}{1 - \theta}$$

Setting $U(\theta) = 0$ and solving for θ yields $\hat{\theta} = r/n$. Its variance is given by the inverse of the Fisher information

$$
\begin{aligned}
E\left(-\frac{\partial^2 \ln \theta}{\partial \theta^2}\right)\bigg|_{\theta=\hat{\theta}} &= \frac{n}{\hat{\theta}(1-\hat{\theta})} \\
&= \frac{n}{\left(\frac{r}{n}\right)\left(\frac{s}{n}\right)} \\
&= n^3/rs
\end{aligned}
$$

Thus $\text{var}(\hat{\theta}) = rs/n^3$. It also leads to a significance test based on the likelihood ratio (LR):

$$
\begin{aligned}
G^2 &= 2\ln[\mathcal{L}(\hat{\theta})/\mathcal{L}(0.5)] \\
&= 2[r \ln(\hat{\theta}) + s \ln(1-\hat{\theta}) - n \ln(1/2)] \\
&= 2[r \ln(r/n) + s \ln(s/n) - n \ln(1/2)] \\
&= 2[r \ln r + s \ln s - n \ln(n/2)]
\end{aligned}
$$

which under the null hypothesis $H_0 : \theta = 1/2$ has a one-tailed chi-squared distribution on 1 df. The reason the test is one-tailed is that the null value $\theta = 1/2$ lies on the boundary of the parameter space (Self and Liang, 1987), as discussed in Chapter 4. The *lod score* (lods) is essentially the same test, without the 2 and using logs to the base 10:

$$
\begin{aligned}
\text{lod}(\theta) &= \log_{10}[\mathcal{L}(\hat{\theta})/\mathcal{L}(0.5)] \\
&= r \log(r) + s \log(s) - n \log(n/2) \\
&\sim G^2/4.6
\end{aligned}
$$

Typical shapes of lod score curves are shown in Figure 7.11 for several pedigrees separately, together with their sum. In pedigree A (with $r > s$), the curve is monotonically increasing; such pedigrees provide evidence against linkage. In pedigree B (with $r = 0$), the curve is monotonically decreasing; such families provide strong evidence in favor of linkage, since there are no recombinants at all. In pedigree C (with $0 < r < s$), the curve attains a maximum between $\theta = 0$ and 0.5; such families provide evidence in favor of linkage, but since there is at least one recombinant, they also provide infinite evidence against the hypothesis that $\theta = 0$, that is, the marker locus cannot be the disease susceptibility locus itself (assuming that there are no typing errors and no ambiguous trait genotypes). The aggregate lod score curve typically attains a single maximum between 0 and 0.5 and diverges to

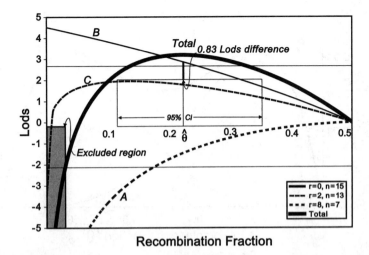

Figure 7.11 Illustrative likelihood curves for several hypothetical families (A, B, C) and the sum over all families, showing the maximum likelihood estimate and its 95% confidence limits.

minus infinity at $\theta = 0$. The highest point on the curve is the MLE of θ, and its 95% confidence limits are obtained by finding the values of θ for which $\text{lod}(\hat{\theta}) - \text{lod}(\theta) = 0.83$. (Historically, geneticists have traditionally reported *1-lod* confidence limits corresponding to the range of θ within 1 lod of the maximum; these limits actually have 96.8% coverage.)

Let us revisit Figure 7.4 in the situation where grandparents are untyped, so that we do not know whether $r = 1, s = 4$ or $r = 4, s = 1$. Since the two possibilities are equally likely, the likelihood for this pedigree would be proportional to

$$\frac{1}{2}[\theta(1 - \theta)^4 + \theta^4(1 - \theta)]$$

which is bimodal, with maxima at approximately 0.21 and 0.79 (Fig. 7.12). If the aggregate information from all families indicated that $\theta \approx 0.5$, then families such as those shown in Figure 7.4 would contribute little additional information (indeed, they would tend to increase the variance of $\hat{\theta}$). If instead the aggregate data suggested that $\theta \approx 0$, then this family would be quite informative, since the second term in its likelihood contribution would be very small in comparison with the first; that is, we would strongly favor the interpretation $r = 1, s = 4$ over $r = 4, s = 1$. However, the likelihood approach still treats this family appropriately, acknowledging the (small) possibility that $r = 4, s = 1$. To ignore this possibility and score the family as a definite $r = 1, s = 4$ would introduce a bias away from the null (unless $\theta = 0$).

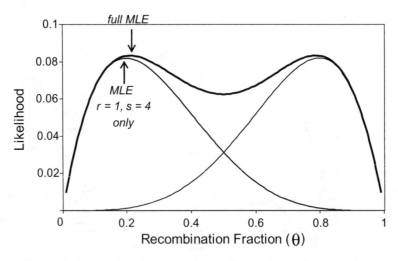

Figure 7.12 Likelihood functions for the pedigree shown in Figure 7.4 if all grandparents were untyped. The two thin lines show the likelihood contributions for the two possible phases, yielding $\hat{\theta} = 0.20$ for $r = 1, s = 4$; the heavy line shows the correct likelihood contribution summing over the two phases, yielding $\hat{\theta} = 0.21$.

Next, consider Figure 7.5, where a similar uncertainty confronts us due to not knowing whether the three unaffected sibs are carriers and, if they are carriers, their phase. Assuming that the gene is a fully penetrant recessive, the three possibilities $d \mid d$, $d \mid D$, and $D \mid d$ are equally likely. For sibs 2 and 3, these three possibilities lead to zero, one, and two recombinants (in different orders); for sib 4, the first possibility leads to zero recombinants and the other two to one recombinant each. The overall likelihood for this family is then proportional to

$$(1 - \theta)^2 \times [\theta^2 + \theta(1 - \theta) + (1 - \theta)^2]^2 \times [2\theta(1 - \theta) + (1 - \theta)^2]$$

where $(1 - \theta)^2$ represents the likelihood contribution for sib 1, $[\theta^2 + \theta(1 - \theta) + (1 - \theta)^2]^2$ for sibs 2 and 3, and $[2\theta(1 - \theta) + (1 - \theta)^2]$ for sib 4.

We now develop the likelihood approach in some generality. First, suppose that all pedigree members are typed at the marker locus and their phases can be determined. The likelihood for the pedigree is then constructed in the same way as described in Chapter 6, with only two differences: first, it is now necessary to distinguish the two phases of the heterozygote genotype $d \mid D$ and $D \mid d$; and second, the transition probabilities $\Pr(G \mid G_f, G_m)$ are now functions of the marker genotypes M and θ, obtained by multiplying the paternal and maternal transmission probabilities given in Table 7.1.

Letting $\omega = (\mathbf{f}, q)$ denote the segregation parameters (the specification of which will be discussed in the next section), we would write the *prospective* likelihood (ignoring ascertainment for the time being) as

$$
\begin{aligned}
\mathcal{L}(\theta, \omega) &= \Pr(\mathbf{Y} \mid \mathbf{M}) \\
&= \sum_{\mathbf{g}} \prod_i P_{\mathbf{f}}(Y_i \mid G = g_i) \\
&\quad \times \begin{cases} P_q(G = g_i \mid M_i) \\ P_\theta\left(G = g_i \mid M_i, g_{f_i}, g_{m_i}, M_{f_i}, M_{m_i}\right) \end{cases}
\end{aligned}
\tag{7.3}
$$

The first factor is the penetrance function, with parameters $\mathbf{f}$. For the second factor, the upper contributions (for founders) are the usual Hardy-Weinberg population genotype probabilities unless the two loci are in linkage disequilibrium (i.e., there is an association between the alleles at the two loci), while the lower contributions (for nonfounders) are the transition probabilities given in Table 7.1. Most linkage analysis assume linkage equilibrium, because one would not generally expect significant linkage disequilibrium at distances of greater than 1 cM except in a recently admixed population; we will revisit this point in Chapter 10. This term depends on a set of population allele frequencies $\mathbf{p}$ for the marker locus, which must either be estimated from the data or specified from other literature. If all founders are typed, they have no influence on the estimation of other parameters. If there are untyped founders, misspecification of these allele frequencies (or heterogeneity due to population stratification) or the presence of linkage disequilibrium can adversely affect the performance of the method. Below we discuss the possibility of simultaneously estimating these parameters with the recombination fraction (joint segregation and linkage analysis). The summation is now taken over all combinations of the *four* possible genotypes for each subject. As before, this summation can be efficiently computed using the Elston-Stewart peeling algorithm.

Now suppose that some individuals are untyped or that one cannot determine the phase of the marker genotypes. One must then expand the summation in Eq. (7.3) to include all possible combinations of *joint* marker-disease genotypes that are compatible with the observed marker data (or equivalently, over all possible combinations of joint genotypes, adding a second penetrance function to indicate whether the marker genotypes and marker phenotypes are compatible). Suppose that the marker locus has only two alleles. Then there are 16 possible joint genotypes, although only 10 of them are distinguishable (Table 7.1). For a marker locus with A alleles, a total of $A(2A + 1)$ distinguishable joint genotypes are possible for each individual. The computational demands for evaluating the summation over all possible genotypes can thus become quite burdensome, even using the Elston-Stewart algorithm.

Partly because of the computational demands of linkage analysis, one seldom attempts to maximize the likelihood over all parameters simultaneously or even to search iteratively for the maximum with respect to the parameter of primary interest, θ. Instead, the standard practice is to fix the segregation parameters ω at values determined by a previous segregation analysis and then evaluate the likelihood over a predetermined grid of values of θ. Since the likelihood is a smooth function of θ, this generally gives an adequate picture of the entire likelihood, at least as a function of θ. Conventionally, the values of $\theta = 0.4, 0.3, 0.2, 0.1, 0.05, 0.01, 0.001$, and 0 are used, so that investigators working independently can pool their results, since the overall loglikelihood for all data is simply the sum of the loglikelihoods for each study separately (Morton, 1955).

An attractive alternative to parametric linkage analysis (which requires specification of the mode of inheritance, penetrances, and allele frequencies) is based on a parameterization of the likelihood suggested by Risch (1990a). He showed that the probability that any pair shares zero, one, or two alleles IBD at the disease locus is a function of the recurrence risks λ_R defined in Chapter 5 (the ratio of the risk to a relative of type R of an affected individual divided by the marginal population risk), which can be estimated from epidemiologic studies of familial aggregation without specification of a particular genetic model. For example, for affected sib pairs, these probabilities are $z_0 = 1/4\lambda_s$, $z_1 = \lambda_o/2\lambda_s$, and $z_2 = \lambda_m/4\lambda_s$, where s indicates siblings, o offspring, and m MZ twins. Under an additive model, $\lambda_o = \lambda_s$ and $\lambda_m = 2\lambda_s - 1$, so this reduces to $\mathbf{z} = (1/4\lambda, 1/2, (2\lambda - 1)/4\lambda)$ (Hauser et al., 1996). Risch gives expressions for the probability of the observed marker data at a pair of flanking loci $\mathbf{M}$ in relation to $\mathbf{z}$ and location x of the disease gene relative to the markers. The likelihood is then written as

$$\ell(x) = \sum_{i=1}^{N} \ln \left(\frac{\Pr(\mathbf{M}_i \mid \mathbf{z}, x)}{\Pr(\mathbf{M}_i \mid \mathbf{z}_0, x)} \right)$$

where $\mathbf{z}_0 = (1/4, 1/2, 1/4)$. The approach is thus nonparametric in the sense of not requiring specification of a particular genetic model, only the observed recurrence risks, but it does provide an estimate of location as well as a lod score.

Joint segregation and linkage analysis and the Mod score

Another reason for not estimating all parameters jointly is that the heavily loaded pedigrees that are the most informative for linkage are seldom a representative sample of all families, or even of those identified through a definable population-based ascertainment scheme and extended following the rules of sequential sampling of pedigrees. Therefore, any attempt to estimate the segregation parameters from such highly selected families is likely to lead to seriously biased estimates. For this reason, these parameters are often fixed at values determined by segregation analyses of other, more representative, series of families.

Suppose, however, that we do in fact have a population-based series of families. Then it is possible to conduct *joint segregation and linkage analysis,* whereby one estimates the segregation parameters (penetrances and allele frequency) at the disease locus jointly with the recombination fraction. Although computationally more demanding than pure linkage analysis with fixed segregation parameters, this is feasible and has been implemented in such programs as the Genetic Analysis Package. Gauderman et al. (1997a) and Gauderman and Faucett (1997) compared the power of separate versus joint segregation and linkage analyses and concluded that the latter tended to be consistently more efficient. However, even though the parameters are estimated rather than fixed at some assumed value, one must still assume a particular *form* for the model, for example that there is only a single disease locus. If the basic model form is misspecified, joint segregation and linkage analysis can be as misleading as assuming an incorrect set of model parameters. And of course, for joint analysis to be possible at all, the data must be population-based in such a way that ascertainment correction is possible.

The difficulty with joint segregation and linkage analysis is ascertainment correction. As shown in Eq. (6.10), the real likelihood is

$$\Pr(\mathbf{Y} \mid \mathbf{M}, Asc) = \frac{\Pr(Asc \mid \mathbf{Y}) \Pr(\mathbf{Y} \mid \mathbf{M})}{\Pr(Asc \mid \mathbf{M})}$$

under the assumption that ascertainment depends only on the disease phenotypes, not on the marker data (a reasonable assumption, since the marker data are generally collected after ascertainment). The term $\Pr(\mathbf{Y} \mid \mathbf{M})$ is the likelihood given in Eq. (7.3), involving a summation over all possible genotype vectors (including marker genotypes for untyped individuals and phase indicators). The denominator $\Pr(Asc \mid \mathbf{M})$ additionally requires summation over all possible $\mathbf{Y}$ vectors that would have led to the ascertainment of the pedigree, a formidable calculation indeed! Instead, one could use a *retrospective* likelihood, $\Pr(\mathbf{M} \mid \mathbf{Y})$, that more accurately reflects the study design; we are given a set of already ascertained families and obtain the marker data on them. By conditioning of the observed phenotypes, we thus have automatically taken into account the way in which they were ascertained. Using

Bayes' formula, we can represent this calculation as

$$
\begin{aligned}
\mathcal{L}_R(\theta, \omega) = P_{\theta,\omega}(\mathbf{M} \mid \mathbf{Y}) &= \frac{P_{\theta,\omega}(\mathbf{Y} \mid \mathbf{M}) P_{\mathbf{p}}(\mathbf{M})}{P_\omega(\mathbf{Y})} \\
&= \frac{P_{\mathbf{p}}(\mathbf{M}) \sum_{\mathbf{G}} P_{\mathbf{f}}(\mathbf{Y} \mid \mathbf{G}) P_{q,\theta}(\mathbf{G} \mid \mathbf{M})}{\sum_{\mathbf{G}} P_{\mathbf{f}}(\mathbf{Y} \mid \mathbf{G}) P_q(\mathbf{G})}
\end{aligned}
\tag{7.4}
$$

where the factor $P_{\theta,\omega}(\mathbf{Y} \mid \mathbf{M})$ in the numerator is the same as in Eq. (7.3). Note also that the denominator does not depend on θ.

Equation (7.3) (suitably adjusted for ascertainment) and Eq. (7.4) are functions of both θ and ω, and thus either could be used to estimate both sets of parameters. In linkage analysis, θ is the parameter of primary interest and ω is viewed as a vector of *nuisance parameters*. The standard method for constructing likelihood ratio tests in the presence of nuisance parameters is to maximize the likelihood separately under the null and alternative hypotheses (Rao, 1973). Let $(\hat{\theta}, \hat{\omega})$ denote the global MLE and let $(\theta_0, \tilde{\omega})$ be the MLE restricted to the null hypothesis value of the parameter of interest, θ_0. Then the likelihood ratio test

$$
G^2 = 2 \ln \frac{\mathcal{L}(\hat{\theta}, \hat{\omega})}{\mathcal{L}(\theta_0, \tilde{\omega})}
\tag{7.5}
$$

asymptotically has a chi-square distribution with degrees of freedom equal to the dimensionality of θ (assuming that the number of nuisance parameters remains fixed as the sample size increases). To avoid having to maximize the likelihood twice, it is tempting to consider solving only for $\hat{\omega}$ or $\tilde{\omega}$. Now it is certainly true that $\mathcal{L}(\theta_0, \tilde{\omega}) > \mathcal{L}(\theta_0, \hat{\omega})$ and also that $\mathcal{L}(\hat{\theta}, \hat{\omega}) > \mathcal{L}(\hat{\theta}, \tilde{\omega})$. Hence, using $\tilde{\omega}$ in both numerator and denominator would understate the true likelihood ratio, while using $\hat{\omega}$ in both places would overstate it. Of course, it is $\tilde{\omega}$ that is obtained by a simple segregation analysis, so the standard procedure of treating estimates from a prior segregation analysis would appear to be somewhat conservative, as confirmed by the simulation studies of Gauderman and Faucett (1997).

An alternative approach does neither of these, but instead maximizes the likelihood *ratio* itself:

$$
MODS(\theta) = \max_\omega \frac{\mathcal{L}(\theta, \omega)}{\mathcal{L}(\theta_0, \omega)} = \max_\omega \frac{P_{\theta,\omega}(\mathbf{Y} \mid \mathbf{M})}{P_\omega(\mathbf{Y})} = \max_\omega \frac{P_{\theta,\omega}(\mathbf{M} \mid \mathbf{Y})}{P(\mathbf{M})}
\tag{7.6}
$$

By maximizing over ω, the mod score depends only on θ. It is not immediately obvious what the statistical properties of the mod score are as a significance test of $H_0 : \theta = \theta_0$ or as an estimator of either θ or ω. This question is dealt with in some depth by Hodge and Elston (1994), who show that the value of θ that maximizes the mod score provides a consistent estimator of both θ and ω (provided that the genetic model for the disease is correctly specified and ascertainment depends only on the trait values) and furthermore that the estimator of θ is fully efficient, although the estimator of ω is not necessarily fully efficient. In particular, if the null hypothesis $\theta = \theta_0$ is true, the mod score provides no information about ω. For this reason, the significance test of H_0 is also valid (i.e., has the correct test size), although it may be somewhat less powerful than the likelihood ratio test given in Eq. (7.5) (Williamson and Amos, 1990). This is a powerful result, because it provides a means of estimating penetrance and allele frequencies even from families that were not ascertained in any systematic manner, and it also provides valid tests and estimators of θ even when the genetic model is unknown. Kraft and Thomas (2000) provide further discussion of retrospective and prospective likelihoods in the context of association studies (see Chapter 11).

Figure 7.13 illustrates the application of the mod score approach to the Breast Cancer Linkage Consortium data to estimate penetrance in these heavily loaded pedigrees (Easton et al., 1993). Even though these families were selected on the basis of having a large number of cases, the retrospective likelihood should provide a consistent estimator of these penetrance functions, assuming that these penetrances are homogeneous across the population and the families were not selected on the basis of marker information. The former assumption could be violated if other genes or environmental

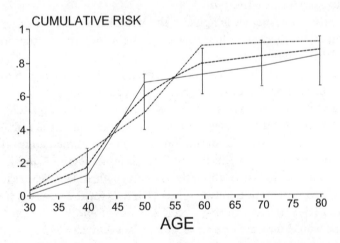

Figure 7.13 Estimates of penetrance from the Breast Cancer Linkage Consortium families using the mod score approach. (From Easton et al., 1993)

factors contributed to the breast cancer risk and aggregate within families, as seems likely; in that case, these families would tend to be at higher risk than the general population, whatever their *BRCA1* genotypes, and this would lead to some overestimation of the penetrance of this gene in the general population, although it would still be an appropriate estimate for similar high-risk families. The latter assumption could be violated if the analysis were restricted to the linked families in an attempt to reduce the impact of genetic heterogeneity, as this would be a form of selection on the basis of marker information; Siegmund et al. (1999a) have shown that this can also yield an overestimation of penetrance. A better approach would be to explictly include an unlinked gene in the analysis, as done by Antoniou et al. (2000) and Ford et al. (1998). In a subsequent analysis (not shown), Easton et al. (1995) found that an allelic heterogeneity model gave a much better fit to the data by allowing for two possible classes of mutation, one of which conferred a high risk of breast cancer (a cumulative risk to age 60 of 62%) and a relatively low risk of ovarian cancer (11%), the other conferring a much lower risk of breast cancer (39%) but a high risk of ovarian cancer (42%). Subsequently, they speculated that these differences might be correlated with the location of the mutation within the gene.

Multipoint linkage and ordering loci

So far, we have discussed linkage to a single marker locus (*two-point linkage*). Greater power can be obtained using *multipoint linkage,* in which two or more marker loci are used simultaneously. The primary aim of such analyses is to identify *flanking markers,* which are on opposite sides of the disease locus and thus help localize the gene.

Suppose, first, that we are given a set of marker loci whose order has not yet been established. The first task might be to determine the most likely order of these markers. Perhaps the simplest approach to this problem is first to estimate $\hat{\theta}_{ij}$ and $\mathrm{lod}(\hat{\theta}_{ij})$ for all pairs of loci i and j by a series of two-point linkage analyses and then to determine the order that leads to the highest overall likelihood (see the example in Khoury et al., 1993, pp. 293–294).

A more powerful approach is to analyze all the markers simultaneously, considering each possible ordering one at a time, and then adopt the order that maximizes the overall likelihood. For example, Figure 7.14 illustrates a pedigree that is informative about the ordering of three loci. We see that there is a single recombination between loci C and D for the paternal haplotype of subject III-2. If the ordering were CDE (panel A), then this individual's genotype would indicate one CD recombinant and zero DE recombinants. The second ordering, CED (panel B), would also lead to a single recombinant, CE, and is therefore just as likely as the first. On the other hand, if the

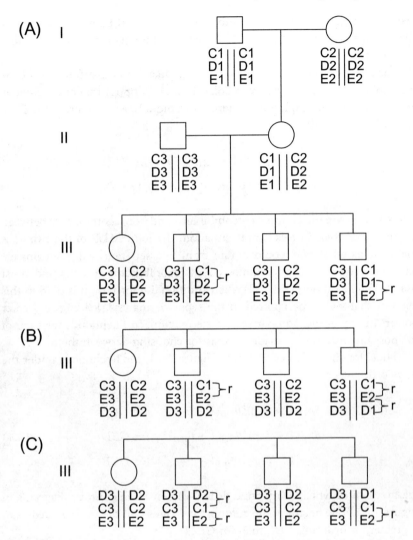

Figure 7.14 Hypothetical pedigree illustrating three-point linkage under three possible orderings of the loci. (Adapted from Khoury et al., 1993)

ordering were *DCE* (panel C), there would have to be two recombinants, one *DC* and one *CE*. Thus, for this subject, the ordering *DCE* appears to be less likely than the other two.

Now consider subject III-4, who has haplotype *C1 D1 E2*. That would be a double recombinant under ordering *CED* but only one under the other two orderings. Thus, across all subjects, there would be a total of two recombinants for ordering CDE and three recombinants for both of the other two orderings.

For any given ordering (say, CDE), the likelihood is a function of the recombination fractions between adjacent loci. Suppose that one were able to determine all the haplotype assignments uniquely, as in Figure 7.14. Then the likelihood would be

$$\mathcal{L}(\theta_{CD}, \theta_{DE}) \propto (\theta_{CD})^{r_{CD}}(1 - \theta_{CD})^{s_{CD}} \times (\theta_{DE})^{r_{DE}}(1 - \theta_{DE})^{s_{DE}}$$

$$\propto (\theta_{CD})^{1}(1 - \theta_{CD})^{3} \times (\theta_{DE})^{1}(1 - \theta_{DE})^{3}$$

where r and s are the counts of recombinants and nonrecombinants between the indicated loci. In this simple situation, the joint MLE of the two θs is the same as what one would obtain from two separate two-point linkage analyses. However, if one cannot count recombinants directly and must use the full likelihood (Eq. 7.3), then additional information is used in this analysis that would be ignored in the separate analysis, leading to greater power. In any event, comparison of the maximized likelihoods for each of the possible orderings provides a basis for choosing between them.

Thus, for the pedigree shown in Figure 7.14, the likelihoods under the three orderings are

$$\theta_{CD}(1 - \theta_{CD})^{3}\theta_{DE}(1 - \theta_{DE})^{3} \quad \text{for } CDE$$

$$\theta_{CE}^{2}(1 - \theta_{CE})^{2}\theta_{ED}(1 - \theta_{ED})^{3} \quad \text{for } CED \qquad (7.7)$$

$$\theta_{DC}(1 - \theta_{DC})^{3}\theta_{CE}^{2}(1 - \theta_{CE})^{2} \quad \text{for } DCE$$

the first two of which are plotted as two-dimensional contour diagrams in Figure 7.15. The height of the contours indicates that the overall maximum is greater for ordering CDE than for CED.

Now suppose that we wish to determine the location of an unknown disease gene G relative to a set of markers (say C, D, E) whose ordering and recombination fractions have already been established. We now consider each possible placement of the disease locus relative to the markers ($GCDE$, $CGDE$, $CDGE$, $CDEG$) and compute the likelihood as a function of the location x_D relative to the flanking markers, holding the marker locations fixed. For example, suppose that we were considering the order CDE in the above example. Then the likelihood would be treated as a function of x in $\mathcal{L}[\theta_{CD}(x), \theta_{DE}(x)]$ where, under the Haldane map function,

$$\theta_{CD}(x) = \left(1 - e^{-2|x_C - x|}\right)/2$$

$$\theta_{DE}(x) = \left(1 - e^{-2|x - x_E|}\right)/2$$

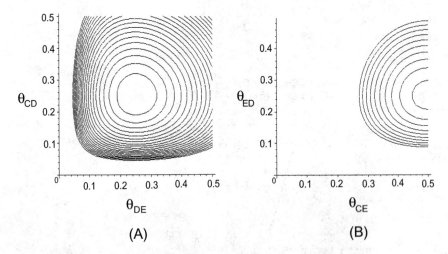

(A)

(B)

Figure 7.15 Three-point linkage. Likelihoods for the pedigree 7.15 under the orderings (A) CDE and (B) CED. The corresponding χ^2 tests for the natural log of these functions are (A) $\chi^2 = 10.12$ and (B) $\chi^2 = 7.16$, where $\theta = 0.5$.

Substituting these in the Eq. (7.7) and normalizing by dividing by the likelihood for D being completely unlinked to C and E $(\theta_{CE}^2 (1 - \theta_{CE})^2 0.5^4)$ produces the one-dimensional plot shown in Figure 7.16, where x_C is arbitrarily located at $x = 0$ and locus E is assumed to be located 20 cM away (corresponding to $\theta_{CE} = 0.165$). This figure shows that the D locus is more likely located between C and E than on either side.

Figure 7.17 illustrates the map function estimated for the *BRCA1* gene relative to five markers on chromosome 17q. The lod scores do not diverge to zero at either marker, indicating the absence of any unequivocal recombinants in this region. If extended further, the lod score curves eventually become negative.

Figure 7.16 Multipoint linkage of the pedigree shown in Figure 7.15, treating the location of marker D as unknown against a known map of loci C and E spaced $\theta = 20$ cM apart.

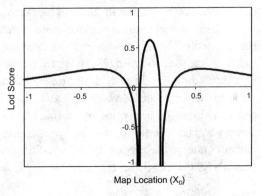

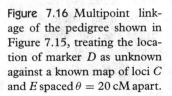

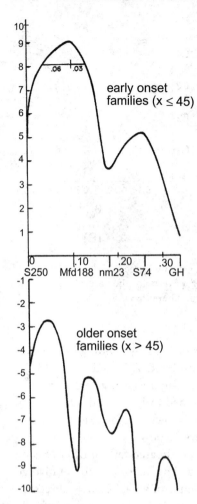

Figure 7.17 Multipoint analysis of linkage between breast and ovarian cancer and the region of chromosome 17q12-q23 between D17S250 and GH. The top curve represents the scores for the seven families in which average age at breast cancer diagnosis is ≤45 years; the lower curve represents lod scores for the 16 families in which average age at breast cancer diagnosis is >45 years. (Reproduced with permission from Hall et al., 1992)

Multipoint mapping is computationally intensive and is currently feasible only for a small number of markers in simple pedigrees of unlimited size or for an arbitrarily large number of markers in simple pedigrees of modest size. These two situations require quite different algorithms: the former is based on the Elston-Stewart peeling described in Chapter 6, extended to multiple loci following Eq. (7.3), where **g** now represents a multilocus genotype, including the disease locus and all the marker loci; the latter is based on a *Hidden Markov Models* approach (Lander and Green, 1987), which proceeds locus by locus, incorporating all the pedigree information simultaneously, conditional on the IBD probabilities for the previous locus. The current state of the art for the Elston-Stewart approach is implemented in the LINKAGE (Lathrop et al., 1984, 1986) and VITESSE (O'Connell and

Weeks, 1995) programs. The current state-of-the-art for the Hidden Markov Models approach is implemented in the MAPMAKER/SIBS (Kruglyak and Lander, 1995) and GENEHUNTER (Kruglyak et al., 1996) programs. The latter supports both parametric and nonparametric approaches to linkage analysis. The following subsection provides a technical explanation of the Lander-Green approach, which the nonmathematical reader can skip. The important point is that, even though the two algorithms look quite different, they are closely related, doing essentially the same calculation—in the Elston-Stewart algorithm, one individual at a time for all loci at once; in the Lander-Green algorithm, one locus at a time for all individuals at once.

The Lander-Green Hidden Markov Models algorithm. The Lander-Green algorithm relies on the fundamental principle that loci are conditionally independent of each other, given the IBD status of their immediately flanking loci. Likewise, the posterior probability of the IBD status at any given locus depends only on the available marker information at that locus and is independent of the marker information at other loci, conditional on the IBD status of the flanking loci. Thus, one can represent the joint probability of the IBD status of all loci simply by multiplying the conditional probabilities of each locus given the preceding one and the conditional probabilities of IBD status at each locus given the available marker information at that locus. On page 182, we showed that for a single marker locus A and a disease locus B at a recombination fraction of θ, one could represent the IBD probabilities at B given the available marker information at A as $\pi_B = \mathbf{Q}_A \mathbf{T}_{AB}$. Now suppose that there was also another marker, C, on the other side of B. Then the natural extension of this approach would be $\pi_B = \mathbf{Q}_A \mathbf{T}_{AB} \mathbf{T}_{BC} \mathbf{Q}_C$. (There is no need for a term $\mathbf{Q}_B$ because the alleles at the disease locus B are not observed.) Continuing in this way, the general calculation of the IBD probability at an arbitrary location x along a chromosome as a function of a string of marker data at L loci, with the disease locus between markers $\ell - 1$ and ℓ, can be described as

$$\pi_x = \Pr(\mathbf{Z}_x \mid \mathbf{M}, x) = \mathbf{1}\mathbf{Q}_{1,\ell-1}\mathbf{T}_{\ell-1,x}\mathbf{T}_{x,\ell}\mathbf{Q}_{\ell,L}\mathbf{1}$$
$$\text{where } \mathbf{Q}_{\ell,m} = \mathbf{Q}_\ell \mathbf{T}_{\ell,\ell+1}\mathbf{Q}_{\ell+1}\cdots\mathbf{Q}_{m-1}\mathbf{T}_{m-1,m}\mathbf{Q}_m$$

(7.8)

Here $\mathbf{Q}_{\ell,m}$ represents the result of all these matrix multiplications between loci ℓ and m inclusive—for example, all those from the first marker to the immediately flanking marker on the left and from the immediately flanking marker on the right to the last marker (Fig. 7.18).

As developed on page 182, the calculation of $\mathbf{Q}$ and $\mathbf{T}$ were restricted to a single sib pair, but there is nothing in principle precluding extension of

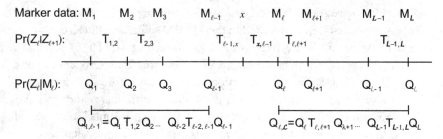

Figure 7.18 Schematic representation of the Lander-Green hidden Markov models approach to calculation of multipoint IBD probabilities.

these calculations to larger pedigrees. All that is required is to extend the definition of the IBD status indicator variable Z to a vector $\mathbf{Z}$ of possible IBD configurations for all the nonfounders, as in the examples of sibships of size three and four described earlier. The corresponding IBD probabilities are denoted $\Pi(\mathbf{Z}_x)$. The calculations follow the same principles as those described earlier, now involving sums over all possible combinations of marker alleles for all untyped founders and over all possible segregation indicators for all nonfounders. In practice, these calculations can become very intensive, even for moderate-sized pedigrees. The practical limitation for the current incarnation of GENEHUNTER is that $2N - F$ must be <16, where N is the number of nonfounders and F is the number of founders.

The vector of IBD configuration probabilities $\Pi(\mathbf{Z}_x)$ is computed using only the marker information, but none of the phenotype information for the disease. These probabilities can then be used in any of the parametric or nonparametric linkage analysis methods described above. For example, in the affected pair method, one could compute a score $S_{\text{pairs}}(\mathbf{Z}_x)$ for each possible IBD configuration vector $\mathbf{Z}_x$ as the number of pairs of alleles from distinct affected pedigree members that are IBD. This score is averaged over all possible inheritance vectors weighted by the probabilities $\Pi(\mathbf{Z}_x)$. It is then normalized by subtracting its mean and dividing by its standard deviation, computed under the null hypothesis of a uniform distribution of inheritance vectors. These normalized scores Z_i for each pedigree are finally combined to produce the NPL$_{\text{pairs}}$ score $\sum_{i=1}^{N} Z_i/\sqrt{N}$ (Kruglyak et al., 1996). (Alternatively, any set of weights such that their sum of squares add to 1 could be used; for further discussion, see Kong and Cox, 1997.) Since each of the Z_i has been standardized to unit variance, the NPL score also has zero mean and unit variance under the null hypothesis of no linkage. A somewhat more complicated scoring function can be used to exploit larger sets of affected relatives within each pedigree rather than just pairs (Whittemore and Halpern, 1994). The resulting statistic has been dubbed NPL$_{\text{all}}$ (Kruglyak et al., 1996). Sengul et al. (2001) compared five different statistics and concluded that the NPL_{all} generally performed quite well, although not necessarily the best in all situations examined. Kruglyak et al. (1995) described yet another application of the approach for homozygosity mapping.

For parametric analysis, we note that the likelihood can be represented in terms of the location x and the segregation parameters $\omega = (\mathbf{f}, q)$ as

$$\mathcal{L}(x, \omega) = \sum_{\mathbf{g}} \Pr(\mathbf{Y} \mid \mathbf{G}_x = \mathbf{g}) \Pr(\mathbf{G}_x = \mathbf{g} \mid \mathbf{M})$$

$$= \sum_{\mathbf{z}} \Pr(\mathbf{Y} \mid \mathbf{Z}_x = \mathbf{z}; \omega) \Pi(\mathbf{Z}_x = \mathbf{z})$$

where

$$\Pr(\mathbf{Y} \mid \mathbf{Z}_x = \mathbf{z}; \omega) = \sum_{\mathbf{a}} \sum_{\mathbf{s} \mid \mathbf{z}} \Pr(\mathbf{Y} \mid \mathbf{G}(\mathbf{s}, \mathbf{a}); \mathbf{f}) \Pr(\mathbf{a}; q) \qquad (7.9)$$

and $\mathbf{G}(\mathbf{s}, \mathbf{a})$ denotes the vector of genotypes corresponding to a particular configuration of founder alleles $\mathbf{a}$ and segregation indicators $\mathbf{s}$. By this formulation of the likelihood, all the parametric assumptions about penetrance and allele frequency are subsumed in the vector of probabilities $\Pr(\mathbf{Y} \mid \mathbf{Z}_x = \mathbf{z})$, which can then be combined with the vector of IBD probabilities $\Pi(\mathbf{z}_x)$ computed once only from the marker data.

Genome-wide scans

Exclusion mapping. The process of gene mapping can be thought of as a sequential trial with well-defined stopping rules chosen to minimize the risk of false positive and false negative conclusions. Having demonstrated by segregation analysis that there appears to be a major gene for a particular disease, one then begins to search for it, initially looking over the entire genome. As evidence begins to accumulate, one narrows down the search by excluding certain regions with highly negative lods as unlikely to include any gene with greater than some specified minimum heritability of interest. (Of course, one can never reject the possibility that there might be a gene at any given location with an arbitrarily small effect; Kruglyak and Lander [1995] illustrate how GENEHUNTER can be used to compute exclusion lod scores for various specifications of effect size λ_s.) Further searching in these regions would be a waste of resources (unless, of course, the genetic model was misspecified, in which case one could obtain spurious evidence against linkage even if a major gene were located in the region). Naturally, one focuses one's efforts in regions that previous studies have suggested as promising (positive lods). Once the accumulated evidence becomes positive enough, one wishes to claim a "significant" result, but not until one has effectively ruled out the possibility of chance, considering the large number of tests being considered. Having established a significant linkage, one can again stop testing that marker, focusing one's energy instead on searching for even more closely linked markers in the same region, hoping to find additional recombinants that can narrow down the excluded region even further.

Operationally, this process is reflected in the historical guidelines that a lods of −2 is considered convincing evidence against linkage and +3 (corresponding to a conventional p-value of 0.0001 for a single one-tailed test) as convincing evidence in favor of linkage (Fig. 7.19). (For an X-linked locus, a threshold of +2 is used instead.) These numbers were derived from the theory of sequential analysis, using the argument about the prior probability of linkage described below (Morton, 1955). In particular, Morton showed that these choices lead to a power of 99% and a 5% false positive rate. These guidelines were originally derived for two-point linkage for a single marker at a fixed recombination fraction. With modern multipoint methods, dense marker maps, and the possibility of complex diseases with multiple genes

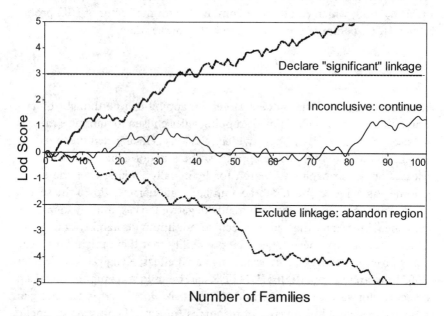

Number of Families

Figure 7.19 Hypothetical realizations of the accumulation of lod scores over time, assuming true linkage (upper curve), a gene of some given magnitude not linked to the marker (bottom curve), or no gene (middle curve). The conventional stopping rules of Morton (1955) are shown as horizontal dotted lines.

involved, more restrictive criteria are needed. Lander and Kruglyak (1995) have proposed a guideline of a lods of 3.3 or for the nonparametric statistic NPL of 3.6. Witte et al. (1996), Curtis (1996), and the rejoinder following it discuss these criteria further. Hauser et al. (1996) have provided some guidelines for conducting genome scans using Risch's (1990a) mode-of-inheritance-free method of affected sib pair analysis described above. They recommend that one exclude from further consideration any region with lod scores less that -2 at the smallest effect of interest and investigate further any region with maximum lod scores greater than 1; such investigation could include typing other families, other members of existing families, additional markers, or additional analyses.

If one were sure that there was a major gene to be found, then in principle, as some regions become excluded, the threshold for excluding other regions should rise, since the gene one is looking for must be located somewhere else (Edwards, 1987). For complex diseases, exclusion mapping is more difficult because a region may contain a gene that is segregating only in a subset of families, so that the overall lod score at a linked marker is negative even though some families contribute positive lods. Ott (1999, §12.4) suggests that only regions with an overall lod score of less than -2 and a heterogeneity lods of less than $+2$ (with the proportion linked maximized separately at each location) be excluded.

Prior probability of linkage. Smith (1959) argued that since there are 22 autosomes, the prior probability that any two randomly chosen loci would be found on the same chromosome is about $1/22$ or about 0.05. Since the chromosomes are not the same size, this probability is actually a bit larger, 0.054 (Renwick, 1971). Given that the two loci are on the same chromosome, Smith assumed a uniform distribution for θ between 0 and 0.5. This was done purely for mathematical convenience and is unlikely to be realistic, since even at moderate distances recombination is likely to be essentially free. Nevertheless, given such assumptions, one can then compute the posterior distribution of θ given a set of data, as summarized in the likelihood function. Ott (1999, §4.2) illustrates the calculations with an example in which a single observed recombinant out of 12 informative meioses (leading to a maximum lod score of 2.11, corresponding to an LR of 128.5 or $p = 0.002$) translates into a posterior probability that $\theta < 0.5$ of only 72%. A lods of about 3 would be required to produce a posterior probability of linkage of at least 95%.

Sequential designs for marker testing. Considering the size of the human genome, finding an unknown disease gene is like finding a needle in a haystack! Since each chromosome is effectively divided into many independent linkage groups, a very large number of markers needs to be tested to have any hope of detecting linkage, unless one is very lucky. Some sort of sequential strategy therefore seems appropriate. Elston et al. (1996) have suggested a two-pass strategy in which one first tests the most widely spaced array of markers that would span the entire genome (i.e., offer reasonable power for detecting linkage for any locus between adjacent markers). A very liberal significance level (e.g., $p < 0.20$) could be used to identify candidate regions at this stage, since any "hits" would be confirmed by further testing. Around each hit, one would then screen a more finely spaced array of markers at a more conservative significance level, possibly continuing on to even a third level of testing. Optimal selection of marker spacing and significance levels to maximize the power of the design, subject to a constraint on the total cost and the overall Type I error rate, has been described and is implemented for two-point linkage in affected sib pair designs in the S.A.G.E. procedure DESPAIR. Table 7.9 provides a typical comparison; for this combination of parameters, the optimal design turns out to require 164 sib pairs with two intermediate markers for each marker that achieves an initial significance level of $\alpha = 0.076$. This is about half the sample size and half the cost of a single-stage design. Use of parametric and/or multipoint methods and larger pedigrees would doubtless substantially improve power overall, but DESPAIR might still provide some reasonable guidance about marker spacing and other design choices. Korczak et al. (1995), Nemesure et al. (1995), and Brown et al. (1994) describe other variants of this general approach for sib pairs, nuclear families, and extended pedigrees (using the affected-pedigree-member method), respectively.

The approaches described above use the entire sample at each stage of the process in what has been called a *grid tightening* strategy. An alternative strategy is to use only a portion of the sample in the initial screen, following up promising results using the entire sample. Such an approach was first suggested for association studies (Sham, 1994; Sobell et al., 1993) and investigated for affected sib pair analysis by Holmans and Craddock (1997).

Table 7.9 Illustrative Results from the DESPAIR Program in the S.A.G.E. Package

Number of Intermediate Markers (k)	Number of Sib Pairs (n)	Initial Significance Level (α)	Total Cost $(\times 1000)$
4	155	0.085	142
3	160	0.080	135
2	164	0.076	128
1	193	0.052	138
0	370	0.005	250

Note: These results assume a final significance level $\alpha = 0.0001$, power $1 - \beta = 80\%$, $\lambda_s = 5$, heterogeneity $h = 40\%$, marker heterozygosity $f = 75\%$, an initial 20 cM panel (166 markers), a ratio of subject to genotype costs $R = 172$, and a Kosambi map function.

This strategy has the advantage of reducing the genotyping costs for the large number of markers required in the first stage while exploiting power of the full sample at the later stage(s). Combining the two approaches, Holmans and Craddock concluded that the optimal strategy entailed testing half of the sample with a coarse grid of markers at the first stage and not typing parents until the second stage.

Genetic heterogeneity

For reasons that are not well understood, it has been observed that the recombination rate differs for mothers and fathers and that the ratio θ_f/θ_m varies from region to region of the genome. There is also some indication that θ may vary by age of the parents. Several linkage programs allow one to evaluate the likelihood over a two-dimensional grid of values of (θ_f, θ_m). The likelihood ratio test relative to $\theta_f = \theta_m = 0.5$ has a chi-square distribution on 2 df, which can be partitioned into two 1 df tests, the standard test of $\bar{\theta} = 0.5$ and the test of homogeneity $\theta_f = \theta_m$. (See Ott, 1999, §9.1–9.2, for further details.)

Another form of heterogeneity refers to variation in recombination rates between families (beyond what would be expected by chance). There are two important models that have been used to test for this form of heterogeneity.

In the first case, we assume that all families are linked but that there may be variation between them in their average recombination fractions (perhaps due to age or other unknown factors). Thus, we wish to test the null hypothesis that $\theta_i \equiv \bar{\theta}$ for all families $i = 1, \ldots, I$. The two tests that are most commonly used to test this hypothesis are the M-test (Morton, 1956) and the B-test (Risch, 1988). The M-test is a straightforward LR test for homogeneity, comparing the likelihoods for the common θ model against the sum of likelihoods for each family computed separately. This test has asymptotically a chi-square distribution on $I-1$ df; here *asymptotically* refers to the number of meioses per family becoming large (but not as the number of families becomes large, keeping the number of meioses per family fixed). The B-test assumes that the θ_i have a Beta distribution and tests the variance of that distribution against 0 as a chi square on 1 df. This test is more powerful, provided that the assumed distribution is correct. Details are provided in Ott (1999, §10.3).

The second form of heterogeneity arises when some families are linked and some are not, the linked families being assumed to have a common value of θ. Such a model arises naturally if there could be other genes that produce the same phenotype, so that some families might be segregating the particular gene linked to the marker under study (all with essentially the same recombination fraction), while other families' hereditary disease is due to other unlinked genes. Letting α denote the proportion of families that are linked, the likelihood contribution for each family is then a mixture of contributions under both 0.5 and θ,

$$\mathcal{L}_i(\alpha, \theta) = \alpha \mathcal{L}_i(\theta) + (1 - \alpha)\mathcal{L}_i(0.5)$$

The *Admixture* or *A*-test (Hodge et al., 1983; Ott, 1983) is simply the LR test comparing the joint MLE to the restricted MLE at $\alpha = 1, \tilde{\theta}$ (i.e., assuming that all families are linked), tested as a one-tailed chi square on 1 *df*. (The reason the test is one-tailed is again that $H_0 : \alpha = 1$ lies on the boundary of the parameter space, larger values being meaningless [Self and Liang, 1987].) The A-test can also be used as a test of linkage in the presence of homogeneity, the only difference being that the null hypothesis is now $\theta = 0.5$ rather than $\alpha = 1, \tilde{\theta}$ (note that at $\theta = 0.5$ the likelihood is independent of α). The likelihood ratio now has a complex distribution as a mixture of chi squares. Faraway (1993, 1994) has shown that this distribution is reasonably approximated as half the probability of the maximum of two independent 1 *df* chi squares. Alternatively, the null distribution can be generated by a randomization test.

For affected sib pairs, it is not possible to test for heterogeneity, because a mixture distribution with proportion α having parameter (π_0, π_1, π_2) and proportion $1 - \alpha$ having parameter $(1/4, 1/2, 1/4)$ cannot be distinguished from a homogeneous trinomial distribution with parameter $(\bar{\pi}_0, \bar{\pi}_1, \bar{\pi}_2)$. However, in principle, it would be possible given sibships with multiple affected members, since the likelihood could then be expressed in terms of the Π_is for each sibship i's IBD configurations, as discussed on page 185:

$$\mathcal{L}(\alpha, \pi_2) = \prod_i \left(\alpha \Pi_i(\pi_2) + (1 - \alpha)\Pi_i\left(\frac{1}{4}\right) \right)$$

In practice, however, the parameters α and π in this likelihood appear to be very highly correlated, at least for sibships with only three or four affecteds, so that the test has very little power. This simply reflects the fact that tests of linkage heterogeneity generally require large pedigrees.

In the first report of the linkage of breast cancer to chromosome 17q, Hall et al. (1990) noted the much stronger evidence of linkage in families with younger average ages of diagnosis. Figure 7.20 shows the cumulative lod scores as a function of average age, with a peak if one includes only ages up to 47 and increasing evidence against linkage at older ages.

The Breast Cancer Linkage Consortium (Easton et al., 1993) used the *A*-test to examine heterogeneity for breast and ovarian cancer. Figure 7.21 shows the likelihood contours for breast-ovarian and pure breast cancer

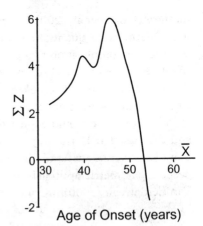

Figure 7.20 Linkage of D17S74 to breast cancer in families based on the autosomal dominant model. Cumulative lod scores ($\sum Z$) are shown for all families for which the mean age of breast cancer diagnosis (M) is less than or equal to the age represented on the x-axis. (Reproduced with permission from Hall et al., 1990)

families as a function of the location of *BRCA1*, x, and the proportion of linked families α. The MLE of α was 1.0 (95% CI 0.72–1) for families with at least one ovarian cancer but only 0.45 (95% CI 0.25–0.70) for breast cancer-only families. Among the latter group, $\hat{\alpha} = 0.67$ for those with an average age at diagnosis under 45 and 0.72 for those with at least five cases.

Special circumstances. Some alterations of these procedures may be required in some situations. For example, we discuss the phenomenon of imprinting in Chapter 12. Strauch et al. (2000) have described an extension of parametric and nonparametric linkage analysis methods to allow for parent-of-origin effects by allowing for separate penetrances for heterozygotes, depending on whether the mutant allele came from the father or the

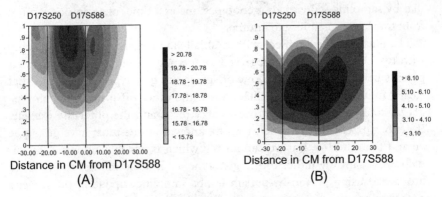

Figure 7.21 Contour plot showing the heterogeneity lod scores by location and proportion of linked families, α, for the 57 breast-ovary families (A) and the 153 breast-only families (B) from the Breast Cancer Linkage Consortium. (Reproduced with permission from Easton et al., 1993)

mother. Hanson et al. (2001) discuss similar extensions of variance components methods for quantitative traits.

Another complication that can arise involves linkage to the pseudoautosomal region of the sex chromosomes (Chapter 2). Because males are more likely to receive the allele linked to the Y chromosome from their fathers, whereas females are more likely to receive the allele linked to the father's X chromosome, one would expect increased IBD sharing by same-sex pairs and decreased IBD sharing by opposite-sex pairs, regardless of whether there is a disease susceptibility allele in the region at all. Ott (1986) proposed a parametric approach to deal with this problem, while Dupuis and Van Eerdewegh (2000) provided a nonparametric multipoint approach.

Gibbs sampling methods

The computational burden in likelihood methods is considerably larger for linkage analysis than for segregation analysis and grows rapidly with the number of alleles, the number of loci, and pedigree size and complexity (especially if many individuals are untyped). Even with a single locus, seldom is joint segregation and linkage analysis feasible. Gibbs sampling, as described in Chapters 4, 5, and 6, offers a potentially attractive solution. For markers with only two alleles, one can proceed as described earlier, now sampling joint marker-disease genotypes for each individual, conditional on their phenotypes and the current assignment of joint genotypes for their immediate relatives (Thomas and Cortessis, 1992). However, polymorphic markers involve additional complications not present in segregation analysis. It is quite possible that the set of marker genotypes that are compatible with the measured marker phenotypes will be subdivided into disjoint sets (*islands*), such that by sampling individuals' genotypes one at a time, one can never move from one legal possibility to another.

To illustrate the problem with multiallelic markers, consider a sibship with two offspring, having observed genotypes *ab* and *cc*, and with their parents being untyped. Since one offspring has genotype *cc*, we know that each parent must carry a *c* allele. Since the other offspring has genotype *ab*, we know that one parent must carry the *a* and the other the *b* allele. If neither parent is typed, we therefore know that one must have genotype *ac* and the other *bc*, but we cannot tell which is which. Suppose that initially we assign the father to the genotype *ac* and the mother to *bc*. If we proceeded using person-by-person Gibbs sampling, updating the father's genotype conditional on the mother's and offsprings' genotypes, the only possible assignment would be *ac*, and likewise the only possible assignment for the mother would be *bc* (conditional on the father). Hence, even in an infinite number of iterations of this process, one could never get to the alternative assignment with their genotypes switched. In this simple case, one could update the pair of genotypes jointly (here, conditional only on their offspring's genotypes), but more complex examples can easily be constructed in which such joint updating schemes would fail.

Several solutions to this problem have been suggested. One approach is to update the entire vector of genotypes for each pedigree simultaneously, but this is possible only if the pedigree structure is peelable so that one can compute the full conditional distribution of joint genotypes given phenotypes and marker data to sample from. If it is possible, however, this would allow more complicated models, such as multipoint linkage, multilocus models, models with polygenic terms, or joint segregation and linkage analysis models, to be fitted. For multipoint linkage, this strategy of updating each pedigree's genotypes at a single locus at a time, conditional on the current assignment of genotypes at flanking loci, can mix poorly if the markers are tightly linked. To remedy this problem, Thompson and Heath (1999) described an approach involving alternating updates of genotype vectors for entire pedigrees locus by locus with updates of entire multilocus genotypes person by person—in a sense, combining the peeling and hidden Markov models approaches in an MCMC fashion. Of course, this still requires the pedigree structures to be single-locus peelable, but it does offer a means to fit complex multipoint models to arbitrarily large pedigrees, a problem that is currently intractable by maximum likelihood methods.

Sheehan and Thomas (1993) were the first to point out the irreducibility problem with multiallelic markers and proposed an approach of *relaxing* the marker penetrance function by setting the zero probabilities to some small number so as to allow occasional incompatibilities between marker phenotypes and the assigned marker genotypes. This permits the chain to eventually explore all possible genotype configurations, but only the *legal* configurations are used in tabulating the statistics of interest. The more the penetrances are relaxed, the more efficiently the chain explores the genotype space but the higher the proportion of assignments that must be rejected as illegal. A similar idea was explored by Lin et al. (1993) and Lin (1995) using a *heated Metropolis algorithm,* which raises the full conditional probabilities to a power to improve mixing. To avoid the problem of having to eliminate illegal configurations, they introduced a *companion chain* approach, in which two Markov chains are run in parallel, one under the true model and one under the heated model, allowing the two to swap when both are in a legal state. Only the results of the legal chain are used in tabulating the statistics of interest. The performance of this approach can be considerably improved by relaxing only a minimal subset of penetrances needed to achieve irreducibility, which can be identified by identifying the pedigree structure in advance (Lin et al., 1994). Geyer and Thompson (1995) extended this idea further by using *Metropolis coupled MCMC*, in which a whole series of Markov chains are run in parallel, with varying degrees of heating to improve mixing within and between chains.

This remains an active area of research, although efficient algorithms remain elusive. The current state of the art is a program called LOKI created by Heath (1997), which conducts multipoint linkage analysis in pedigrees allowing for an unknown number of trait loci. At each iteration, the locations of each locus are allowed to move around, their segregation parameters are updated, and new loci can be added to the model or existing loci removed, using the technique of *reversible jump* MCMC (Green, 1995). Lee and Thomas (2000) provide simulation results of the performance of this approach for a variety of single-locus and multilocus disease models. Similar methods of *quantitative trait locus (QTL)* mapping have been developed in experimental genetics (Bink et al., 2000; Satagopan et al., 1996). Sheehan (2000) and Waagepeterson and Sorensen (2001) provide reviews of other recent developments. Sillanpää and Corander (2002) review these methods in the context of Bayesian model averaging.

Design Issues

Power and sample size

Affected pair method. The power of the affected pair method depends on a number of factors, including the number of pairs, their relationships, the genetic model and the magnitude of the relative risk, the true recombination fraction, and the degree of polymorphism in the marker locus. In general, the stronger the genetic risk and the more polymorphic the marker, the greater the power. In this section, we show how to compute power for a given genetic model by first determining the expected proportion $\bar{\pi}$ of alleles shared IBD under the alternative hypothesis and then evaluating the noncentrality parameter λ for the chi-square trend test (the expected chi-square per number of affected pairs N). The power $1 - \beta$ for a given value of N, or the sample size needed to obtain a given degree of power, is then approximately the solution to the equation $\lambda N = (Z_{\alpha/2} - Z_{1-\beta})^2$. More precisely, the variance of the proportion of alleles shared IBD is larger under $H_0 : \theta = 0.5$ than under $H_1 : \theta = \theta_0$; denote these standard deviations by s_0 and s_1, respectively, and the corresponding difference in proportions by Δ, all of which can be computed by systematic enumeration of all possible combinations of parental and offspring joint genotypes. Then, to compute power for a given sample size or the sample size required to attain a given

Table 7.10 Sample Size Requirements for the Affected Sib Pair Method: Number of Affected Pairs N Required for a Dominant Fully Penetrant Disease Susceptibility Locus with a Fully Informative Marker

θ	λ	$N_{\alpha=0.05, 1-\beta=0.95}$
0.00	0.5000	22
0.10	0.2048	53
0.20	0.0648	168
0.30	0.0128	851
0.40	0.0008	13,613
0.50	0.0000	∞

power, one solves the equation

$$\sqrt{N} = \frac{s_0 Z_{\alpha/2} + s_1 Z_{1-\beta}}{\Delta}$$

for N or $1 - \beta$. For example, for a rare dominant, fully penetrant disease susceptibility locus with a fully informative marker (i.e., so highly polymorphic that it is likely that the IBD status can be inferred unambiguously), we need consider only the transmission from a single parent. It is easy to see, then, that the probability that a sib pair shares a marker allele from that parent is $\pi = (1 - \theta)^2 + \theta^2$. Hence, the noncentrality parameter is $\lambda = 2(\pi - 1/2)^2 = (1 - 2\theta)^4/2$. The corresponding sample size requirements are provided in Table 7.10.

In general, to compute $\mathrm{E}(\bar{\pi} \mid H_1)$, we use some of the quantities derived on page 182, together with the disease model. Letting Z^A denote the IBD status at the disease locus and Z^B the IBD status at the marker locus, we seek $\Pr(Z^B = b \mid \mathbf{Y})$, which we compute by combining terms of the form $R_a = \Pr(\mathbf{Y} \mid Z^A = a)$ and $T_{ab} = \Pr(Z^A = a \mid Z^B = b)$. The former is given by Eq. (7.9) and the latter by Eq. (7.2). [For this purpose, we do not need terms of the form of $Q^B = \Pr(G^B \mid Z^B)$ because we have not yet obtained any marker data; indeed, the point of the calculation is to consider all possible marker data that could be collected!] Combining these together, we obtain

$$\begin{aligned}
\pi_b = \Pr(Z^B = b \mid \mathbf{Y}) &= \frac{\Pr(\mathbf{Y} \mid Z^B = b)\ \Pr(Z^B = b)}{\Pr(\mathbf{Y})} \\
&= \frac{\sum_a \Pr(\mathbf{Y} \mid Z^A = a)\ \Pr(Z^A = a \mid Z^B = b)\ \Pr(Z^B = b)}{\sum_{a,b} \Pr(\mathbf{Y} \mid Z^A = a)\ \Pr(Z^A = a \mid Z^B = b)\ \Pr(Z^B = b)} \\
&= \frac{\sum_a R_a T_{ab} \pi_b^0}{\sum_{ab} R_a T_{ab} \pi_b^0}
\end{aligned}$$

Table 7.11 Identical by Descent (IBD) Probabilities for Sibships

Disease Concordance	Probability of Outcome	Probability of Sharing Alleles			E(IBD)
		0	1	2	
Both Unaffected	0.96317	0.24939	0.50000	0.25061	0.50061
Discordant	0.03406	0.28475	0.50000	0.21525	0.46525
Both Affected	0.00277	0.03625	0.50000	0.46375	0.71375

where $\pi^0 = (1/4, 1/2, 1/4)$ are the null IBD probabilities. The noncentrality parameter for the 1 df trend test in proportions is then $\lambda = 2(\pi_2 - \pi_0)^2$.

For example, for an additive model with penetrances of $\mathbf{f} = (0.01, 0.50, 0.99)$, a disease allele frequency of $q = 0.01$, and a recombination fraction of $\theta = 0.001$, brute force evaluation of this expression yields the IBD probabilities for sibships in relation to their disease status shown in Table 7.11. It is evident that concordant affected pairs have much higher probabilities of sharing alleles IBD, while concordant unaffected pairs have only trivially higher sharing probabilities, and discordant pairs have lower sharing probabilities than expected under the null hypothesis. Nevertheless, we might consider using discordant pairs in a test for linkage. We can use these numbers to compute the sample sizes that would be needed in the same way as described above. For affected pairs the noncentrality parameter is $\lambda = 2 \times (0.46375 - 0.03635)^2 = 0.367$, while for discordant pairs it is only $2 \times (0.21525 - 0.28475)^2 = 0.00966$. To achieve a significance level of $\alpha = 0.001$ with 90% power ($Z_{\alpha/2} - Z_{1-\beta} = 4.57$), we would therefore require $4.57^2/0.367 = 58$ affected pairs but $4.57^2/0.00966 = 2164$ discordant pairs. Thus, it is evident that concordant pairs would be much more efficient than discordant pairs, at least for this combination of parameters, despite the greater availability of the latter (more than 12-fold in this case—3.4% compared with 0.28% of all sibships in the population). One could also perform a two-sample chi-square comparison of affected vs a sample of discordant pairs (page 187), as suggested by Guo and Elston (2000). One would not generally expect that this test would improve power, but it would provide some protection against bias if, for example, IBD probabilities could not be determined with certainty. Proceeding in a similar way as above, the noncentrality parameter for this chi-square test, comparing $N/2$ concordant with $N/2$ discordant pairs, is $0.283N$, so we would require a total of $4.57^2/0.283 = 74$ pairs (37 of each type)—more than would be needed using just affected pairs but a tempting solution if affected pairs were in short supply.

Lod score methods. The power of lod score analyses is more difficult to compute analytically except where direct counting is possible. In that case, one would compute the expected numbers of recombinants and nonrecombinants under the postulated model and hence the expected lods. Power (or sample size) would then be computed as described in the previous paragraph or, better, using exact methods for the Binomial distribution as described by Breslow and Day (1980).

For example, consider how many informative meioses n are needed if the true $\theta = \theta_0$. The likelihood is $\mathcal{L}(\theta) = \text{Binom}(r \mid n, \theta)$, so the likelihood ratio chi square is

$$G^2 = 2\ln[\mathcal{L}(\hat{\theta})/\mathcal{L}(1/2)] = 2[r\ln\theta + (n-r)\ln(1-\theta) + n\ln 2]$$

Substituting $E(r) = n\theta_0$, we get

$$E(G^2) = 2[E(r\ln\theta) + E((n-r)\ln(1-\theta)) + E(n\ln 2)]$$
$$= 2n[\theta_0\ln\theta_0 + (1-\theta_0)\ln(1-\theta_0) + \ln 2]$$

which tends to $2n\ln(2) = 1.39n$ as $\theta \to 0$. Now a lods of 3 corresponds to $G^2 = 13.84$, so roughly $n = 10$ informative meioses are needed to attain this level. In general, to estimate power, one would solve the equation $nE(G^2 \mid \theta_0) = (Z_{\alpha/2} + Z_{1-\beta})^2$, where for a lods of 3, $Z_{\alpha/2} = \sqrt{13.84}$. Table 7.12 illustrates the results of this calculation for various values of θ_0.

For general likelihood calculations, one must usually resort to simulation to assess the power of a study. The program SLINK (Ploughman and Boehnke, 1989) will do the necessary calculations for a set of pedigrees that have already been collected, including their disease phenotypes and which members are available for typing, to evaluate whether the family is likely to be informative for linkage. The program generates a large number of possible sets of marker data for each family, given the number of alleles, their frequencies, and a postulated value of θ, and evaluates the lods for each set. The average lods for each family, known as the ELODS, or the probability that lod > 3 (or any other value), can then be readily obtained and used to decide whether it is worth the effort of obtaining marker data. These data can also be used to evaluate the overall power of the study, given various strategies for selecting families to pursue. For further details, see Khoury et al. (1993, §9.3.1) or Ott (1999, §8.7).

Table 7.12 Sample Size Requirements for the Direct Counting Method: Number of Informative Meioses n Required as a Function of θ_0

θ_0	$E(G^2 \mid \theta_0)/n$	$n_{\text{lod}=3}$	$n_{95\%\text{power,lod}=3}$
0.01	1.274	11	23
0.1	0.736	19	40
0.2	0.385	36	75
0.3	0.165	84	175

The algorithm is essentially as follows:

1. By peeling, compute

$$\Pr(Y_2, \ldots, Y_n \mid G_1 = g_1), \ldots, \Pr(Y_{i+1}, \ldots, Y_n \mid G_i = g_i)$$

at the trait locus g.

2. Generate sampled trait genotypes by the *gene dropping:*

$$g_1 \sim \Pr(G_1) \Pr(Y_1 \mid G_1) \Pr(Y_2, \ldots, Y_n \mid G_1)$$
$$\cdots$$
$$g_i \sim \Pr\big(G_i \mid G_{m_i}, G_{f_i}\big) \Pr(Y_i \mid G_i) \Pr(Y_{i+1}, \ldots, Y_n \mid G_i)$$

3. Generate marker genotypes by gene dropping conditional on **g**:

$$m_1 \sim \Pr(m_1 \mid G_1)$$
$$\cdots$$
$$m_i \sim \Pr\big(m_i \mid (G_{m_i}, m_{m_i}), (G_{f_i}, m_{f_i}), G_i; \theta_0\big)$$

4. Compute the lod score for this realization of **g,m** and the observed **g**, using only the marker data on subjects who are available for genotyping.
5. Repeat steps 1–4 many times to assemble a distribution of lods and tabulate $\Pr(\text{lod} > 3)$ or $E(\text{lod})$.

If no pedigree data have yet been assembled, one could use a similar approach to generate random disease and vital status information under a given segregation model for a fixed pedigree structure and then offer these simulated pedigrees to SLINK. Alternatively, one could simulate marker and disease data simultaneously (Gauderman, 1995). The SIMLINK program also has an option to simulate marker data conditional on some already available marker information; in this way, families that are more likely to be linked can be identified, as well as the individual members who are likely to be the most informative.

Selection bias and misspecification

We noted earlier that heavily loaded pedigrees are often sought for linkage analysis, with little concern for their representativeness. Thus, joint estimation of both segregation and linkage parameters would be biased, even if it were computationally feasible. As a result, segregation parameters are often fixed at values estimated from other (it is hoped) population-based data sets. What happens if these parameters are misspecified?

Fortunately, numerous simulation studies (e.g., Clerget-Darpoux et al., 1986; Freimer et al., 1993; Greenberg, 1989; Hodge and Greenberg, 1992;

Neuman and Rice, 1990; Williamson and Amos, 1990) have demonstrated that linkage analysis is relatively robust to misspecification of the segregation parameters and that in most instances, the effect is to bias θ toward 0.5 and reduce the power. The major exception is misspecification of the dominance assumption, which can lead to bias away from the null. However, published simulation studies have considered a rather limited range of misspecification models, ignoring, for example, environmental effects and $G \times E$ interactions, linkage disequilibrium, and disease-related selection bias. Although it seems likely that most forms of misclassification are more likely to lead to false negative rather than false positive linkages, it is quite likely that it could lead to premature exclusion of regions from further consideration. For further discussion, see Ott (1999, §11).

The intuition to support the general robustness of linkage analysis even with selected samples rests on the assumption that markers and disease genes are independently distributed in the population (i.e., no linkage disequilibrium). If this is the case, then families could be ascertained or extended in a biased fashion with respect to disease, provided that knowledge of their marker status is not used in the sampling, so that the cosegregation of the two would be unaffected. Of course, if the same families are to be used for segregation analysis or for testing characterization of the penetrance and frequency of candidate genes, then population-based samples are essential.

Fine Mapping and Cloning of *BRCA1*

As the search for a gene is narrowed, fewer recombinants will be observed between the marker and the disease gene. Even in a large family study, the resolution of linkage analysis is usually no better than 1 million bp (1 cM) (Boehnke, 1994; Atwood and Heard-Costa, 2003). Eventually, one must abandon procedures that involve estimating population parameters and, instead, further narrow the candidate region based on observations of *convincing* recombinants in single individuals. This technique is referred to as *meiotic mapping*.

Linkage mapping and meiotic mapping are both *genetic* (as opposed to *physical*) mapping techniques. Distance on genetic maps is measured in recombination units (cM) between genetic markers. The first genetic map of the entire human genome, completed in 1987 by the Centre d'Étude du Polymorphisme Humaine (CEPH), was based on the pattern of inheritance of 403 markers in a panel of 21 three-generation families. This was a relatively low-resolution map, with an average distance of 10–15 cM between markers. The genetic map released by Génethon in 1994 contained more than 2000 microsatellite markers with an average distance of 2.9 cM between them. In contrast, the first comprehensive SNP survey, carried out by the SNP Consortium (Reich et al., 2002), listed 1.42 million markers, yielding an average density of 0.002 cM (about 1 SNP per 2000 bp). Such high-resolution maps, in which distances are measured in terms of base pairs (rather than recombination units), are called *physical maps*.

Using meiotic mapping, genes can often be localized to a region of several hundred kilobases. The first step in meiotic mapping is to construct haplotypes from the available marker data for all pedigrees that may be linked to the gene. Haplotypes are constructed by examining the pedigree structure and the marker data and, for each individual, identifying the maternal and paternal alleles at each locus. This process is often complicated by the presence of multiple copies (which are not IBD) of the same marker segregating in a family and by lack of DNA on some family members.

The second step in meiotic mapping is to examine the pedigree to identify the haplotype that is shared by most of the cases. Cases who do not share this haplotype are assumed to be *sporadics*. Among cases who do share the high-risk haplotype (the *nonsporadic* cases), we hope to observe recombination between a marker locus and the disease gene. A recombination event is indicated by finding regions of the haplotype that are not shared by all of the nonsporadic cases.

An important caveat is that the recombinant must be convincing. If there is some suspicion that the case in which the recombination is observed is not due to the gene, then the observed recombinant will be unconvincing. Table 7.13 summarizes the information on critical recombinants identified by the Breast Cancer Linkage Consortium in relation to the three markers surrounding the peak in the multipoint linkage analysis shown in Figure 7.22 (not every family was typed at the central marker D17S579). *BRCA1* was eventually found in the region distal to D17S579 and proximal to D17S588. Although there were two recombinants suggesting that it was on the other side of this marker, one could have been a sporadic case and the other an unlinked family.

Table 7.13 Critical Recombinants with Respect to Three Markers Identified by the Breast Cancer Linkage Consortium

Location	Number of Recombinants	Total Lod Score
Distal to D17S250	7	3.14
Distal to D17S250 and proximal to D17S579	1	0.82
Distal to D17S579 and proximal to D17S588	2	5.32
Proximal to D17S588	8	10.16

Source: Easton et al. (1993).

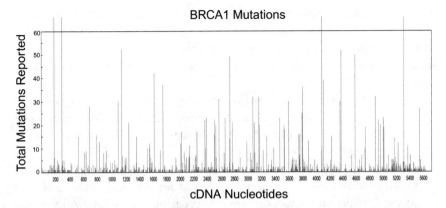

Figure 7.22 Mutations in *BRCA1* from the Breast Cancer Information Core as of July 30, 2001. The length of the vertical lines shows the number of times each mutation has been reported at the indicated location.

As the candidate region is narrowed down by observing convincing recombinants, more markers are targeted to the remaining candidate region. For reasons of efficiency, one usually continues to type only those families in which recombinants are observed, although one may also want to type families in which the haplotypes are still ambiguous.

Haplotypes can also be used to identify regions that are shared by apparently unrelated cases who may be descended from a common ancestor bearing a disease mutation, as described in Chapter 10. One can think of this technique as merging the many small pedigrees available for study into one or more very large ancestral pedigrees (whose structure is unknown), thereby increasing the number of recombination events "observed."

The cloning of *BRCA1* was reported by Miki et al. (1994) 1 year after the report of the Breast Cancer Linkage Consortium, using physical mapping techniques. Further linkage analyses finally concentrated the linkage signal to a region of about 600 kb between markers C17S1321 and D17S1325 (Neuhausen et al., 1994). This was done using a physical map constructed for the purpose comprising overlapping yeast artificial chromosomes (YACs), P1, bacterial artificial chromosomes (BACs), and cosmid clones. Once this region was localized, a detailed transcript map was created using 65 candidate expressed sequence tags (ESTs). These expressed sequences were sequenced in individuals from kindreds that were linked to markers in the region. Three expressed sequences were eventually combined into a single transcription unit. This transcription unit was located in the center of the candidate region surrounding D17S855, strongly suggesting that it could be *BRCA1*. A full-length cDNA for the gene was constructed from cDNA clones, hybrid-selected sequences, and amplified PCR products. The gene was found to contain 22 exons, spanning a total of 1863 amino acids, distributed over an interval of roughly 100 kb of genomic DNA. BLAST searches (scans of genomic databases to recognize known sequences similar to a given sequence) identified a characteristic feature similar to zinc-finger domains.

To establish that this gene really was *BRCA1*, it was necessary to show that affected individuals in the linked families carried mutations in the gene that were not shared by other members of these kindreds and were rare in the general population. Eight kindreds were selected for this purpose that either had high lod scores or demonstrated haplotype sharing for at least three affected members. In the initial screen for mutations, the gene was sequenced for one individual carrying the predisposing haplotype from each of the kindreds. Four of the eight were found to carry a mutation in the coding region—a different mutation in each kindred—and one was found to have a loss of transcript, presumably due to a promoter-region mutation that had still not been identified at the time of publication (Table 7.14). Five common polymorphisms that were not associated with breast or ovarian cancer were also found.

From the four kindreds in which mutations were found, several additional individuals, including both carriers and noncarriers of the predisposing haplotype, were then also screened for mutations. In every kindred, the mutation was found only in individuals carrying the linked haplotype. The kindreds in which mutations were not found all had low lod scores, indicating that they may not in fact be linked to *BRCA1;* indeed, a note added in proof indicated that one of the remaining three families appeared to be linked to *BRCA2*. Using allele-specific oligonucleotides (ASOs), the same mutations were screened for in a random sample of the Utah population, and none of the four mutations were found even once.

Table 7.14 Predisposing Mutations in *BRCA1* Found in Affected Individuals from Eight Kindreds Linked to the Region

Kindred	Total Cases	Lod Score	Codon	Mutation Nucleotide Change	Mutation Coding Effect	Frequency in Control Chromosomes
2082	31	9.49	1313	$C \rightarrow T$	Gln $\rightarrow$ Stop	0/170
2099	22	2.36	1775	$T \rightarrow G$	Met $\rightarrow$ Arg	0/120
2035	10	2.25	N/A	?	Loss of transcript	N/A
1901	10	1.50	24	−11 bp	Frameshift or splice	1/180
1925	4	0.55	—	—	—	—
1910	5	0.36	1756	Extra C	Frameshift	0/162
1911	8	−0.20	—	Linked to *BRCA2*		—
1927	5	−0.44	—	—	—	—

Mutations were associated with a wide range of phenotypes. In kindred 2082, which has the only mutation leading to premature truncation of the protein, there were 22 ovarian cancers—an extraordinarily high number given the rarity of this disease—but the mean age of breast cancer was older than in the other kindreds. The other four kindreds segregating *BRCA1* mutations had on average only 1 ovarian cancer per 10 breast cancers, but a high proportion of breast cancers occurred in the late 20s to early 30s. In kindred 2035 with the presumed regulatory mutation, 80% of the cases occurred under age 50. Kindred 1910, with the 1 bp insertion, had four cases of bilateral breast cancer, and in every case both tumors were diagnosed within a year of each other. Nevertheless, each of the four kindreds included at least one female carrier who lived to age 80 without developing cancer, indicating that these mutations are not fully penetrant. (As we shall see in Chapter 11, population-based penetrance estimates are more typically in the range of 40%–65% penetrance by age 70.)

Miki et al. (1994) concluded that they had identified a "strong candidate" for *BRCA1* primarily on the basis of having found a gene (*1*) that was located within the region found to be linked to familial breast and ovarian cancer and (*2*) that contained frameshift, nonsense, and regulatory mutations that cosegregate with the predisposing haplotypes in these families and are rare in the general population. They warned, however, that "the large size and fragmented nature of the coding sequence will make exhaustive searches for new mutations challenging"—a forecast that has certainly proved true. Nevertheless, by the following year, a large international collaborative effort (Shattuck-Eidens et al., 1995) had already identified 38 distinct mutations (63 in total) by sequencing a series of 1086 unrelated individuals drawn from a combination of high-risk and population-based families. Two of these (*185delAG* and *5382insC*) were found relatively frequently and have subsequently been shown to have unusually high prevalence in Ashkenazi Jews. The Breast Cancer Information Core (http://www.nhgri.nih.gov/Intramural_research/Lab_transfer/Bic/) currently lists a total of 864 distinct mutations in 3856 reports, of which 498 have been reported only once each (Fig. 7.22).

The cloning of *BRCA2* was reported the following year by Wooster et al. (1995). The intense efforts to characterize these two genes, which have continued to the present, will be described in Chapter 11. Meanwhile, conflicting evidence for the existence of additional breast cancer susceptibility genes continues to accumulate (Antoniou et al., 2001; Cui et al., 2001) and will be also be discussed in Chapter 11.

The labor-intensive physical mapping techniques used to clone *BRCA1* and *BRCA2* have undergone rapid evolution in the past decade with the wealth of genomic sequence data now available from the Human Genome

Project. Although linkage analysis will likely still be useful for coarse mapping of disease genes, fine mapping is now mainly done by scanning genomic databases for known or suspected gene sequences and identifying polymorphic sites in these regions, which can then be tested for association in the investigators' own samples using the techniques to be described in Chapter 9 or using linkage disequilibrium mapping, as described in Chapter 10. Some authors have even proposed dispensing with linkage analysis entirely and looking for genes by whole genome association scans (Risch and Merikangas, 1996). Such a search might require testing over a million polymorphisms, which still poses formidable laboratory and data analysis challenges but will eventually become feasible. We will discuss the prospect for such methods in Chapters 10 and 12.

Conclusions

Historically, the primary means of locating major disease genes—absent a lucky guess about a possible candidate gene based on its known function—has been linkage analysis. This techniques relies on recombination, so each chromosome the offspring receives from a parent consists of segments derived from both grandparents. Hence, by finding markers that are transmitted within families in a manner that parallels the transmission of the trait, one can obtain an estimate of the general location of the gene responsible for the trait. This can be done using parametric lod score methods or nonparametric sib pair methods. A typical genome scan will begin with a sparse map of markers (say, spaced on average at 10 or 20 cM intervals), looking for regions of suggestive linkage, and then narrow down on these regions with additional markers and/or additional families. This technique was used by the Breast Cancer Linkage Consortium to localize *BRCA1* and subsequently *BRCA2*, using extended pedigrees with many cases of breast (especially early-onset cases) or ovarian cancer. Subsequent positional cloning and physical mapping techniques ultimately led to the identification of these two genes.

It is well recognized that linkage analysis is most effective for localizing relatively rare genes with very high penetrance, particularly those for classical Mendelian single-gene traits. Statistical power can be very limited for complex traits, which may involve common polymorphisms with modest penetrance, multiple genes, environmental factors, or complex interactions. The techniques of linkage disequilibrium mapping and candidate gene association analysis described in the remainder of this book may prove to be more effective for finding genes involved in complex diseases.

8

Principles of Population Genetics

In the next four chapters, we will consider the use of association studies for three purposes: (*1*) to further localize the region containing a causal gene; (*2*) to test associations with potential candidate genes; and (*3*) to characterize such genes once they have been established as causally related to disease.

Suppose that through the process of linkage analysis, we have narrowed down the search for a particular gene to a small region. We might then consider trying to find the gene by looking at a number of specific loci in the region that have already been identified. Some may be genes whose function has already been characterized and could plausibly be related to the disease in question. Since the region under study is now quite small, we do not expect to find recombinants, so linkage analysis is unlikely to be informative. How do we tell whether a particular locus contains the gene we are looking for?

One method we might try is to look for *allelic association* with the trait under study. This is a tendency for particular alleles or genotypes to be associated with the trait—for example, higher prevalence of the alleles among those affected by a dichotomous trait. Unless the gene is fully penetrant, we would not expect a one-to-one correspondence between the trait and alleles, but a causal gene must show some degree of association. However, association does not necessarily imply causation. In addition to the usual epidemiologic concerns (confounding, selection bias, etc.), we must consider the phenomenon of *linkage disequilibrium (LD)*.

This chapter provides a brief introduction to some of the concepts of population genetics on which the subsequent chapters will rely. Because many of the techniques of association analysis use *unrelated* individuals rather than families, it is important to understand something about the distribution of genes in populations as they evolve over time from drift, selection, mutation, and recombination. (I highlight the word *unrelated* because it is believed that all humans are ultimately descended from a common ancestor, and indeed, it is these unobserved ancestral relationships that are exploited in the techniques of LD mapping.) The chapter also introduces the concept of LD, by which associations with polymorphisms that are not themselves causal risk factors for the trait under study can arise and be used to further localize the trait gene at a finer level of resolution than may be possible by linkage analysis. Chapter 9 covers the various population-based and family-based designs that can be used for testing associations with candidate genes or markers that are in LD with causal genes. Chapter 10 describes a variety of methods based on LD that can be used for fine mapping of disease genes. Chapter 11 surveys the studies that can be done to *characterize* a gene once it has been cloned, for example to estimate its age-specific penetrance, mutation frequency, and interactions with other genes or environmental exposures.

This chapter starts with the variation in gene frequencies at a single locus over time in populations, developing in greater depth the concept of the Hardy-Weinberg equilibrium that was introduced in earlier chapters. We then consider two loci jointly and take up the concept of LD, statistical measures of LD, its origins and evolution over time, and estimation of the LD parameter. Next, we explore the evolution of haplotypes—sequences of alleles at a series of linked loci on a single chromosome. The chapter concludes with a discussion of coalescent trees for a single locus and ancestral recombination graphs for multiple loci—tools that will be useful for LD mapping in Chapter 10. For a more thorough introduction to this subject, the reader can consult the concise primer by Hartl (2000) or the more extensive textbooks by Hartl and Clark (1997) and Bolding et al. (2001).

Distribution of Genes at a Single Locus

Hardy-Weinberg equilibrium in large populations

We begin by considering a diallelic locus with alleles a and A with population frequencies $1 - q$ and q, respectively. Earlier chapters relied extensively on the result that if the two copies of the gene that an individual carries are inherited independently, then the number of copies of the A allele will follow a binomial distribution, $\text{Binom}(2,q)$, that is, that the probabilities of the three possible genotypes (aa, aA, AA) will follow the Hardy-Weinberg law: $((1-q)^2, 2q(1-q), q^2)$. The fundamental theorem is that in large, homogeneous, randomly mating populations, these probabilities are preserved from generation to generation and, further, that in nonhomogeneous but randomly mating populations, they are established in a single generation after

Table 8.1 Expected Frequency of an Allele Transmitted from an Individual Sampled from a Population in Hardy-Weinberg Equilibrium

Parental Genotype	Genotype Probability	Probability of Transmitting A	Joint Probability
aa	$(1-q)^2$	0	0
aA	$2q(1-q)$	$1/2$	$q(1-q)$
AA	q^2	1	q^2
Total	1	—	q

mixing. The proof of the first of these claims is quite simple. The alleles transmitted from one parent will have probabilities given in the second column of Table 8.1. Thus, if the parent's genotype is randomly sampled from a population in Hardy-Weinberg equilibrium with A allele frequency q, he or she can be expected to transmit the A allele with probability q. Since both parents transmit alleles independently, it follows that the offspring generation will also have genotype probabilities given by the Binom$(2,q)$ distribution.

Now to prove the second part of the claim, suppose that the father and mother come from different populations, with allele frequencies q_f and q_m, respectively. Following the above argument, the father will transmit the A allele with probability q_f and the mother with probability q_m, so the genotype probabilities in the offspring (F1) generation will not be in Hardy-Weinberg equilibrium but instead will be as shown in the second column of the Table 8.2. Now consider what will happen in the second generation. If the F1 generation mates at random, each member will be expected to transmit to his or her offspring (the F2 generation) an A allele with probability $\bar{q}$, and hence, as above, the F2 generation will have a Binom$(2,\bar{q})$ genotype distribution, again in Hardy-Weinberg equilibrium.

The assumption of random mating says that the probability that any pair of individuals mates is unrelated to their genotype (except, of course, for the X chromosome) or their ethnic origin. Needless to say, this is seldom strictly true in practice, as couples tend to mate within their ethnic group and are likely to select mates with compatible traits (such as height), some of which

Table 8.2 Expected Frequency of an Allele Transmitted from an Individual Sampled from the F1 Generation of an Admixed Population

Parental Genotype	Genotype Probability	Probability of Transmitting A	Joint Probability
aa	$(1-q_f)(1-q_m)$	0	0
aA	$(1-q_f)q_m + q_f(1-q_m)$	$1/2$	$[(1-q_f)q_m + q_f(1-q_m)]/2$
AA	$q_f q_m$	1	$q_f q_m$
Total	1	—	$(q_f + q_m)/2 \equiv \bar{q}$

may be influenced by specific genes. Such nonrandom mating is commonly ignored in many genetic analyses of chronic disease traits, for which its effect may be negligible. Nevertheless, to the extent that it occurs, its major effect is to slow down the rate of convergence to Hardy-Weinberg equilibrium (and LD, as discussed below) rather than to distort the equilibrium distribution.

Genetic drift in finite populations

To derive the results above, we have relied on the assumption that the mating populations are large. In small populations, these results will still be true in expectation, but the allele frequencies will vary from generation to generation simply as a result of chance. We now show that in finite populations, the expected value of the allele frequency will remain constant, but its variance will increase from one generation to the next. This means that in generation, there is a nonzero probability that one allele or the other might not be transmitted to *any* offspring, in which case that allele becomes extinct and the other becomes *fixed*. In fact, with certainty (absent mutation and selection), one allele or the other will eventually become extinct, and the probability that it is the A allele that disappears turns out to be simply $1 - q$. At first blush, this might seem to contradict the claim that in expectation, the allele frequency remains constant, until one realizes that with probability q the allele frequency will eventually become 1 and with probability $1 - q$ it will become 0; hence in expectation, the allele frequency remains $q \times 1 + (1 - q) \times 0 = q$.

These results are most easily demonstrated using a simplified representation of a constant, finite, homogeneous, randomly mating population, with only two alleles and no mutation or selection, known as the *Wright-Fisher model* in honor of Sewell Wright and Ronald Fisher, who were the first to investigate the phenomenon of drift in the 1930s. Suppose that at the beginning, the population consists of N alleles, of which some proportion $q_0 = x_0/N$ are A alleles and the remainder are a alleles. Suppose that generations occur at discrete intervals, always containing exactly N alleles. Thus, each offspring is generated from the parent distribution by sampling an allele a or A with probability $1 - q_t$ or q_t, so the probability of observing x_1 A alleles in the first generation will be $\text{Binom}(N, q_0)$. The expected value of x_1 is thus Nq_0 and its variance is $Nq_0(1 - q_0)$, or equivalently, the expectation of $q_1 = x_1/N$ is equal to q_0 and its variance (conditional on x_1) will be $q_0(1 - q_0)/N$. In particular, the probability that the A allele will be extinguished in the first generation is $(1 - q_0)^N$ and the probability that the a allele will be extinguished is q_0^N. Since $\text{E}(q_1 \mid q_0) = q_0$ and exactly the same argument can be made for each successive generation, it follows that the expected value of the allele frequency will remain constant over time, while its variance gets larger and larger, eventually reaching the maximum possible value of $p(1 - p)$ (corresponding to q being either 0 or 1). Calculation of its full probability distribution is more complicated, however. For the tth generation, we would have to compute the probability distribution for x_t by summing over all possible realizations of x_{t-1}:

$$\Pr(x_t) = \sum_{x_{t-1}=0}^{N} \Pr(x_{t-1}) \times \text{Binom}\left(x_t \,\middle|\, \left(\frac{x_{t-1}}{N}\right), N\right) \tag{8.1}$$

This does not allow any simple closed form expression, although direct calculation is straightforward, and by recursion, the probability distribution can be computed for any subsequent generation, as illustrated for the case $N = 10$ and $q_0 = 0.1$ in Figure 8.1. In the first generation, the distribution of allele frequencies is a simple Binomial with $q = 0.1$ and $N = 10$. Thereafter the distribution becomes increasingly dispersed, with $\Pr(x = 0)$ (i.e., the A allele becoming extinct) tending to 0.9 and the $\Pr(x = 10)$ (i.e., the A allele becoming fixed) tending to 0.1, while all intermediate values $x = 1, \ldots, 9$ gradually disappear.

In general, we are only interested in loci that show some polymorphism today, since genes that are completely *conserved* cannot be responsible for

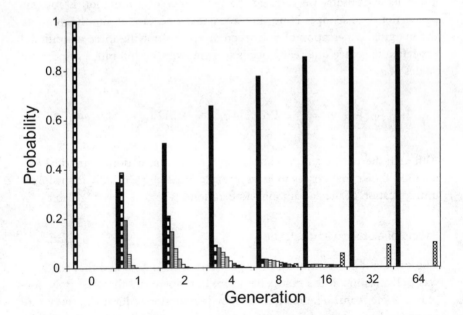

Figure 8.1 Drift in allele frequencies in a population of size $N = 10$ with an initial allele frequency of $q_0 = 0.1$, that is, a single copy of the A allele in the first generation. Each block shows the distribution of allele frequencies at different generations after the initial mutation.

variation in disease risks and are uninformative about other causal genes in their neighborhood. Thus, it is relevant to inquire about the *conditional* distribution of q given that $0 < q < 1$. Again, this has no simple closed form expression, but it is readily computed using the recursion relation described above. In particular, a simple recursion can be derived for the conditional expectation of q given nonextinction as

$$E(q_t \mid q_t > 0, q_{t-1}, n) = \frac{\sum_{x_t=1}^{n} (x_t/n) \text{Binom}(x_t \mid q_{t-1}, n)}{\sum_{x_t=1}^{n} \text{Binom}(x_t \mid q_{t-1}, n)} = \frac{q_{t-1}}{1 - (1 - q_{t-1})^n}$$

In a similar way, we can compute the conditional expectation of q given polymorphism as

$$E(q_t \mid 0 < q_t < 1, q_{t-1}, n) = \frac{q_{t-1}\left(1 - q_{t-1}^{n-1}\right)}{1 - (1 - q_{t-1})^n - q_{t-1}^n}$$

which is very similar to the previous formula until q approaches 0.5, after which the first formula will continue to rise to the asymptote of 1.0, while the second will approach the asymptote of 0.5. This is the basis of Fisher's observation that *common alleles are older*. Indeed, until the curve begins to attain its asymptote, we see that the prevalence of a mutation is roughly proportional to its age. Note, however, that one cannot simply compute the marginal expectation of q_t by recursively multiplying these conditional expectations, since one really needs to sum over the full range of possible values of q_{t-1}:

$$E(q_t \mid q_t > 0, n) = \sum_{x_{t-1}=0}^{n} \Pr(x_{t-1} \mid q_{t-1} > 0, n)\, E(q_t \mid q_t > 0, q_{t-1}, n)$$

Although there is no simple expression for this summation, numerical calculation shows that it rises to its asymptote much more rapidly than simple multiplication of the conditional expectations.

Effects of mutation and selection

The calculations illustrated in the previous section assumed that the gene was polymorphic at the first generation, but where did that first polymorphism come from? The obvious answer is mutation. Although a very rare event (perhaps of the order of 10^{-4} to 10^{-9} per meiosis, depending on the nature of the mutation), this is one of the driving forces of evolution. Suppose that we continue to assume for the time being that there are only two alleles, a and A, with mutation rates μ_1 from a to A and μ_2 from A to a.

If both of these mutation rates are nonzero, neither allele can become extinct because new mutations can be formed at any time. It is easy to show that the frequency of the A allele will eventually converge to a beta distribution with parameters μ_1 and μ_2, which has expectation $\mu_1/(\mu_1 + \mu_2)$ and variance $\mu_1\mu_2/(\mu_1 + \mu_2)^2(\mu_1 + \mu_2 + 1)$.

Now suppose that each new mutation is unique and occurs only once (the *infinitely many alleles* model), and suppose that these mutations arise as a Poisson process with rate μ per meiosis. Let a index the set of A_t distinct alleles in a population at generation t and let $\mathbf{q}_t = (q_1, \ldots, q_{A_t})$, $\sum_a q_a = 1$ denote the frequencies of each of these alleles, sorted in descending order by the time since they first arose. As before, the allele frequencies will vary from generation to generation due to drift, with probability $(1 - q_a)^N$ that allele a will become extinct in any given generation, thereby decreasing A_t. On the other hand, a new allele may arise by mutation with probability $N\mu$, thereby increasing A_t. On average, one would therefore expect that the number of alleles circulating in the population would eventually attain a state of stochastic equilibrium, with an expectation that depends on μ (Fig. 8.2A). This equilibrium distribution is given by the Ewens sampling formula,

$$\Pr(A, \mathbf{q}) = \frac{A!}{\mu_{(A)}} \prod_{a=1}^{A} \left(\frac{\mu}{a}\right)^{Nq_a} \frac{1}{Nq_a!}$$

where $\mu_{(A)} = \mu(\mu + 1) \cdots (\mu + A - 1)$. Derivation of this result is beyond the scope of this book (see, e.g., Ewens, 1979), but two of its basic implications are worth mentioning: first, $A - 1$ has roughly a Poisson distribution with a mean that increases with μ (Fig. 8.2B); second, for any given A, the expected values of q_a will be proportional to their ages, with a proportionality constant that also depends on $N\mu$.[1] This leads to a distribution of allele frequencies that is somewhat lopsided—one or two common alleles and others appearing very infrequently (Fig. 8.2C). However, we emphasize that the relationship between age and prevalence is only statistical, not deterministic, and that there can be very wide scatter around that relationship (Fig. 8.2D).

So far, we have not mentioned the other main force of evolution—natural selection. The theory derived above is neutral with respect to mutation; that is, it assumes that any new mutation is as likely to be transmitted to the next

[1] It is not possible to estimate N and μ separately, so in the population genetics literature, their product is generally treated as the parameter of interest, conventionally denoted $\theta = 4N\mu$. We will avoid this notation to avoid confusion of θ with the recombination rate elsewhere in this book.

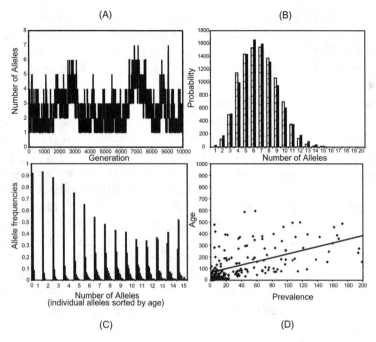

Figure 8.2 Simulation of the infinitely many alleles model in a population of $N = 1000$ with $\mu = 0.0002$: (A) Stochastic process of the number of alleles by generation, showing a pattern of increases by mutation and decreases by extinction of rare alleles. (B) Equilibrium distribution of the number of alleles (observed (solid bars) and fitted Poisson approximation (hatched bars)). (C) Conditional mean of the allele frequencies **q** for each value of A. (D) Relationship between age of mutations and their prevalence, based on every 100th generation between generation 5000 and 10,000 from panel A, omitting the most common allele (which was never extinguished in this simulation and retained high prevalence).

generation as any existing mutation. Clearly, many mutations are deleterious: they may be incompatible with life or produce diseases early enough in life to interfere with reproductive fitness. For genes involved in late-onset diseases, however, some polymorphisms may indeed be evolutionarily neutral. And let us not forget that some mutations can be beneficial, leading to evolutionary progress. Generally speaking, deleterious mutations are rare if there is significant selection against them. Some deleterious recessive mutations are relatively common, however. This can arise from the phenomenon of heterozygote advantage. The most familiar example of this is sickle cell anemia, a recessive trait with high prevalence in people of African descent. The mutation has retained its high prevalence in this population as a result of the protection it confers in the heterozygote state against malaria, a disease that is also endemic to Africa.

To understand this phenomenon quantitatively, let ϕ_0 denote the ratio of the probability that an individual with the aa genotype survives to reproduce relative to that for an individual with the Aa genotype, and let ϕ_2 denote the corresponding relative fitness of the AA genotype. If the genotype frequencies at birth in the parental generation are (Q_{aa}, Q_{Aa}, Q_{AA}), then at reproduction they will be $(\phi_0 Q_{aa}/\Phi, Q_{Aa}/\Phi, \phi_2 Q_{AA}/\Phi)$, where $\Phi = \phi_0 Q_{aa} + Q_{Aa} + \phi_2 Q_{AA}$. Hence, in large populations, the probability that each parent will transmit the A allele is $q' = (Q_{Aa}/2 + \phi_2 Q_{AA})/\Phi$ and the genotype probabilities at the next generation will be $((1-q')^2, 2q'(1-q'), q'^2)$. Now, if $\phi_0 < 1$ and $\phi_2 > 1$, it is easy to see that at each generation, q' will become larger, so that eventually the a allele will vanish; conversely, if $\phi_0 > 1$ and $\phi_2 < 1$, the A allele will vanish. If both ϕ_0 and ϕ_2 are greater than 1, then either the a or the A allele will vanish, depending on whether the initial q is greater or less than $q_{eq} = (\phi_2 - 1)/(\phi_0 + \phi_2 - 2)$. Only if both ϕ_0 and ϕ_2 are less than 1 will a new state of equilibrium be attained with allele frequency q_{eq}. This is the condition of heterozygote advantage.

Of course, in reality, both mutation and selection are likely to be in play and the eventual equilibrium level depends on the balance of these two opposing forces. Suppose, for example, that we allow only mutations from a to A with probability $(1 - q)\mu$, and suppose that we set $\phi_2 = 1, \phi_2 > 1$. Then the new equilibrium level can be shown to be $q_{eq} = \mu\phi_2/(\phi_2 - 1)$.

Distribution of Genes at Two Loci

Linkage disequilibrium is the tendency for alleles at two linked loci to be associated in the general population. As a consequence, an allele at a particular locus may appear to be associated with a disease, but only because it is associated with a mutant allele at the causal locus, not because it has anything to do with the disease directly. How does this phenomenon arise?

In a theoretically infinite population that has been randomly mating for eons and in the absence of new mutation and selection, one would expect the process of recombination to have led to independent distributions of alleles at any pair of loci (this claim is explored more rigorously below). Thus, if a candidate locus is not the causal gene but is only linked to it, one would not normally expect there to be any association between the disease and alleles at the locus. Within one family, the D allele might be associated with marker allele m, while within another family, the D allele might be associated with marker allele M (Fig. 8.3A). In both families, the two alleles tend to segregate together, implying tight linkage, yet across families, the two loci appear to be independently associated. Thus, it is possible for a gene to be tightly linked to a causal gene but not show LD. Conversely, it

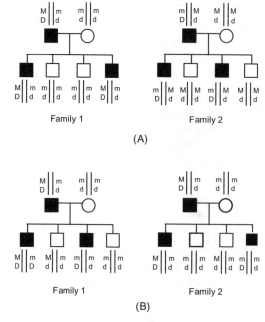

Figure 8.3 Illustrative examples of linkage versus association under dominant inheritance. (A) Perfect linkage ($\theta = 0$) and no association ($\delta = 0$). (B) Perfect association ($\delta = \delta_{max}$) and no linkage ($\theta = 0.5$).

is also possible for there to be a population association between alleles at loci that are not linked—possibly not even on the same chromosome—as a result of admixture or chance, for example (Fig. 8.3B). Such associations are of no real interest. In the remainder of this section and in the following two chapters, we will be concerned with pairs of loci that show both linkage *and* association. Linkage disequilibrium can arise in a variety of ways and will tend to decay over time at a rate that depends on the recombination rate. We begin by describing a number of alternative parameters that can be used to measure LD, discuss its sources and evolution, and conclude this section with methods for estimating LD. Chapter 10 discusses the extent of LD predicted to exist across the human genome and relevant empirical observations.

Consider two linked diallelic loci, A and B, with mutant allele frequencies q and p, respectively, and cross-tabulate the alleles that occur on the same chromosome (Table 8.3). There are a variety of ways one might

Table 8.3 Haplotype Probabilities for Two Loci in Relation to Their Marginal Allele Frequencies and the Disequilibrium Parameter

Haplotype	a	A	
b	$x = (1 - p)(1 - q) + \delta$	$y = (1 - p)q - \delta$	$1 - p$
B	$z = p(1 - q) - \delta$	$w = pq + \delta$	p
	$1 - q$	q	1

characterize the departure from linkage equilibrium in this table, that is, parameters measuring LD. For epidemiologists, the most familiar measure is the odds ratio $R = xw/yz$ or the noncentrality parameter for the chi-square test $\lambda = (xw - yz)^2/q(1 - p)p(1 - q)$. However, neither of these parameters leads to simple expressions for the evolution of LD over time, so the canonical measure of LD has become the difference between observed and expected, $\delta = w - pq = xw - yz$. In a 2×2 table, all four differences between observed and expected are necessarily equal in absolute magnitude, with opposite signs on the main and off diagonals. Because of the constraint that no cell can be negative, the range of possible values is bounded by

$$\delta_{\max} = \begin{cases} \min[q(1 - p), (1 - q)p] & \text{if } \delta > 0 \\ \min[(1 - p)(1 - q), pq] & \text{if } \delta < 0 \end{cases} \tag{8.2}$$

Hence, it is appealing to use the rescaled parameter $\delta' = |\delta|/\delta_{\max}$, which ranges between 0 and 1. Another measure that is widely used is $r^2 = \delta/q(1 - q)p(1 - p)$ (also denoted Δ^2), which also is adjusted for the marginal allele frequencies and is easily seen to be the noncentrality parameter for the chi-square test; that is, Nr^2 has a chi-square distribution on 1 df. Lewontin (1988) provides a general discussion of alternative measures of LD.

For associations between loci with more than two alleles, say n and m, respectively, there are more degrees of freedom to summarize. Letting P_{ij} denote the observed frequency for haplotype ij (expressed as a proportion, i.e., $\sum P_{ij} = 1$), $E_{ij} = p_i q_j$ the corresponding expected frequency under LD, and $\delta_{ij} = P_{ij} - E_{ij}$, the natural generalization of δ is $\Delta^2 = \sum_{ij} \delta_{ij}^2$. However, there are many more constraints and hence no simple scaled measure like δ'. An appealing standardized measure is the noncentrality parameter for the chi square, $W = \sqrt{\sum_{ij}(P_{ij} - E_{ij})^2/E_{ij}}$. NW^2 has a chi-square distribution on $(n - 1)(m - 1)$ degrees of freedom. The corresponding scaled parameter is $W' = W/\sqrt{nm - 1}$ (Cohen, 1988). Hedrick (1987) reviews the properties of many other methods of standardization and concludes that the only one that is not heavily dependent on the marginal allele frequencies is Lewontin's (1964) D':

$$D' = \sum_{ij} p_i q_j \delta'_{ij} = \sum_{ij} p_i q_j \frac{|\delta_{ij}|}{\delta_{\max,ij}}$$

where $\delta_{\max,ij}$ is the maximum possible value of δ_{ij} given p_i and q_j, as defined earlier.

When more than two loci are considered jointly, there are many more possible ways to describe the patterns of LD. For example, with three loci, there are eight possible haplotypes, whose frequency might be represented in terms of three marginal allele frequencies, three pairwise δs, and one three-way LD parameter (say η) as follows:

$$P_{ijk} = p_i^A p_j^B p_k^C + \delta_{ij}^{AB} + \delta_{ik}^{AC} + \delta_{jk}^{BC} + \eta_{ijk}^{ABC}$$

subject to the constraint that $\sum_{\ell=0}^{1} p_\ell^L = 1$ for $L = A, B, C$, $\delta_{00} = -\delta_{01} = -\delta_{10} = \delta_{11}$ for all three pairwise LD coefficients; likewise, all the ηs are equal or opposite in sign so that each margin sums to zero. As the number of loci increases, the number of possible higher-order LD coefficients rises, although only the lowest few may be important in practice. Nevertheless, the haplotype frequencies themselves may be more useful than this way of representing them, particularly if only a few of the many possible haplotypes actually occur with any frequency. Indeed, early observations indicate that the human genome appears to be broken up into well-defined *haplotype blocks*, with limited haplotype diversity within blocks and high rates of recombination between them, as described in Chapter 10.

In this chapter, we consider only the haplotype distributions for two or more genes, which could be markers or disease susceptibility loci. In the next chapter, we describe other measures of LD when the disease locus is unobserved and we wish to estimate the association between a disease phenotype and a marker that is in LD with a causal locus.

Origins of linkage disequilibrium

Linkage disequilibrium can occur for a number of reasons, including random drift in allele frequencies, leading to chance associations in finite populations; natural selection for or against a particular combination of alleles; nonrandom mating based on joint genotypes; mixtures of subpopulations with different allele frequencies; and mutation or founder effects.

Founder mutations. Let us focus for the moment on the last of these explanations. Suppose that a new mutation was introduced into the population at some point in the recent past. That mutation would have occurred on a single chromosome and would then be transmitted to descendants along with the alleles that happened to be on the same chromosome, at least until recombinations occur. Thus, for many generations, the mutant allele would be associated with certain alleles at linked loci, and the strength of that association would diminish over time as a function of the recombination rate. Thus, generations later, the strength of the LD is inversely a measure of the distance between the loci. Of course, this presumes that the mutation was transmitted to offspring and through the process of drift expanded to sufficient prevalence to account for a significant burden of disease in present-day descendants of the affected founder.

Table 8.4 Expected Distribution of Haplotypes Under Population Admixture

	Population 1		Population 2		Total	
	a	A	a	A	a	A
b	0.01	0.09	0.81	0.09	0.41	0.09
B	0.09	0.81	0.09	0.01	0.09	0.41

Some isolated populations may have been founded by a very small number of individuals. Because of their small size, there could have been chance associations between many pairs of loci, whether linked or not, including mutations that may have occurred many generations before the founding of the isolate.

Admixture. Suppose instead that the study population consists of a mixture of two subpopulations with A and B allele frequencies $p_1 = q_1 = 0.9$ and $p_2 = q_2 = 0.1$, and that the two loci were independently distributed within each subpopulation. Then, in a 50-50 mixture of the two populations, we would expect to observe the distribution of haplotypes presented in Table 8.4. Thus, we see an apparently very strong LD in the total population that is entirely an artifact of population stratification. It is also worth noting that admixture will also produce a distortion of the Hardy-Weinberg equilibrium. In this example, assuming that the two founding populations were in Hardy-Weinberg equilibrium with genotype probabilities $(0.01, 0.18, 0.81)$ or vice versa, in the mixed population the genotype probabilities would be $(0.41, 0.18, 0.41)$, a far cry from the expected distribution $(0.25, 0.50, 0.25)$!

Selection. We have seen how selection can lead to a distortion of the genotype probabilities from Hardy-Weinberg equilibrium at a single locus and can act as a counterbalancing force to that of new mutation. The situation is considerably more complex in the case of two loci. If there is no linkage, it is reasonable to assume that in the absence of epistasis, the effects of selection by two genes would be approximately the same as the product of their marginal effects on each locus separately. Thus, only in the case of an epistatic interaction between the two linked genes would one expect selection to be a source of LD (Kelly and Wade, 2000). Such an interaction would have to be strong to maintain LD over a distance of more than 1 cM between the loci. Other selection mechanisms that have been suggested as a source of LD are balancing selection (e.g., within the major histocompatibility complex [MHC] region [Abecasis et al., 2001]) or selective sweeps, in which a rare, favorable mutation is quickly swept to fixation (Kaplan et al., 1989).

Decay of linkage disequilibrium

Now consider the transmission of haplotypes from parent to offspring. Suppose that a parent has genotype $ab \mid AB$. The offspring will receive haplotypes ab or AB with probability $(1 - \theta)/2$ and haplotypes aB or Ab with probability $\theta/2$. According to Table 8.3, the probability of the parent having this genotype is xw. By summing similar terms over all possible parental genotypes, we could compute the probability distribution for the offspring's genotypes. It is easily shown that the marginal allele frequencies remain unchanged (p and q—this is just a reflection of Hardy-Weinberg equilibrium) and the LD parameter is reduced by $(1 - \theta)$. Hence, after T generations, an initial δ_0 has decayed to

$$\delta(T) = \delta_0(1 - \theta)^T \tag{8.3}$$

Proof: Let us consider all 16 possible combinations of haplotype pairs for a single parent, and consider the probability that each combination would lead to the transmission of the AB haplotype (Table 8.5), where x, y, z, and w are the population probabilities of the four haplotypes. Some of these probabilities reflect only a single possible transmission, either nonrecombinant (e.g., $AB \mid ab \rightarrow AB$) or recombinant (e.g., $Ab \mid aB \rightarrow AB$), hence depending on θ. Others reflect two distinct possible events with probabilities $\theta/2$ and $(1 - \theta)/2$ (e.g., $AB \mid Ab \rightarrow BA$ or AB, respectively), hence adding to $1/2$. Thus, the total probability from all these cells becomes

$$\begin{aligned} \Pr(AB \text{ transmitted}) &= (w^2 \times 1) + (2 \times wy \times 1/2) \\ &\quad + (2 \times wz \times 1/2) + (2 \times wx \times (1 - \theta)/2) \\ &\quad + (2 \times yz \times \theta/2) \\ &= w(w + y + z + x) - \theta(wx - yz) \\ &= w - \theta\delta \end{aligned} \tag{8.4}$$

Table 8.5 Probability That an Individual with Indicated Paternal and Maternal Haplotypes Transmits the AB Haplotype

Paternal Haplotype	Haplotype: Probability:	*Maternal Haplotype*			
		AB w	Ab y	aB z	ab x
AB	w	1	$1/2$	$1/2$	$(1 - \theta)/2$
Ab	y	$1/2$	0	$\theta/2$	0
aB	z	$1/2$	$\theta/2$	0	0
ab	x	$(1 - \theta)/2$	0	0	0

Table 8.6 Expected Decay of an Initial Disequilibrium in Large Populations as a Function of Distance and Number of Generations Since Admixture

θ	Number of Generations (T)						
	5	10	20	50	100	1000	10,000
0.0001	1.00	1.00	1.00	1.00	0.99	0.90	0.37
0.001	1.00	0.99	0.98	0.95	0.90	0.37	0.00
0.01	0.95	0.90	0.82	0.61	0.37	0.00	0.00
0.05	0.77	0.60	0.36	0.08	0.01	0.00	0.00
0.10	0.59	0.35	0.12	0.01	0.00	0.00	0.00
0.20	0.33	0.11	0.01	0.00	0.00	0.00	0.00

since $x + y + z + w = 1$ and $\delta = wx - yz$. In a similar way, we can show that y and z are increased by $\theta\delta$ and x is decreased by $\theta\delta$. Thus, the marginal probabilities $w + y, w + z, y + z, y + x$ are unchanged and the expected value of each cell under linkage equilibrium (E, the product of the margins) is the same as for the parental generation. Thus, writing $w = E + \delta$, the corresponding cell in the next generation becomes $w' = w - \theta\delta = E + (1 - \theta)\delta$, and the disequilibrium parameter $\delta' = w' - E$ is reduced by a multiplicative factor of $(1 - \theta)$. Since this same process occurs in each generation, after T generations the initial δ is reduced by a factor of $(1 - \theta)^T$.

Table 8.6 and Figure 8.4 illustrate the expected rate of decay of the initial disequilibrium between any pair of loci. Of course, this argument relies on an assumption of a large population, so that random drift in allele frequencies at either locus can be ignored; we have also ignored mutation and selection. Following the earlier arguments about drift for a single locus, in small populations we need to be concerned with the expected value of the LD parameter conditional on both loci being polymorphic in the present-day population. If, for example, the initial association arose as a result of a

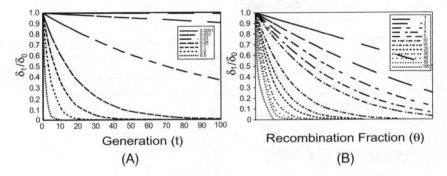

Figure 8.4 Expected decay of an initial disequilibrium (δ_t/δ_0) (A) as a function of the number of generations t for various recombination fractions θ and (B) as a function of θ at various times t.

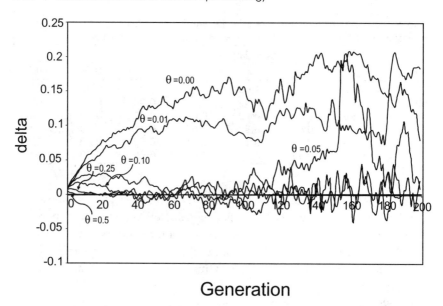

Figure 8.5 Simulation of linkage disequilibrium in a population of $N = 100$ haplotypes over a range of values of θ.

single founder mutation, this would generate substantial LD today only if that mutation had expanded to a substantial prevalence. In this case, $\delta_0 = (1/N)(1-p)$; even though it is equal to δ_{max}, it is still small in magnitude due to the $1/N$ factor. This process is difficult to address analytically, but again, it can be explored by simulation (Fig. 8.5). Basically, what one expects to see is two countervailing tendencies: the increase in marginal allele frequencies at both loci, conditional on the loci being polymorphic today, and the decline in the extent of LD due to recombination at rate $(1 - \theta)$. This will generally lead to a pattern of δ initially *increasing* due to expansion in p, followed by decline due to recombination. Of course, either mutation or selection could distort these patterns further. In any event, the process is highly variable, not to mention variability in the magnitude of the initial LD, so that one might not see a clear pattern of decay in LD with distance from a causal gene. We will explore statistical tools for trying to localize genes using LD in Chapter 10.

Estimation of linkage disequilibrium

In most of the designs we will be considering in the next chapter, independent individuals are studied, so without their parents it is not possible to determine the phase of the double heterozygotes, that is, to count the

Table 8.7 Expected Genotype Distribution Under Linkage Disequilibrium in Relation to the Haplotype Probabilities Given in Table 8.3

	aa	aA	AA
bb	$X = x^2$	$R = 2xy$	$Y = y^2$
bB	$S = 2xz$	$V = 2xw + 2yz$	$T = 2yw$
BB	$Z = z^2$	$U = 2zw$	$W = w^2$

haplotypes in Table 8.3 directly. It is instructive to consider the joint distribution of *genotypes*, shown in Table 8.7.

The most useful information about LD comes from the double homozygotes, (X, Y, Z, W), from whom we could estimate

$$\hat{\delta} = \sqrt{XW} - \sqrt{YZ}$$

directly. However, if one or especially both mutant alleles are rare, double homozygotes will be extremely rare and this estimate may be highly unstable. There is additional information in each of the other cells, which will also differ from their expected value. This information can be captured by maximum likelihood (Hill, 1974), using the multinomial likelihood $\mathcal{L}(p, q, \delta) = \prod_{ij} P_{ij}(p, q, \delta)^{N_{ij}}$, where P_{ij} is the predicted value for the joint genotype probabilities given in Table 8.7 and N_{ij} are the observed haplotype counts.

An even simpler method is to use the *expectation-maximization (E-M) algorithm*. For all cells except V, we can count directly the number of copies of each of the four possible haplotypes (ab, Ab, aB, AB) and represent them as

$$\begin{pmatrix} (2,0,0,0) & (1,1,0,0) & (0,2,0,0) \\ (1,0,1,0) & (r,s,s,r) & (0,1,0,1) \\ (0,0,2,0) & (0,0,1,1) & (0,0,0,2) \end{pmatrix}$$

where r and s are given by

$$r = \frac{[(1-p)(1-q) + \delta](pq + \delta)}{[(1-p)(1-q) + \delta](pq + \delta) + [(1-p)q - \delta][p(1-q) - \delta)]}$$

and $s = 1 - r$. One then proceeds iteratively, starting with an initial guess at p, q, and δ, (say, $\delta = 0$ and the marginal allele frequencies assuming Hardy-Weinberg equilibrium), computing x and y, counting the expected number of haplotypes x, y, z, and w, and finally deriving updated estimates of p, q, and δ. This process is then repeated until convergence occurs. Thus, using the weights in the array above, we would estimate x, for example, as $2X + R + S + r(p, q, \delta)V$, and likewise for the other cells. Then we would

Table 8.8 Illustrative Example of the First Iteration of the Expectation-Maximization Algorithm for Estimation of Haplotype Frequencies and δ for Two 2-Allele Loci, A and B, with True $p = 0.4$, $q = 0.3$, and $\delta = 0.15$

	True	Initial Guess	Next Iteration Estimate
p	0.4	0.5	0.4
q	0.3	0.5	0.3
δ	0.15	0	0.075
ab	0.57	0.25	0.4950
aB	0.03	0.25	0.1050
Ab	0.13	0.25	0.2050
AB	0.27	0.25	0.1950

$$r = 0.5 = \Pr(H = (aB/Ab) \mid G = (aA, bB))$$

HAPLOTYPE CODING

		Scores Per Observation			Total Scores		
	Frequency	aB	Ab	AB	aB	Ab	AB
$ab \mid ab$	0.3249	0	0	0	0	0	0
$ab \mid aB$	0.0342	1	0	0	0.0342	0	0
$aB \mid aB$	0.0009	2	0	0	0.0018	0	0
					0	0	0
$ab \mid Ab$	0.1482	0	1	0	0	0.1482	0
$ab \mid AB$	0.3078						
$aB \mid Ab$	0.0078						
aA, bB	0.3156	0.5	0.5	0.5	0.1578	0.1578	0.1578
$aB \mid AB$	0.0162	1	0	1	0.0162	0	0.0162
					0	0	0
$Ab \mid Ab$	0.0169	0	2	0	0	0.0338	0
$Ab \mid AB$	0.0702	0	1	1	0	0.0702	0.0702
$AB \mid AB$	0.0729	0	0	2	0	0	0.1458
				Next Iteration of Haplotype Frequencies			
					0.4950	0.1050	0.2050	0.1950

update the parameters by

$$p = (y + w)/2N$$

$$q = (z + w)/2N$$

$$\delta = w/2N - pq$$

This procedure is illustrated in Table 8.8 for some hypothetical genotype data generated under $p = 0.4$, $q = 0.3$, $\delta = 0.15$ and starting the E-M estimation with $p = q = 0.5$, $\delta = 0$. These values produce an initial estimate of $r = 0.5$, which is used to score the double heterozygote genotypes appropriately. This leads to immediate convergence of the estimates of p and q (this phenomenom is a consequence of the Hardy-Weinberg principle) and a first-iteration estimate of $\delta = 0.075$, exactly one-half the true value. Subsequent estimates, hereafter using $p = 0.4$ and $q = 0.3$, are 0.118, 0.136, 0.141, ..., gradually converging to the true value of 0.15.

The E-M algorithm is easily applied to the estimation of frequencies for multi-locus haplotypes (Excoffier and Slatkin, 1995). Suppose that we observe a random sample of L-locus genotypes $\mathbf{G}_i = (G_{i1}, \ldots, G_{iL})$ for a set of subjects i and we wish to estimate the frequencies Q_h corresponding to haplotypes $\mathbf{H}_h = (H_{h1}, \ldots, H_{hL})$ in the population from which they were sampled. In the E-step of the E-M algorithm, we estimate for each subject the probabilities of all possible haplotype resolutions,

$$E_{ihk} = \Pr[(\mathbf{H}_h, \mathbf{H}_k) \mid \mathbf{G}_i] = \frac{I[\mathbf{G}_i \sim (\mathbf{H}_h, \mathbf{H}_k)] Q_h Q_k}{\sum_h \sum_k I[\mathbf{G}_i \sim (\mathbf{H}_h, \mathbf{H}_k)] Q_h Q_k} \quad (8.5)$$

where $I(\mathbf{H} \sim \mathbf{G})$ is an indicator function for the compatibility of haplotype pair $(\mathbf{H}_h, \mathbf{H}_k)$ with genotype $\mathbf{G}$. In the M-step, the population frequencies are then updated by

$$Q_h = \sum_{i=1}^{N} \sum_k (E_{ihk} + E_{ikh})/2N$$

This approach works well for small numbers of loci, for which it is possible to systematically enumerate all possible haplotype configurations (e.g., for 10 SNP loci there would be $2^{10} = 1024$ possible haplotypes and $2^{H_i - 1 + 2M_i}$ possible haplotype resolutions for any individual's genotypes, where H_i is the number of heterozygous loci and M_i is the number of missing loci). For longer haplotypes, the computational burden becomes unmanageable unless the space of possible haplotypes is restricted in some way (e.g., to the most common ones or to the set of obligatory haplotypes determined by homozygous individuals). In this case, MCMC methods are very effective. For each individual, one samples a possible haplotype resolution with probability given by Eq. (8.5) and then updates the haplotype frequencies using the current frequencies of haplotype assignments. The sampling for each subject can be done without having to enumerate all possible haplotype assignments by using the Metropolis-Hastings method, proposing (say) a flip of the alleles at a single locus or a single segment and then accepting or rejecting the proposal with probability $Q_{h'} Q_{k'} / Q_h Q_k$. Morris et al. (2003) use a similar MCMC approach but reduce the dimensionality of the Q vector by log-linear modeling. Several authors (Chiano and Clayton, 1998; Liu et al., 2001; Niu et al., 2002; Stram et al., 2003; Thomas et al., 2001) have extended these general approaches for using multilocus haplotypes in LD mapping using case-control samples, as will be discussed further in Chapter 10.

Although not currently cost-effective for large-scale epidemiologic studies, new "conversion" technologies may soon make it unnecessary to use statistical methods to infer haplotypes from conventional unphased genotype data. These methods allow the isolation of somatic cell hybrids containing single haplotypes. Douglas et al. (2001) investigated the information gain for haplotype frequency estimation using these methods and found a 1.3–4.8 fold gain for haplotypes of 2–6 SNPs, respectively (averaging over various haplotype frequencies).

Estimates of LD tend to be upwardly biased in small samples (Terwilliger and Weiss, 1998). In part this follows simply from the fact that the various definitions constrain the parameter to be nonnegative, so that the expectation of the estimated parameter includes a component due to the sampling variance of the estimator; for example, $E(\hat{r}^2) = r^2 + \text{var}(\hat{r}^2)$. This should be borne in mind when interpreting some of the evidence on the extent of LD in the human genome presented in Chapter 10.

Evolution of Haplotypes

To this point, we have considered only a single locus or a pair of loci. We now consider the evolution of the entire segment of a chromosome surrounding some location of interest x, say the location of a causal mutation we are trying to find. Suppose that an individual has inherited this mutation from some ancestor T generations ago. We would expect that this person would likely also have inherited intact an entire segment of the ancestral haplotype bearing that mutation as well. How long would we expect that segment to be? Assuming that recombinations occur randomly as a Poisson process on the real line at rate 1 per Morgan per meiosis, this question is tantamount to asking, what is the probability that no crossovers have occurred throughout that segment? Thus, the probability of no recombinations between x and some location x_R to the "right" of x over T generations is simply $\exp[-(x_R - x)T]$; likewise, the distribution of shared segments on the "left" is also negative exponential with rate T, where x is measured in Morgans. Hence, the total length L of a shared segment surrounding x, $x_R - x_L$ will have the distribution of a sum of two exponentials, which is a gamma with shape parameter 2 and scale parameter $2T$, written as $\Gamma(2, 2T)$:

$$\Pr(x_R - x_L \mid x, T) = e^{-(x_R - x_L)T}(x_R - x_L)(2T)^2$$

a highly skewed distribution, with mean $1/T$.

We can invert this calculation to obtain the distribution of the time to a common ancestor for a pair of haplotypes as a function of their shared length surrounding a particular location. As discussed in the following section, the *coalescent prior* for the time to a common ancestor in a population of constant size at any particular location has a negative exponential distribution with parameter $2N$, where N is the number of haploid "individuals." It is convenient to write this distribution as $T \sim \Gamma(1, 1/(2N))$, because then we see that this is the conjugate prior for the likelihood of shared length given above, so by Bayes' formula, $\Pr(T \,|\, L) \propto \Pr(L \,|\, T) \Pr(T) = \Gamma(3, 2L + 1/(2N))$.

Now suppose that we observe chromosomes at only a discrete set of markers at locations $x_i, i = -L, \ldots, R$, and suppose that the segment we observed to be identical to the ancestral haplotype runs from markers $-\ell$ to r. Then the probability of this event would be the probability of no recombinations between markers $-\ell$ and r times the probability of recombinations between $-\ell - 1$ and $-\ell$ and between r and $r + 1$:

$$g(T, \ell, r) = e^{-(x_r - x_\ell)T} \left[1 - e^{(x_\ell - x_{-\ell-1})T} \right] \left[1 - e^{(x_{r+1} - x_r)T} \right] \quad (8.6)$$

Of course, it is possible that some of the identity between the observed segment and the ancestral one could be by state and not by descent; conversely, some differences could be due to new mutations at marker loci. The real likelihood of the observed haplotype sharing thus entails a summation of such terms over all subintervals within $(-\ell, r)$ containing x, weighted by their probability of sharing the segments outside these intervals by chance (a function of the allele frequencies and their serial correlations); see McPeek and Strahs (1999) for details. Also, as discussed in Chapter 10, recombinations do not occur as a homogeneous Poisson process due to interference and *hot spots*. A fuller treatment of this topic will be deferred to Chapter 10, where we discuss the use of shared haplotypes as a tool for fine mapping.

Ancestral Inference

Coalescent trees

The idea of the *coalescent*, introduced by Kingman (1982), is central to the theory of population genetics and underlies many of the methods for LD mapping discussed in Chapter 10. The basic idea is simple: in any sample from a finite population, all genes are ultimately derived from a common ancestor. The coalescent provides a mathematical theory to describe the probability distribution of the time to the *most recent common ancestor (MRCA)* and the ancestral relationships among any sets of members of the sample. Here the basic assumption is that alleles are transmitted intact over generations except for mutation (i.e., without recombination). It is thus generally applied to the analysis of very short sequences, for which we might postulate a process of drift under the infinitely-many-alleles model discussed earlier. *Ancestral recombination graphs (ARG)* will extend this approach to models incorporating recombination.

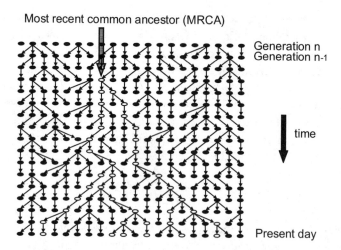

Figure 8.6 Wright-Fisher model of the transmission of alleles between generations. The open ovals represent a sample from the present generation (shown in the bottom row) and their ancestors. Note how many of the lines of descent have either become extinct or are not represented in the sample.

The intuition behind the coalescent is shown in Figure 8.6, where each row represents one generation and the dots each represent one haploid individual, with lines indicating each individual's offspring. Suppose that we take a random sample of individuals from the present day (the bottom row), indicated by the open circles, and trace back their lineages; we see that they eventually coalesce to a common ancestor MRCA. The filled circles, representing individuals who are not ancestors of anyone in the sample (some may have no ancestors in the entire present-day population) can be eliminated from further consideration, yielding the simplified tree structure represented in Figure 8.7. Here the height of the lines indicates the ages of

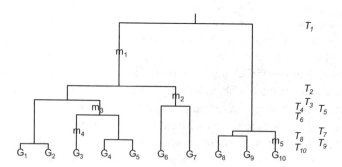

Figure 8.7 A coalescent tree: horizontal line indicate coalescences at times T_n; m's indicate mutations.

the various coalescent events in generations. If we now measure the genotypes for the 10 individuals in the present-day sample $(G_1, \ldots, G_{10})$ and find that they are not all the same, we can presume that the differences must be due to mutations, shown by the letters $m_1, \ldots, m_5$ superimposed on the tree structure. Thus, G_1–G_7 all carry the m_1 mutation, which distinguishes them from G_8–G_{10}, but some of these also carry additional mutations, while others (e.g., G_1 and G_2) are identical.

Let N denote the size of the population of alleles and suppose that we have a sample of size $n < N$ from that population. For any pair of alleles, the probability that they have a common parent is $1/N$ and the number of such pairs that could be formed within the sample is $_nC_2 = \binom{n}{2} = n(n-1)/2$. Hence, the number of generations to the first coalescence T_n has a negative exponential distribution with rate $_nC_2/N$. At this point there will remain $n-1$ distinct alleles and $_{n-1}C_2$ possible pairs, which will coalesce with an expected time of $E(T_{n-1} - T_n) = N/_{n-1}C_2$, and so on, until the entire sample has coalesced to the common ancestor. This last coalescence will occur with an expected time of N generations, for a total expected time to the MRCA of $N \sum_{t=0}^{n-1} 1/_{n-t}C_2 = 2(1 - 1/n)^N$; thus, half of the total coalescence time will on average be required for that last coalescence, and most coalescences will have occurred quite recently. The probability distribution for the time to the MRCA for an entire set of individuals is thus a sum of exponential distributions with differing parameters and has no simple closed-form expression. However, for any given pair of individuals, the time to their common ancestor is simply a negative exponential distribution with parameter $2N$, as discussed in the previous section.

Of the $\prod_{t=2}^{n} {}_tC_2$ possible such trees that could be formed, how do we choose between them? For this purpose, we need to exploit the similarity of the n observed haplotypes $\mathbf{G}$ in the present generation. Let Λ denote a particular topology of the tree and let $\mathbf{T} = (T_1, \ldots, T_n)$ the vector of associated coalescence times. The likelihood of the tree is then given by summing over all possible locations of the sets of mutations $\mathbf{M}$ and all possible haplotypes of the common ancestor, $\mathbf{G}_0$

$$\mathcal{L}(\Lambda, \mathbf{T}, \mu) = \sum_{\mathbf{M}} \sum_{\mathbf{G}_0} I[\mathbf{G} = \mathbf{G}(\mathbf{G}_0, \mathbf{M}, \Lambda)]$$
$$\times \Pr(\mathbf{G}_0) \Pr(\mathbf{M} \mid \mathbf{T}; \mu) \Pr(\mathbf{T} \mid \Lambda) \Pr(\Lambda)$$

where the first factor is simply an indicator for the compatibility of the observed haplotypes with the assumed ancestral haplotype, mutation locations, and tree topology. The factor $\Pr(\mathbf{M} \mid \mathbf{T}; \mu)$ describes the model for mutation, which might, for example, involve a 4×4 set of parameters μ for each of the possible mutations from one base to another. Calculation of this likelihood requires essentially the same peeling approach as that described in Chapter 6.

Because the space of possible coalescent trees is so large, it is generally not feasible to enumerate every possible topology systematically, so MCMC or importance sampling methods are used instead. A typical approach uses the Metropolis-Hastings algorithm, proposing a minor alteration to the structure of the tree—say, by detaching one branch and reattaching it somewhere else, reassigning times for the affected branches conditional on their new locations—and then deciding whether to retain the new structure by comparing the likelihoods of the new and old structures, $L(\Lambda', \mathbf{T}')/L(\Lambda, \mathbf{T})$ (see, e.g., Griffiths and Tavaré, 1997; Kuhner et al., 1995).

An alternative to coalescent theory, which is based on principles of evolutionary biology, is phylogenetic inference, which aims simply to produce hierarchical clusters from multivariate data based on some choice of a distance metric between observations. This approach has been widely applied to DNA sequence data to infer ancestral origins of species, for which coalescent methods would not be appropriate since different species do not interbreed. Hey and Machado (2003) provide a comparison of the two approaches in the context of structured human populations, where the assumption of random mating would also not apply. Flemming et al. (2003) applied a method of phylogenetic inference due to Huelsenbeck et al. (2001) to data on *BRCA1* exon 11 sequences in 57 mammalian species to identify codons evolving under positive selection. They concluded that selection is acting most strongly on the role of *BRCA1* in DNA repair and on this basis identified 38 missense polymorphisms in concerved regions and 3 in rapidly evolving regions that would be priority candidates for breast cancer susceptibility.

Ancestral recombination graphs

To incorporate recombination, we modify the graphical structure of the coalescent to add recombination events. Moving up the graph (backward in time), a join represents the coalescence of two haplotypes to a common ancestor, as before; a split represents a recombination of two haplotypes from different ancestral origins. We further annotate the graph by the location along the chromosome where these recombination events occurred: the segment from 0 to x derived from the left branch of the join and the segment from x to the end of the segment derived from the right branch of the join. The resulting structure is known as an *ancestral recombination graph (ARG)*, as shown in Figure 8.8.

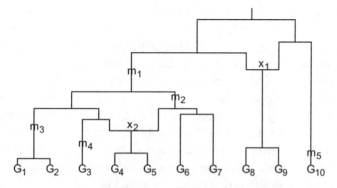

Figure 8.8 An ancestral recombination graph. As before, moving up the graph, a join indicates a coalescence to a common ancestor; here a split indicates a recombination of two segments from different ancestors; m's indicate mutations, and x's indicate locations of recombinations.

At a level at which there are n_t branches, coalescence events will occur at rate $_{n_t}C_2/N$ and recombinations at rate $\theta n_t/N$, where θ is the total length of the segment under consideration. Thus, the expected time to the next event of either type is $N/(_{n_t}C_2 + \theta n_t)$, and given that an event occurs, the probability that it is a coalescence is $(n_t - 1)/(n_t - 1 + \theta)$. Thus, the number of distinct events can either increase or decrease, and it is not as obvious as for the coalescent that this process will eventually converge to a common ancestor. It does, however, as proven by Griffiths and Marjoram (1997); the proof entails noting that the rate of coalescence is quadratic in n_t, so that for large n_t, coalescent events will be more common than recombinations. As before, the likelihood of an ARG involves summation over all possible locations of mutations and haplotypes of the common ancestor, and MCMC methods are used to explore the set of possible ARGs.

The use of coalescent and ARG methods for fine mapping of genes will be described in Chapter 10.

Conclusions

Whereas linkage analysis relies on recombination, leading to associations between marker alleles and a trait *within families*, the techniques to be described in the following chapters rely on LD, meaning associations between marker alleles and a trait *between unrelated individuals in the general population*. In outbred populations, detectable LD tends to be limited to very short intervals between loci—on the order of tens of thousands of base pairs—due to the breakup of haplotypes at each generation caused by recombination, although it can extend much further in recently admixed populations. In this chapter, we have described the effect of drift, selection, and mutation on the distribution of alleles in populations, the origins and decay of LD over time, and the evolution of haplotype segments shared by individuals descended from a common ancestor. Coalescent theory is a particularly powerful approach for modeling these processes and will be applied to mapping disease genes by allelic associations in Chapter 10. Before we can discuss the use of multiple tightly linked markers in this way, however, we need to consider associations of disease with a single locus, which could be either a candidate gene or a marker in LD with a candidate gene.

9

Testing Candidate Gene Associations

Suppose that by linkage analysis we have localized the chromosomal region where we believe a disease gene is located. Association studies can then be used for three main purposes:

- To further localize the region where the gene might be found by looking for additional markers that are in strong LD with the still unidentified gene (*LD mapping*).
- To test the hypothesis that a particular gene that has already been identified in the region could be the disease gene we are looking for by determining whether polymorphisms in that gene are associated with the disease. Such *candidate gene association studies* are usually limited to those for which we already have some knowledge about their biological function and a plausible mechanistic hypothesis for their relevance to the disease.
- To estimate the risk associated with an already established causal gene and other factors affecting its penetrance (*gene characterization*).

The fundamental study designs and statistical analysis methods for testing associations between genetic polymorphisms and a disease are essentially the same for any of these purposes and are developed in the rest of this chapter, where we are concerned primarily with the limited objective of testing to see if such an association exists, whether with a marker, a candidate gene, or an already cloned gene. The next chapter will further develop the use of associations with markers for LD mapping, while in Chapter 11 we will explore the use of association studies for gene characterization. This chapter is limited to testing associations with a candidate gene or a single marker locus at a time; Chapter 10 discusses testing associations with multilocus haplotypes.

Depending on the context, association studies can be used to test several different hypotheses. First, one might be interested in testing whether a gene has a direct causal effect on the disease (i.e., $H_0 : OR_G = 1$). However, it is not generally possible for association studies with unrelated individuals to distinguish this possibility from the case of the gene under study being in LD with another truly causal gene and having no direct effect of its own. Indeed, it is not even possible to distinguish strong linkage and weak LD from weak linkage and strong LD (Whittaker et al., 2000). Hence, hypotheses for association studies are generally expressed in terms of a two-locus model, with M being the marker being studied and G an unobserved causal locus. [The case of M being directly causal would correspond to perfect linkage and disequilibrium, $p = q$, $\theta = 0$, and $\delta = \delta_{max} = q(1 - q)$.] The validity of the various family-based procedures described below depends on which of several null hypotheses we are interested in testing: $H_0 : \theta = 1/2$ and $\delta = 0$ (the case of complete ignorance a priori); $H_0 : \theta = 1/2$, $\delta \neq 0$ (whether a gene already known to be associated with the disease is also linked to it); or $H_0 : \delta = 0$, $\theta < 1/2$ (whether a gene in a region already known to be linked to the disease is also associated with the disease, i.e., is in LD with the gene). Before we discuss the various design options and their methods of analysis, it is therefore worth while to begin by discussing the distribution of genes in relation to phenotypes in populations and in families.

Distributions of Genes in Affected and Unaffected Individuals

Homogeneous populations

The previous chapter described measures of LD between two observable loci (there denoted A and B), which could be either marker or disease susceptibility loci. In this chapter, we consider the association between a disease phenotype Y and a marker genotype M, which could be either a candidate gene itself or a marker linked to a candidate gene G. For the most part, we will assume that both loci are diallelic, with alleles m, M at the marker locus and d, D at the disease locus. Since it is generally not possible to determine with certainty the disease genotype G, let alone the phase, the data are represented in the form of a 2×3 contingency table (Table 9.1).

Table 9.1 Marker Genotype Distribution for Cases and Controls in Relation to Marker-Disease Haplotype Frequencies in Table 8.7

Marker Genotype	Controls	Cases
mm	$D_0 = x^2(1 - f_0) + 2xy(1 - f_1)$ $\qquad + y^2(1 - f_2)$	$C_0 = x^2 f_0 + 2xy f_1 + y^2 f_2$
mM	$D_1 = 2xz(1 - f_0) + 2(xw + yz)(1 - f_1)$ $\qquad + 2yw(1 - f_2)$	$C_1 = 2xz f_0 + 2(xw + yz) f_1$ $\qquad + 2yw f_2$
MM	$D_2 = z^2(1 - f_0) + 2zw(1 - f_1)$ $\qquad + w^2(1 - f_2)$	$C_2 = z^2 f_0 + 2zw f_1 + w^2 f_2$

These probabilities are computed as follows:

$$C_m = \Pr(M = m \mid Y = 1)$$

$$= \frac{\Pr(Y = 1, M = m)}{\Pr(Y = 1)}$$

$$= \frac{\sum_g \Pr(Y = 1 \mid G = g) \Pr(G = g, M = m)}{\sum_g \Pr(Y = 1 \mid G = g) \Pr(G = g)}$$

$$= \frac{\sum_g f_g \Pr(G = g, M = m)}{\sum_g f_g \Pr(G = g)}$$

$$D_m = \frac{\sum_g (1 - f_g) \Pr(G = g, M = m)}{\sum_g (1 - f_g) \Pr(G = g)}$$

where the genotype probabilities in these expressions are functions of p, q, δ given by

$$\Pr[G = (g_1, g_2), M = (m_1, m_2)] = \Pr(g_1, m_1) \Pr(g_2, m_2)$$
$$+ \Pr(g_1, m_2) \Pr(g_2, m_1)$$

and the haplotype probabilities $\Pr(g, m)$ are as shown in Table 8.3. None of these quantities depends directly on the recombination rate θ, although as discussed in Chapter 8, δ decays with time as a power of $1 - \theta$.

Next, we count the number of copies of the m and M alleles in cases and controls and array them as in Table 9.2. (Later in this chapter we will describe an alternative way of assembling this table based on alleles transmitted and not transmitted to cases from their parents.) Table 9.3 lists a number of alternative measures that have commonly been used to define LD in this situation.

Although perhaps the most widely used measure in epidemiology, the OR ψ (sometimes called λ) does not lend itself to simple algebraic expressions in terms of the underlying genetic parameters. It does, however, have the attractive feature of being the only one of these measures that is independent of the marginal allele and disease frequencies. It also shares the important

Table 9.2 Counting the Number of Allele Copies in Cases and Controls

Marker Allele	Controls	Cases
m	$n_1 = 2D_0 + D_1$	$n_3 = 2C_0 + C_1$
M	$n_2 = D_1 + 2D_2$	$n_4 = C_1 + 2C_2$

Table 9.3 Measures of Linkage Disequilibrium (LD) for Disease Phenotype by Marker Associations

Symbol	Formula	Perfect LD	Reference
δ^*	$\dfrac{n_1 n_4 - n_2 n_3}{n_1(n_3 + n_4)}$	$n_3 = 0$	(Levin, 1953)
Q	$\dfrac{n_1 n_4 - n_2 n_3}{(n_1 n_4 + n_2 n_3)}$	$n_2 = 0$ or $n_3 = 0$	(Yule, 1900)
$\Delta = r$	$\dfrac{n_1 n_4 - n_2 n_3}{\sqrt{(n_1 + n_2)(n_3 + n_4)(n_1 + n_3)(n_2 + n_4)}}$	$n_2 = 0$ and $n_3 = 0$	(Hill and Weir, 1994)
D'	$\dfrac{n_1 n_4 - n_2 n_3}{(n_1 + n_3)(n_3 + n_4)}$	$n_3 = 0$	(Lewontin, 1964)
d	$\dfrac{n_1 n_4 - n_2 n_3}{(n_1 + n_2)(n_3 + n_4)}$	$n_2 = 0$ and $n_3 = 0$	(Kaplan and Weir, 1992)
ψ	$\dfrac{n_1 n_4}{n_2 n_3}$	$n_2 = 0$ and $n_3 = 0$	(Edwards, 1963)

property with d and Q of being unaffected by the use of different sampling fractions for cases and controls. With the exception of ψ, all these measures have the same numerator, $D = n_1 n_4 - n_2 n_3$, the only difference being the denominators that standardize them in different ways. For example, the denominator for D' is $D_{\max}$, the largest possible difference given the marginal frequencies, as described earlier for $\delta_{\max}$ (Eq. 8.2); thus, the maximum possible absolute value of D' is 1. For a rare disease, $D_{\max}$ will take the value indicated in the table. Q is a simple transformation of the OR, $Q = (\psi - 1)/(\psi + 1)$, so that it ranges between -1 and $+1$, which after some simple algebra allows it to be expressed in a form similar to the other measures. δ^* has the same interpretation as the population attributable risk (Thomson, 1981), the proportion of disease attributable to the risk factor, or excess risk divided by population risk. This quantity has also been called P_{excess} (Lehesjoki et al., 1993) and λ (Terwilliger, 1995). (Here δ^* is not the same quantity as the δ defined earlier for the haplotypes themselves.) Δ is equal to the correlation coefficient r and is frequently reported as r^2, which ranges between 0 and 1. d is simply the difference in allele frequencies between cases and controls. Both Δ and d depend on the marker allele frequencies and hence can be difficult to interpret when comparing multiple markers in a region (Hedrick, 1987).

The various measures also differ in the criteria that would define *perfect LD* (i.e., the measure equaling 1 [or infinity for ψ]). For $\Delta(r)$, d, and ψ, both off-diagonal elements of Table 9.2 must be zero, corresponding to the two loci being identical. D' and δ^*, however, only require that all cases carry the variant allele alone, while both alleles can appear in the controls. Q would also yield a perfect LD score if none of the controls carried the variant allele but both appeared in cases. Under the scenario of a recent founder mutation, discussed in Chapter 8, one might expect that both pre-existing marker alleles would be circulating in a population at the time the new mutation arose. Only a single copy of that mutation would exist in the population, and hence it would be in perfect LD with any of the markers on that chromosome (i.e., $n_4 = 1$ and $n_3 = 0$ if the linked marker allele were M), even though the Δ parameter would be less than 1. As the mutation-carrying chromosome is transmitted to descendants, its prevalence might grow by random drift, while recombination would gradually reduce the LD except at the very closest markers. This is the reason parameters like D' are favored for LD mapping over, say, Δ.

Devlin and Risch (1995) provided a comparison of all these measures and concluded that δ^* is the most appropriate measure for fine mapping because it is directly related to θ, is least sensitive to the marker frequencies, and is unaffected by differential case-control sampling. D' produced results similar to δ^*, and Q was the best of the remaining alternatives. Hedrick (1987), Lewontin (1988), and Cordell and Elston (1999) provided some further discussion of these measures. In general, there is no simple algebraic expression for any of these parameters in terms of the penetrances, allele frequencies, and disequilibrium parameter for a general disease model, but relatively simple expressions can be derived by straightforward but tedious algebra for dominant and recessive models with full penetrance or for a multiplicative model of a rare disease ($f_1 = Rf_0$, $f_2 = R^2 f_0$):

Recessive $\quad D' = \delta / p(1 - q)$

Multiplicative $\quad D' = \delta(R - 1)/(1 - q)[1 + (R - 1)p]$

Dominant $\quad D' = \delta(1 - p)/p(2 - p)(1 - q)$

Thus, we see that in all three cases, the measure D' is proportional to δ, with a constant of proportionality that depends on the allele frequencies and (in the case of the multiplicative model) on the relative risk per allele, R. In that model, the multiplicative factor increases with R, eventually attaining as the limiting value that given for the recessive model.

It is instructive to consider the behavior of the *induced risk* with respect to the marker allele, $r_g = C_g/(C_g + D_g)$, and the corresponding odd ratios, $OR_g = r_g(1 - r_0)/r_0(1 - r_g) = C_g D_0/C_0 D_g$. In general, these induced risks by marker genotype will be intermediate between the true disease-locus penetrances. (Intuitively, one might think of the marker locus as a misclassified measure of the disease locus, leading to the familiar dilution effect of nondifferential misclassification.) Table 9.4 illustrates the results

Table 9.4 Expected Penetrances and Relative Risks for a Noncausal Candidate Gene in Linkage Disequilibrium with the Causal Gene (Assuming That $p = q = 0.1$)

Model	f_0	f_1	f_2	δ	r_0	r_1	r_2	$RR_{1:0}$	$RR_{2:0}$	$RR_{2:1}$
	0.01	0.99	0.99	0.00	0.196	0.196	0.196	1.00	1.00	1.00
	0.01	0.99	0.99	0.01	0.176	0.276	0.363	1.56	2.06	1.32
Dominant	0.01	0.99	0.99	0.05	0.095	0.615	0.833	6.47	8.75	1.35
	0.01	0.99	0.99	0.08	0.032	0.893	0.980	28.2	31.0	1.10
	0.01	0.99	0.99	0.09	0.010	0.990	0.990	99.0	99.0	1.00
	0.01	0.01	0.99	0.00	0.019	0.019	0.019	1.00	1.00	1.00
	0.01	0.01	0.99	0.01	0.018	0.027	0.049	1.55	2.77	1.79
Recessive	0.01	0.01	0.99	0.05	0.012	0.036	0.363	3.03	30.4	10.0
	0.01	0.01	0.99	0.08	0.010	0.020	0.804	1.96	79.4	40.6
	0.01	0.01	0.99	0.09	0.010	0.010	0.990	1.00	99.0	99.0

for selected values of the parameters, fixing $p = q = 0.1$ (details of the calculations are provided in the example below). The induced ORs with respect to the marker genotypes are generally much smaller than the corresponding genetic ORs at the disease locus, even where there is strong disequilibrium. Also, in both dominance models, the heterozygote OR is biased away from the null (compared with whichever homozygous genotype it ought to equal). The last line for each model corresponds to perfect disequilibrium, $\delta = \delta_{max}$: in this case, since $p = q$, it follows that $\Pr(dM) = \Pr(Dm) = 0$; that is, the D allele always occurs with the M allele, so the two loci are indistinguishable and thus the marker could indeed be the disease locus.

Worked example. Consider the recessive model with $f_0 = 0.01$, $f_1 = 0.01$, and $f_2 = 0.99$ with marker and disease allele frequencies $p = q = 0.1$ and disequilibrium parameter $\delta = 0.01$. Then the haplotype probabilities are

Haplotype	d	D
m	$x = (0.9)(0.9) + 0.01 = 0.82$	$y = (0.9)(0.1) - 0.01 = 0.08$
M	$z = (0.1)(0.9) - 0.01 = 0.08$	$w = (0.1)(0.1) + 0.01 = 0.02$

and the genotype probabilities are

Genotype	dd	dD	DD
mm	$x^2 = 0.6724$	$2xy = 0.1312$	$y^2 = 0.0064$
mM	$2xz = 0.1312$	$2xw + 2yz = 0.0456$	$2yw = 0.0032$
MM	$z^2 = 0.0064$	$2zw = 0.0032$	$w^2 = 0.0004$

Combining with the penetrances,

$$C_0 = f_0 \Pr(dm, dm) + 2 f_1 \Pr(dm, Dm) + f_2 \Pr(Dm, Dm)$$

$$= f_0 x^2 + 2 f_1 xy + f_2 y^2$$

$$= (0.01)(0.82)^2 + 2(0.01)(0.82)(0.08) + (0.99)(0.08)^2$$

$$= 0.01437$$

$$D_0 = (0.99)(0.82)^2 + 2(0.99)(0.82)(0.08) + (0.01)(0.08)^2$$

$$= 0.79563$$

we obtain

Genotype	Unaffected	Affected	Risk	*RR*
mm	$D_0 = 0.79563$	$C_0 = 0.01437$	$r_0 = 0.0177$	1.00
mM	$D_1 = 0.17506$	$C_1 = 0.00494$	$r_1 = 0.0274$	1.55
MM	$D_2 = 0.00951$	$C_2 = 0.00049$	$r_2 = 0.0492$	2.77

which appear in the second line of the recessive block in Table 9.4. Counting alleles, we obtain

Allele	Controls	Cases
m	$n_1 = 1.766320$	$n_3 = 0.03368$
M	$n_2 = 0.194080$	$n_4 = 0.00592$

The measure $D' = 0.05499$, and Levin's $\delta^* = 0.05604$ (remember, this is a different parameter from the $\delta = 0.01$ for the haplotype LD). The $OR = 1.60$ is a weighted average of the genotype ORs, 1.55 (*mM* vs. *mm*), 2.77 (*MM* vs. *mm*), and 1.79 (*MM* vs. *mM*), with the first receiving the greatest weight because it has the largest sample size.

Ethnically stratified populations

A number of authors (Altshuler et al., 1998; Ewens and Spielman, 1995; Khoury and Beaty, 1994; Khoury and Yang, 1998; Lander and Schork, 1994; Witte et al., 1999) have expressed concern that cohort or case-control designs using unrelated individuals could be susceptible to a form of confounding by ethnicity known in the genetics literature as *population stratification,* since there are often considerable gradients in gene frequency within the broad racial groupings that are generally used for stratification (Cavalli-Sforza et al., 1994), and such variation could be correlated with other unknown risk factors (Fig. 9.1). Although Wacholder et al. (2000, 2002) have

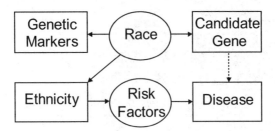

Figure 9.1 Conceptual model for population stratification or confounding by ethnicity: We wish to test the association between "Candidate Gene" and "Disease"; the allele frequency for the candidate gene is determined by "Race," which is also a determinant of other unmeasured "Risk Factors" and hence a confounder. "Genetic Markers" can be used to infer race, but self-reported "Ethnicity" can also be used for this purpose and can also be a surrogate for the other risk factors. (Reproduced with permission from Thomas and Witte, 2002)

questioned the practical importance of these concerns, at least in non-Hispanic white populations of European descent, some populations are highly diverse ethnically, and multiracial individuals are becoming more and more common. The use of family-based controls is therefore appealing because they completely overcome the problem of bias from population stratification, although they may be subject to other problems, such as selection bias due to some cases not having an eligible familial control (Gauderman et al., 1999; Thomas and Witte, 2002; Witte et al., 1999). Later we will review a variety of methods under the general heading of *genomic control* and *structured association* that have been proposed for using a panel of markers unlinked to the candidate genes under study to estimate the extent of stratification in the study population and infer ethnic affiliation.

While allelic association does not necessarily imply that the marker locus is indeed the causal gene, it normally would be interpreted as strong evidence of LD, which in turn would suggest tight linkage. Nevertheless, there are numerous examples in the literature of allelic associations occurring with no evidence of linkage. One classic example is given by Knowler et al. (1988), who showed that confounding by population stratification led to an inverse association between variants in the immunoglobulin haplotype $Gm^{3;5,13,14}$ and NIDDM among residents of the Gila River Indian community. This association was not causal, however, and instead reflected confounding by a population-stratifying factor—degree of Caucasian heritage. In particular, the inverse association actually reflected the association between heritage and $Gm^{3;5,13,14}$ and the inverse association between Caucasian heritage and the risk of NIDDM. When Knowler et al. adjusted for heritage, the inverse association disappeared.

Numerous studies of the purported association between alcoholism and the *A1* allele at the D_2 dopamine receptor locus (*DRD2*) give equivocal results. Initial reports strongly suggested an association, while further studies failed to support this finding. Gelernter et al. (1993) evaluated published studies attempting to replicate the initial association observed by Blum et al. (1990) and found much greater heterogeneity among studies than differences between alcoholics and controls. This result might be explained by population stratification, as there are large ethnic differences in *DRD2* alleles—and a wide range of corresponding allele frequencies among potential population-based controls. Moreover, there is a wide range of ethnic differences in the incidence of alcoholism (Gelernter et al., 1993). The few studies that were restricted to ethnically homogeneous populations did not observe an association (Gelernter et al., 1993). While these examples imply that population stratification might be a serious concern in genetic association studies, the potential magnitude of the bias resulting from this phenomenon remains unclear.

A somewhat different perspective on population stratification is given by a third example. An association has been reported between the $5'FP$ RFLP adjacent to the insulin gene on chromosome 11p and IDDM (Bell et al., 1984). Although this association had been consistently replicated across several populations, standard affected sib pair methods initially gave no evidence of linkage (Spielman et al., 1989). This situation suggested that the association might be due to population stratification and led Spielman et al. (1993) to develop the *transmission/disequilibrium test (TDT)*, described below, which showed highly significant evidence of linkage. It appears that the initial failure of the affected sib pair linkage tests was due to their low power for detecting genes with modest relative risks. Here the use of family member controls helped confirm a population association that could otherwise have been dismissed as due to population stratification.

Families

Some of the designs discussed below entail the use of various comparisons within families, so it is worthwhile to consider first the joint distribution of genotypes in families ascertained through affected cases. Here we are primarily concerned with two types of comparisons: between affected and unaffected siblings and between affected offspring and their parents. First, consider a nuclear family with two offspring, and let G_m, G_f denote the genotypes of the parents and G_1, G_2 the genotypes of the offspring. Assume that we have restricted the sample to affected/unaffected sib pairs, so $Y_1 = 1, Y_2 = 0$. We can then compute the joint distribution of the two sibs' genotypes as

$$\Pr(G_1, G_2 \mid Y_1 = 1, Y_2 = 0) = \frac{\Pr(Y_1 = 1, Y_2 = 0 \mid G_1, G_2) \Pr(G_1, G_2)}{\Pr(Y_1 = 1, Y_2 = 0)}$$

$$= \frac{\sum_{G_m, G_f} \left(\begin{array}{l} \Pr(Y_1 = 1 \mid G_1) \Pr(Y_2 = 0 \mid G_2) \\ \times \Pr(G_1 \mid G_m, G_f) \Pr(G_2 \mid G_m, G_f) \Pr(G_m) \Pr(G_f) \end{array} \right)}{\sum_{G_1, G_2, G_m, G_f} \left(\begin{array}{l} \Pr(Y_1 = 1 \mid G_1) \Pr(Y_2 = 0 \mid G_2) \\ \times \Pr(G_1 \mid G_m, G_f) \Pr(G_2 \mid G_m, G_f) \Pr(G_m) \Pr(G_f) \end{array} \right)}$$

as described in Chapter 5. The observed data would be arrayed as shown in Table 9.5. Of course, if M is not the causal gene, the expected values in this table would need to be computed by summing over the joint marker-disease genotypes of the four individuals, and would then be a function of the marker allele frequencies p, the disequilibrium parameter δ, and the recombination fraction θ, as well as the disease allele frequency q and penetrances $\mathbf{f}$. We will return to methods of analysis of such data later in this chapter.

Now consider a set of parent–offspring trios ascertained through an affected case, $Y_1 = 1$. Because the two parents are symmetric, we can simplify their joint genotypes to six possible parental *mating types: MT = dd × dd, dd × dD, dd × DD, dD × dD, dD × DD, DD × DD*. The joint distribution of the trio's genotypes, conditional on the offspring being affected, is then

$$\Pr(MT, G_1 \mid Y_1 = 1) = \frac{\Pr(Y_1 = 1 \mid G_1) \Pr(G_1 \mid MT) \Pr(MT)}{\sum_{G_*} \Pr(Y_1 = 1 \mid G_*) \Pr(G_*)}$$

Data from such a study might then be presented as a 6×3 contingency table, as shown in Table 9.6. Again, if M is not the causal gene, the calculations entail summation over the three joint genotypes at the two loci.

A somewhat simpler presentation of the data from a case-parent trio study, albeit with some loss of information, involves a tabulation not of genotypes but of alleles that are transmitted to the case compared with the alleles not transmitted (Table 9.7). This representation, based on the

Table 9.5 Presentation of Data from a Sib-Matched Case-Control Design

Case's Genotype	Sibling Control's Genotype		
	mm	mM	MM
mm	n_{00}	n_{01}	n_{02}
mM	n_{10}	n_{11}	n_{12}
MM	n_{20}	n_{21}	n_{22}

Table 9.6 Presentation of Data from a Case-Parent Trio Design

Parental Mating Type	Case's Genotype		
	mm	mM	MM
$mm \times mm$	m_1	0	0
$mm \times mM$	m_{20}	m_{21}	0
$mm \times MM$	0	m_3	0
$mM \times mM$	m_{40}	m_{41}	m_{42}
$mM \times MM$	0	m_{51}	m_{52}
$MM \times MM$	0	0	m_6

Table 9.7 Distribution of Transmitted and Nontransmitted Alleles in Case-Parent Trios in Relation to the Mating Type Counts Given in Table 9.6

Nontransmitted Allele	Transmitted Allele	
	m	M
m	$n_{00} = 2m_1 + m_{20} + m_{21} + m_3$	$n_{10} = m_{21} + m_{41} + 2m_{42} + m_{52}$
M	$n_{01} = m_{20} + 2m_{40} + m_{41} + m_{51}$	$n_{11} = m_3 + m_{51} + m_{52} + 2m_6$

distribution conditional on MT,

$$\Pr(G_1 \mid Y_1 = 1, MT) = \frac{\Pr(Y_1 = 1 \mid G_1) \Pr(G_1 \mid MT)}{\sum_{G_*} \Pr(Y_1 = 1 \mid G_*) \Pr(G_* \mid MT)}$$

forms the basis of the TDT described below.

Worked example (continued). Using the same parameters as in the previous example ($q = 0.1$ and $\mathbf{f} = (0.01, 0.01, 0.99)$), the joint distribution of genotypes at the causal locus in disease discordant sib pairs turns out to be

Case's Genotype	Sibling Control's Genotype		
	dd	dD	DD
dd	0.43600	0.04590	0.00001
dD	0.04590	0.05851	0.00003
DD	0.11957	0.29228	0.00180

and in case-parent trios it is

Parental Mating Type	Case's Genotype		
	dd	dD	DD
$dd \times dd$	0.33136	—	—
$dd \times dD$	0.07364	0.07364	—
$dd \times DD$	—	0.00818	—
$dD \times dD$	0.00409	0.00818	0.40500
$dD \times DD$	—	0.00091	0.09000
$DD \times DD$	—	—	0.00500

which can be summarized in terms of transmitted and nontransmitted alleles as

| Nontransmitted | Transmitted Allele | |
Allele	d	D
d	0.81818	0.98182
D	0.09091	0.10909

We will revisit these data later as we describe various methods of analysis.

Design Options for Association Studies

Associations of disease with candidate genes or markers in LD with causal genes can be tested with any of the standard cohort or case-control designs described in Chapter 4 using unrelated individuals. This section begins with a review of these designs as applied to testing genetic associations and then covers a range of family-based association studies using siblings, parents, or even other pedigree members as controls. Major factors to consider in choosing a design are whether we are looking for a rare mutation with a very large relative risk or a common polymorphism with moderate relative risk, the age distribution of the cases, and whether we wish to study interactions with environmental factors or with other genes. We will defer discussion of interaction effects to Chapter 11, focusing here on basic designs for testing the main effect of a gene on disease risk. After reviewing the basic design options, we provide some more technical details on methods of analysis, which the nonmathematical reader may prefer to skip. We conclude this chapter with a brief discussion of approaches to testing associations with a quantitative trait.

Cohort study designs

The basic principles of the design and analysis of cohort studies of unrelated individuals were discussed in Chapter 4. These are generally ambitious undertakings, particularly if it was necessary to obtain biological specimens from thousands of individuals and store them for decades while waiting for cases to develop. Fortunately for the genetic epidemiologist, there are now quite a few very large cohorts that have been identified for other purposes and have repositories of stored specimens that would allow the subjects to be genotyped for candidate genes of interest (not to mention the baseline information about other risk factors that may also be of interest). Furthermore, because genotypes do not change over time, retrospective assessment of this risk factor, at least, does not create any new difficulties. Langholz et al. (1999a) discuss opportunities and study design issues for doing genetic studies within existing cohorts.

Case-control designs

It should be obvious to most epidemiology students that if the aim of a case-control study is to estimate a population parameter (such as the genetic relative risk), then both the case and the control series need to be representative of their respective populations (or at least similarly biased, something that is difficult to achieve). By *representative,* we mean having expected allele frequencies equal to the true frequency in the respective populations, something that is best achieved by complete enumeration or random sampling. Obtaining representative samples of cases is usually not a problem, at least if there is a population-based disease registry. Finding a representative control series is the major challenge. The rest of this section thus focuses on a number of different approaches to obtaining an appropriate control group (Witte et al., 1999).

Conceptually, any case-control study—whether using unrelated population controls or family member controls—can be thought of as a nested case-control study within some notional cohort, even if that cohort is not explicitly enrolled by the investigator. This concept will help clarify some of the study design and analysis issues discussed below. In particular, it clarifies that the OR estimated by a matched case-control study in which controls are selected from those free of disease at the time each case occurred (*incidence density controls:* Greenland and Thomas, 1982) estimates the incidence rate ratio described in Chapter 4. Lubin and Gail (1984, p. 104) also explain why the appropriate selection of controls should allow individuals who later develop the disease to serve as controls for earlier cases (see p. 67).

Population controls. The most obvious control group is a random sample from the source population of cases, in which case the data would be presented as in Table 9.1 and analyzed using standard epidemiologic methods for unmatched case-control studies (Breslow and Day, 1980)—the odds ratio and chi-square statistics for single categorical variables and logistic regression for continuous or multiple variable, as described in Chapter 4. Thus, exactly the same approaches described in Chapter 5 could be used, with family history being replaced by genotype as the exposure variable. Analysis methods for matched case-control studies were also described in Chapter 4.

Although it ought to be obvious that controls should be carefully sampled from the source population of cases and matched on appropriate confounders, sadly this is often not done well by geneticists (London et al., 1994). Finding a representative control group is particularly difficult in genetics, where (because of population heterogeneity) there may be a wide range of allele frequencies across subgroups and the appropriate way to define these groups may not be apparent. For example, HLA antigens are known to vary widely from one population to another, and even within a racial group to depend on ancestral origin (Cavalli-Sforza et al., 1994). Thus, the usual epidemiologic technique of matching on ethnicity may be inadequate to guarantee representativeness. Whether this matters depends on the usual conditions for confounding. Ancestral origin is a confounder only if it is both associated with gene frequency (which is very likely) and is an *independent* risk factor for the disease, that is, has an influence on disease risks conditional on genotype. Of course, this can happen for many reasons, including other genetic or environmental risk factors. Thus, most of the examples in which noncausal associations have been detected by case-control studies of candidate genes have usually turned out to be due to inadequately matched population control groups.

Genomic control and structured association. Recently, a number of authors have proposed using genomic information to help address the problem of bias due to *cryptic stratification* (i.e., unobserved subdivision of the population into strata with differing allele frequencies and baseline risks of disease) and overdispersion due to *cryptic relatedness* (i.e., unobserved ancestral relationships between individual cases and controls who are treated as independent in the standard chi-square test). In particular, with a panel of polymorphic markers that are not linked to the candidate gene under study, one can attempt to address the issue of population stratification by (*1*) using an overdispersion model to determine a test statistic's appropriate empirical distribution; (*2*) evaluating whether stratification exists; and (*3*) using a latent-class model to distinguish homogeneous subpopulations. The restriction to unlinked genes is intended to avoid the loss of statistical precision due to overadjustment by a correlate of the genes of interest; it is not necessary or desirable, however, to exclude all markers that are associated with the candidate gene but not linked with them, as it is precisely these associations that are needed to control for cryptic stratification.

With regard to the overdispersion approach for addressing population stratification, Devlin and Roeder (1999), Bacanu et al. (2000), and Reich and Goldstein (2001) point out that in the presence of population stratification, the null distribution of the usual chi-square test of the hypothesis of no association between the disease and a candidate gene will tend to be shifted toward higher values, leading to an inflated false positive rate. If one had enough markers that were not causally related to the disease, one could in principle estimate this null distribution simply by tabulating the distribution of the observed test statistics across all the markers and comparing the value for the specific candidate gene to this empiric distribution. In practice, however, the number of markers that would be required to determine significance levels with any precision would be prohibitive, probably even with modern SNP array technologies. However, using population genetics theory, Reich and Goldstein showed that the theoretical null distribution in the presence of stratification was shifted by a multiplicative constant. The size of that constant depends on the details of the population history, which are generally unknown, but the authors suggested that the constant could be estimated from the observed chi-square values for the marker data in the same subjects in which one wishes to test a specific candidate gene. They then proposed an adjusted chi-square test that takes account of the fact that the constant is estimated rather than known with certainty. Some additional complications include the dependence of the constant on allele frequency, suggesting that their procedure should be restricted to the subset of markers with frequencies that are similar to that of the candidate gene being tested.

Simulation studies indicate that their method might perform well with a panel of a few dozen markers. This *genomic control* approach is computationally simple, and simultaneously addresses issues of population stratification bias and overdispersion due to cryptic relatedness; furthermore, it allows for a large number of potential subgroups (i.e., it works well with very-fine-scale substructure) (Devlin and Roeder, 1999). An investigation of power indicates that the genomic control approach can generally be more powerful than the TDT (Bacanu et al., 2000). And it can be undertaken with pooled DNA samples, which can be substantially less expensive than individual genotyping.

In another approach known as *structured association,* Pritchard and Rosenberg (1999) suggest that inference should follow a two-step process: first, one uses a panel of markers to test for stratification; then, one evaluates the candidate gene association only if homogeneity is not rejected. By simulation, they have explored the critical values that should be used at each stage of the inference process and have shown that the method performs well using a panel of a couple of dozen markers. However, they provide no guidance on what the investigator should conclude if the hypothesis of homogeneity is rejected in the first stage. Most epidemiologists would be unhappy to learn that a study they had laboriously conducted should be simply discarded due to the existence of population stratification at a panel of markers!

The third, latent-class approach, entails using genomic information to distinguish subpopulations within which any potential population stratification is minimized. For example, following the above work, Pritchard et al. (2000a) developed a Bayesian approach to estimation of ethnic origins. In a population comprising a mixture of an unknown number of subpopulations without admixture, their approach leads to an estimate of the posterior distribution of the number of such subpopulations and the probability that each individual belongs to any given subpopulation. In the presence of admixture, the method estimates the proportion of an individual's genome that derives from each of the founding populations. Schork et al. (2001) have proposed a similar approach for addressing population stratification. Related work was also presented by Kim et al. (2001), who suggested using phylogenic trees defined by nonlinked SNPs to cluster individuals into homogeneous subgroups. In all of these approaches, once one has an estimate of membership within a particular subgroup, this information can be incorporated into the analysis of a case-control study to obtain an estimate of the candidate gene's effect, adjusted for potential stratification (Pritchard et al., 2000b). Satten et al. (2001) have described a different approach to adjusting for population stratification using molecular markers, based on a maximum likelihood approach to latent class models, summing each individual's likelihood contribution over all possible strata. The naive alternative of adding all the markers as covariates in a multiple logistic regression, although appealing due to its simplicity, has been shown to produce less precise estimates than the Pritchard et al. approach (J. Witte, unpublished data). Pritchard and Donnelly (2001) and Devlin et al. (2001) provided a formal comparison of all the alternative approaches. Hoggart et al. (2003) extended the structured association approach by allowing for the uncertainty in the estimation of individuals' population assignments.

Family member controls. One of the best ways to achieve a match on ancestral origin is to use family matched controls. Penrose (1939) appears to have been the first to suggest using discordant sib pairs for testing association, with some of its earliest applications to testing associations with blood groups (Clarke, 1956; Manuila, 1958), and the design has produced a great deal of interest in the genetics literature since the 1990s. Because siblings are individually matched, a matched analysis, based on a cross-tabulation of the case's and control's genotypes (Table 9.5), is required. If we were to reduce the 3×3 table in the worked example above to a 2×2 table by collapsing the dd and dD genotypes into a single category and comparing it with the DD genotype, we would obtain $n_{10} = 0.41185$ and $n_{01} = 0.000042$, which yields $OR = 9801 = (0.99)(1 - 0.01)/0.01(1 - 0.99)$. Analysis of the full 3×3 table would require the use of conditional logistic regression (see Eq. 4.8), which also allows one to analyze multiple factors and their interactions jointly (Schaid and Rowland, 1998).

   If the sole purpose of the study were to examine candidate gene associations, then there would be little need to match on age, sex, or birth cohort unless there could be differential survival due to these factors. Thus, aunts or any other relatives might be suitable. However, this is generally unwise for several reasons. First, if the candidate gene does indeed have a causal effect, one would expect to see some variation in gene frequency with age due to the *survival of the fittest* effect (even though an individual's genotype obviously does not change over time). Second, if the genotype is to be determined by a phenotypic assay rather than by DNA typing, then there may be differential measurement error by age or other factors. Finally, one is very likely to want to collect environmental data at the same time to examine $G \times E$ interactions. For all these reasons, one would be well advised to match on age and sex, which essentially limits the choice to sibs or cousins (Fig. 9.2). The choice between the two possibilities represents the usual trade-off between bias and efficiency. Sibs are likely to offer a closer match on confounding factors but also tend to be overmatched on the factors of interest, including genotype. Despite the fact that siblings tend to share both genotypes and exposures, it turns out that this design is often *more* efficient for testing $G \times E$ interactions than using unrelated subjects as controls. This paradox will be discussed further in Chapter 11.

A problem with this design is that sibs (other than twins) cannot be matched on both year of birth and age, both of which can be important determinants of environmental factors such as OC use. In order to evaluate exposure over a comparable age range, older sibs are preferable as controls. The standard procedure is to define a *reference age* for each case-control pair

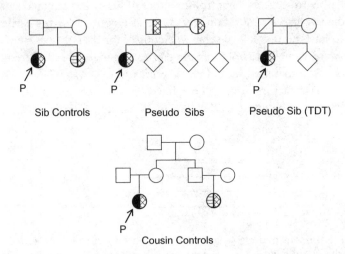

Figure 9.2 Basic family-controlled designs. Left solid symbols indicate the case and left-hatched symbols indicate unaffecteds chosen as controls; right-shaded symbols indicate individuals to be genotyped.

as the age at onset of the case (or some fixed interval prior to it to allow for latency) and then evaluate any time-dependent risk factors at the same age for both case and control. However, the potential exposure periods are systematically earlier in calendar time for older sibs than for cases. This could lead to confounding by secular trends in exposure or to recall bias because controls are remembering events that are more remote from the date of interview. In principle, analytical adjustments are possible that would allow the use of younger siblings as controls; see Kraft and Thomas (2003) for details.

In addition to controlling for time-dependent environmental factors, age at onset itself may contain useful information that would not be exploited in an analysis of disease status alone as a binary phenotype (Li et al., 1998; Li and Hsu, 2000). The standard conditional logistic regression can be thought of as a form of Cox regression stratified by family. Thus, each case is compared to a *risk set* comprising those sibs who had survived to the age of onset of the case. Sibships with multiple cases (n) and controls (m) would thus contribute a separate case versus risk set comparison for each case rather than treating it as an $n : m$ matched set by conditional logistic regression. (However, we will see later that neither of these analyses is strictly valid for testing the null hypothesis of no disequilibrium in the presence of linkage.) Figure 9.3 illustrates the concept of risk sets in a Cox regression analysis of a family-stratified case-control design. Suppose that a sibship has three subjects at risk, two of whom become cases at times t_2 and t_3, while the third has only attained age t_1 by the end of the observation period (or has died of some unrelated cause). Here the first subject would not be eligible to serve as a control for either of his or her affected sibs. The later of the two cases could, however, serve as a control for the earlier case but would have no one left to serve as a control for him or her. Hence, this sibship would contribute only a single pair to the analysis rather than being treated as a 2 : 1 matched set in logistic regression.

Because risk factors are less correlated between cousins than between sibs, there should be greater efficiency for measured factors, at the risk of

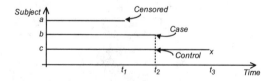

Figure 9.3 Case-control design. Note: even though subject c became a case at time t_3, he or she could still be used as a control for subject b, because he or she was still unaffected at the time t_2 when subject b become affected. However, one does not know for sure if subject a would have actually been disease free at time t_2 and therefore should not use him or her as a control.

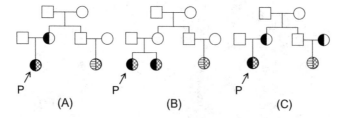

Figure 9.4 Some biased multiple-case family designs.

poorer control of unmeasured confounders. Also, more cousins than sibs are likely to be available as potential controls, so a higher proportion of cases might be informative for this purpose, reducing concerns about unrepresentative case selection. Finally, it may be possible to attain closer matching on age and year of birth for cousins than for sibs. Further subtleties in the use of sibling controls are discussed by Langholz et al. (1999b).

An attraction of family-based case-control designs is the high statistical efficiency they offer, particularly for studying rare major genes, if one restricts the sample to multiple-case families. This must be done with care, however, to avoid introducing bias in the estimates of relative risk. Figure 9.4 illustrates three biased designs: in panels A and B, the case is required to have a positive family history, while the control is not, thereby leading to a positive bias; in panel C, both the case and the control have an affected parent, but the affected mother of the case is also a relative of the control, while the affected mother of the control is not a mother of the case, leading to a bias toward the null. Figure 9.5 illustrates some unbiased designs: all of them involve a comparison of one case with one sibling control who shares a common positive family history (A: sibling; B: parent; C; grandparent). Figure 9.6 illustrates some unbiased designs using cousin controls: in panel A, a cousin pair shares an affected grandparent; in panel B, each cousin has an affected parent who is also a relative of the other cousin; in panel C, a pair of affected sibs is compared with a pair of unaffected sibs. The analysis of this last design would have to treat the two pairs as a $1:1$

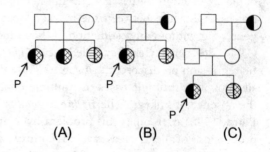

Figure 9.5 Unbiased multiple-case designs using sib controls.

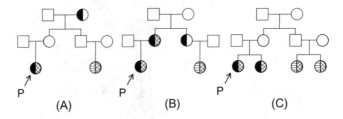

Figure 9.6 Unbiased multiple-case designs using cousin controls.

matched set of pairs rather than as a 2 : 2 matched set of individuals, since other permutations would distort the genetic relationships between them.

The designs discussed so far in this section relate to case-control *pairs*, that is, a single case and a single related control per matched set. However, many sibships may contain multiple cases or multiple sibs who would be eligible to serve as controls. The analysis of such sibships (or larger pedigrees) involves additional complications of two types (Schaid and Rowland, 1998). First, even if the gene under study is the causal risk factor, not simply in LD with a causal gene, there may be other unmeasured risk factors that will induce a dependency between the phenotypes of the subjects. Second, the standard conditional logistic likelihood requires an assumption of *exchangeability* under the null hypothesis of no association. In the presence of linkage, the set of possible permutations of the disease vector are not equally likely, given the marker data, because of sharing of marker alleles IBD. This has led to a number of suggestions for how to deal with these problems. Curtis (1997) suggested that larger sibships should be reduced to case-control pairs by selecting a single case and a single control from each sibship. Provided that the specific alleles are not used for this selection, it is possible to improve on simple random selection by choosing the case at random and then picking the sibling control who shares the fewest alleles with the case.

Others have suggested a variety of tests that would use the entire sibship in various ways. Many of these provide tests of the null hypothesis of no association with a genetic marker in the presence of linkage (i.e., no disequilibrium between the marker locus being tested and the causal gene), but without any estimation of the induced relative risk. Martin et al. (1997) described what they called the *sib TDT,* essentially conditional logistic regression on discordant sibships. While this does use all the data from sibships with multiple cases or multiple controls, the test is valid only in the absence of linkage. The *sibship disequilibrium test (SDT)* (Horvath and Laird, 1998) overcomes this problem by a simple sign test comparing the proportions of alleles in cases versus controls within each sibship. Siegmund and Gauderman (2000) and Siegmund et al. (2001) address this problem in the context of likelihood-based logistic regression methods, but relying on a robust variance estimator to construct valid significance tests and confidence intervals. Martin et al. (2000, 2001) extended the nonparametric approach to general pedigrees, while Kraft (2001) likewise extended the likelihood-based approach to a robust score test for general pedigrees.

Unrelated familial cohort member controls. Another possibility is to select controls from within the entire cohort of family members of the probands, matching on age, year of birth, and other factors but not on family. This design is biased toward the null for estimation of relative risks for environmental or genetic factors if probands are included as cases, but not if the cases are restricted to the familial cases. The basic reason for this is that the cohort will tend to over-represent positive risk factors relative to the source population of the probands but not relative to the source population of all familial cases. Further subtleties of ascertainment bias in this design remain to be investigated. The main advantages of this design appear to be that it overcomes the problem of obtaining close matches on age and year of birth with the case-sib design and that it focuses on the familial cases, who may be more informative for analysis of genetic factors and $G \times E$ interactions. Results would not be generalizable to all cases in the population, however.

The other difficulty with this design is that, like population-based designs involving unrelated individuals, it is subject to bias from population stratification. One possible way to avoid this problem would be to condition the analysis on the parental mating type, for example by including a vector of indicator variables for parental mating type, but of course this would be possible only if the parental genotypes were available. The *genotype decomposition* method (Li and Fan, 2000) is based on constructing two covariates for each member j of sibship i: $Z_{ij}^B = \bar{Z}_i$ (the average genotype coding for the sibship) and $Z_{ij}^W = Z_{ij} - \bar{Z}_i$ (the deviation of member j's genotype coding from the sibship mean). Both covariates are included in a standard Cox regression model in which risk sets are not stratified by family. Thus, fewer cases will have to be discarded because they do not have an age-matched sib control, leading to a more powerful test, and the expectation is that Z^B will adjust for any bias due to population stratification. Thus, inference is based solely on the regression coefficient for Z^W, which has the same interpretation as a within-family log RR parameter as the sib-control and TDT procedures. If the two regression coefficients were constrained to be equal, the resulting estimate would be the same as that from a standard Cox regression; it would be a more efficient estimator but potentially biased due to population stratification. Indeed, a test of $\beta^W = \beta^B$ is thus a test for the presence of confounding by population stratification.

Parental controls and the transmission/disequilibrium test

Perhaps the most appealing way to obtain a matched control group of geno-types is to use the parents. (For obvious reasons, parents are unlikely to be suitable controls for studying environmental effects, but as discussed in Chapter 11, it is still possible to investigate $G \times E$ interactions using this design.) The basic idea was first proposed by Rubinstein et al. (1981) and was later formalized as the *haplotype relative risk (HRR)* method by Falk and Rubenstein (1987). Their procedure entailed an unmatched comparison between the set of cases and the set of hypothetical individuals composed of the two alleles not transmitted by their parents (the case's *anti-self*). How-ever, in this form, this test is biased if $\theta \neq 0$ (Ott, 1989; Schaid and Sommer, 1993) and is potentially susceptible to population stratification bias (Schaid and Sommer, 1994).

There are three important variants of this procedure. In the TDT (Spielman and Ewens, 1996; Spielman et al., 1993; Terwilliger and Ott, 1992), the case is compared against his or her anti-self, as in the HRR, but using the correct matched analysis (Fig. 9.7A). In the *conditional lo-gistic regression (CLR)* method of Self et al. (1991), the case is compared against the three *pseudo-sibs* who have the other three genotypes that could have been transmitted to the real or hypothetical sibs (Fig. 9.7B). The third variant uses Poisson regression (Weinberg et al., 1998) to model the joint distribution of case and parental genotypes shown in Table 9.6.

Under the null hypothesis, the alternative genotypes are equally likely to have been transmitted to the case, so any deviation from this expected distribution in the case is evidence of association with that gene. We show below that under appropriate circumstances, the matched odds ratio esti-mated from these case-control designs estimates the genetic relative risk. The data are arrayed as illustrated in Table 9.7 (here alleles, not individuals'

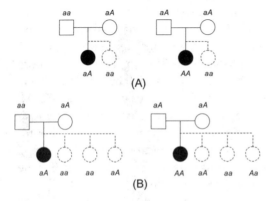

Figure 9.7 Possible compar-isons using parental control. (A) Comparison of an affected case with his or her anti-self having the two alleles not transmitted from the parents. (B) Comparison of an affected case with his three pseudosibs having the other possible genotypes given the parental genotypes.

genotypes, are being tabulated, so each subject contributes two observations to the table).

The standard McNemar estimator for the OR is n_{10}/n_{01} with $\mathrm{var}(\ln OR) = 1/n_{10} + 1/n_{01}$, and the significance test is $(n_{10}-n_{01})^2/(n_{10}+n_{01})$ (Eq. 4.3). We will show momentarily that in a *log additive* model for dominance, $f_G(\beta) = f_0 r_{g_1} r_{g_2} = \exp(\beta_{g_1} + \beta_{g_2})$, the McNemar OR is an estimator of r_g, the relative risk associated with a single copy of the mutant allele. When this is applied to the example data, we obtain an estimate of the $OR = .98182/.09091 = 9.9$, obviously much lower than the true $RR = 99$ for the comparison of the GG genotype against the gg, gG genotypes. The reason is, of course, that the log additive model is not correct for these data, as is evident by computing genotype RRs from the previous table of parental mating type results: for the mating type $gG \times GG$ we get $0.09000/0.00091 = 99$ in comparing offspring genotypes DD versus dD, whereas for the mating type dd versus dD we get $0.07364/0.07364$ in comparing genotypes dD versus dd, both as they should be.

The TDT has been extended to include multiallelic markers (Bickeboller and Clerget-Darpoux, 1995; Kaplan et al., 1997; Sham and Curtis, 1995; Spielman and Ewens, 1996), essentially by the natural generalization of 1 : 1 matched case-control studies to multilevel exposure factors (Breslow and Day, 1980), which can easily be implemented by conditional logistic regression. However, for multiallelic markers, the transmissions from the two parents are not independent when $\delta \neq 0$ (Bickeboller and Clerget-Darpoux, 1995), leading to inflated Type I errors (Cleves et al., 1997). An alternative formulation of this procedure using a randomization test (Kaplan et al., 1997) overcomes this problem, as do the CLR approaches that treat each trio as a separate unit rather than treating the transmissions from each parent as independent. The test has also been extended to tightly linked markers using haplotypes (Clayton, 1999; Clayton and Jones, 1999; Li et al., 2001; Merriman et al., 1998; Seltman et al., 2001; Zhao et al., 2000), essentially treating the haplotypes as multiallelic markers, as described above. However, when the haplotypes cannot be inferred with certainty, one must essentially average either the score (in a randomization test) or a likelihood contribution over the possible haplotype resolutions. Use of multiallelic or multilocus markers can also lead to a multiple comparisons problem, for which Bayesian smoothing (Molitor et al., 2003a; Thomas et al., 2001) or clustering (Molitor et al., 2003b; Seltman et al., 2001) approaches may be helpful.

The most general formulation of a likelihood for this design is by Self et al. (1991), who suggested that a conditional likelihood contribution be formed for each parent–proband triplet comparing the actual genotype of the proband to the set of four possible genotypes G_i^* that could have been transmitted from the parents,

$$
\mathcal{L}(\beta) = \prod_i \Pr\left(G_i \mid Y_i = 1, G_{f_i}, G_{m_i}\right)
$$

$$
= \prod_i \frac{\Pr(Y_i = 1 \mid G_i)\,\Pr\left(G_i \mid G_{f_i}, G_{m_i}\right)}{\sum_{G_*}\Pr(Y_i = 1 \mid G_*)\,\Pr\left(G_* \mid G_{f_i}, G_{m_i}\right)} \tag{9.1}
$$

$$
= \prod_i \frac{R_{G_i}(\beta)}{\sum_{G_i^*} R_{G_i^*}(\beta)}
$$

where $R_G(\beta)$ is the relative risk associated with genotype G. In the special case of a log additive model, this likelihood becomes

$$
\mathcal{L}(\beta) = \prod_i \frac{r_{g_{i1}} r_{g_{i2}}}{\sum_{G_i^*} r_{g_{i1}^*} r_{g_{i2}^*}}
$$

$$
= \prod_i \left(\frac{r_{g_{i1}}}{\sum r_{g_{i1}^*}}\right)\left(\frac{r_{g_{i2}}}{\sum r_{g_{i2}^*}}\right) \tag{9.2}
$$

$$
= \prod_{ij} \frac{r_{g_{ijt}}}{r_{g_{ijt}} + r_{g_{ijn}}}
$$

where g_{ijt} denotes the allele transmitted from parent j of subject i and g_{ijn} denotes the corresponding nontransmitted allele.

This likelihood leads directly to the McNemar OR for the TDT test. In dominant and recessive models, the CLR and TDT tests are not the same. It can be shown that only the CLR approach provides consistent estimation of the genotype relative risks in these models. Another advantage of the CLR approach is that it easily generalizes to multiple alleles or to multiple loci. If there is virtually no recombination between loci (as in the HLA region), then the sum over G^* is still over the four possible *haplotypes* that could be transmitted. If there is recombination, then the number of possible genotypes is much larger, and each must be weighted by its respective probability (a function of the recombination fractions) (Gauderman, 2002b).

The case-parent trio approach depends on the assumptions that both alleles are equally likely to be transmitted (no *meiotic drive*) (Lyttle, 1993) and that survival from fertilization to age at onset does not depend upon genotype (Witte et al., 1999). Including multiple cases from the same nuclear family as independent contributions to either the TDT or the CLR test is valid only in the absence of linkage; otherwise, their contributions are not independent, again leading to an inflation of the Type I error rate (Martin et al., 1997; Schaid and Rowland, 1998). A solution to this problem is to condition on IBD information (Cleves et al., 1997; Lazzeroni and Lange, 1998; Martin et al., 1997; Rabinowitz and Laird, 2000; Siegmund and Gauderman, 2001), but it is not always possible to infer the IBD status with certainty, and conditioning in this way can lead to a loss of power. The robust score (Kraft, 2001) and Wald (Siegmund and Gauderman, 2001) tests discussed earlier for sibships provide somewhat more powerful approaches. Another practical difficulty is that both parents may not be available for genotyping. One approach to this problem is to use the available genotype information on the nuclear family to infer the genotype of the missing parent (Curtis, 1997; Curtis and Sham, 1995); for example if the case has genotype MM and a sibling has genotype mm, then both parents must be Mm. However, restricting the analysis to the subset where the missing genotypes can be inferred can lead to bias. Knapp (1999) described a *1-TDT* test that is valid assuming that parental missingness is *uninformative*, that is, unrelated to the family's true genotypes. Subsequently, Allen et al. (2003) provided more general procedures that do not require uninformative missingness.

The Poisson regression approach is closely related to the CLR approach, being based on a model for $\Pr(G_m, G_f, G_i \mid Y_i = 1)$ rather than $\Pr(G_i \mid G_m, G_f, Y_i = 1)$. Thus, this likelihood depends on the population mating type probabilities, $\Pr(G_m, G_f)$, which are estimated from the data as a vector of nuisance parameters (Weinberg et al., 1998). The resulting estimator turns out to be identical to that from the conditional likelihood approach. However, the flexibility of this approach allows for natural generalization to testing for prenatal effects of maternal genes (Wilcox et al., 1998), imprinting (Weinberg, 1999), $G \times E$ interactions (Umbach and Weinberg, 2000), and maternal–fetal genotype interactions (Kraft and Wilson, 2002; Sinsheimer et al., 2003).

In principle, environmental risk factors and $G \times E$ or $G \times G$ interactions could be incorporated into the RR function. We will discuss these methods further in Chapter 11.

What hypothesis is the transmission/disequilibrium test really testing? The TDT is actually a test of the joint null hypothesis that $\theta = 1/2$ or $\delta = 0$, since we will demonstrate that under either situation, $E(n_{10}) = E(n_{01})$. (Of course, the test could still reject the null by chance in finite samples.) The remainder of this section provides a formal proof of this claim and can be skipped by the less mathematically inclined reader.

Table 9.8 gives the expected values of the cells in Table 9.7 in the case of a recessive disease with no phenocopies (Ott, 1989). This result is derived by first computing the expected distribution of marker/disease genotypes in a single parent of an affected proband, then for each possible genotype

Table 9.8 Expected Distribution of Transmitted and Nontransmitted Alleles Under a Recessive Model

Nontransmitted Allele	Transmitted Allele	
	m	M
m	$E(n_{00}) = (1-p)^2 - (1-p)\delta/q$	$E(n_{10}) = p(1-p) + [(1-\theta-p)\delta/q]$
M	$E(n_{01}) = p(1-p) + [(\theta-p)\delta/q]$	$E(n_{11}) = p^2 + p\delta/q$

computing the probability distribution of possible haplotypes transmitted to the proband, and finally summing over all possible parental genotypes.

Consider the n_{01} cell corresponding to a parental marker genotype mM transmitting allele m. We wish to compute $E(n_{01}) = Pr(M_p = mM, T_p = m \mid Y_o = 1)$, where T_p is the allele transmitted by parent p to offspring o. Because we are assuming a recessive disease, the offspring must have received a D allele at the disease locus, and hence the parent must have either genotype dD or DD. If the parental genotype is dD, then there are two possible haplotype configurations, $md \mid MD$ or $mD \mid Md$, with probabilities xw and yz, respectively. Transmission of the mD haplotype would therefore require a recombinant event in the first case and a nonrecombinant event in the second. If the parental genotype is DD, then the haplotype configuration would be $mD \mid MD$ with probability yw and probability $1/2$ of transmitting mD. Thus the total probability of this cell is $[xw\theta + yz(1-q) + yw]/2q$ (where the q in the denominator comes from conditioning on the fact that the offspring has a D allele and the 2 in the denominator does not appear in the table because each individual receives two alleles). After substituting the expressions for x, y, z, and w as a function of p, q, δ, and some algebraic simplification, we obtain $n_{01} = p(1-p) + [(\theta-p)\delta/q]$, as shown in Table 9.8. Similar reasoning leads to the other cells of the table.

If $\delta = 0$, the terms in square brackets for n_{10} and n_{01} vanish. On the other hand, if $\theta = 1/2$, then these two terms are identical. In either case, the two expectations are equal. Thus, the test would be expected to reject only if *both* conditions are false, that is, that the candidate gene is linked to the causal gene and is in LD with it, hence the name *transmission/disequilibrium test*. One obvious situation in which both conditions would be met is where the candidate is indeed the causal gene; hence $\theta = 0$, $p = q$ and $\delta = p(1-p)$. In this case, the off-diagonal elements become $n_{01} = 0$ and $n_{10} = 1 - p$, so the OR is infinite, as expected because we are assuming a recessive disease with no phenocopies. The beauty of the test is that it is not sensitive to most of the noncausal situations that could lead to disequilibrium in the absence of linkage (e.g., population heterogeneity) or linkage without disequilibrium (distant mutations).

While we have limited this proof to the case of a recessive gene with no phenocopies, similar calculations can be done for other penetrance models, requiring consideration of transmissions from both parents. The general expressions are

$$E(n_{01}) = \frac{f_0(a+b+c)^2 + 2f_1(a+b+c)(d+e+f) + f_2(e+f+g)^2}{f_0(1-q)^2 + 2f_1q(1-q) + f_2q^2}$$

$$E(n_{10}) = \frac{f_0(a+d+e)^2 + 2f_1(a+d+e)(b+c+f) + f_2(b+c+g)^2}{f_0(1-q)^2 + 2f_1q(1-q) + f_2q^2}$$

where $a = xz$, $b = xw(1-\theta)$, $c = yz\theta$, $d = xw\theta$, $e = yz(1-\theta)$, and $f = yw$. Unfortunately, no algebraic simplification is possible in the general case, but it is still possible to show that $E(n_{01}) = E(n_{10})$ under either of the null hypotheses.

Family-based association tests

The general class of *family-based association tests* (*FBATs*) allows information on all available genotypes for parents and multiple siblings to be used jointly. In principle this includes extended pedigrees, although most of this literaure has been developed in the context of nuclear families. The basic idea is to compute the distribution of some appropriate test statistics under the null hypothesis, conditional on the observed phenotypes. The null hypothesis could be no linkage in the presence of association, no association in the presence of linkage, or neither linkage nor association (Horvath et al., 2000, 2001; Laird et al., 2000; Lake et al., 2000; Mokliatchouk et al., 2001; Rabinowitz and Laird, 2000).

Whittemore and Tu (2000) describe a parametric likelihood-based score test framework for FBATs consisting of two statistics, one relating to transmissions of genotypes to nonfounders, the other to the distribution of genotypes in founders. Their test statistic takes the form $T_i = \sum_j u(Y_{ij}) v(M_{ij})$, where u and v are appropriate scoring functions and the summary statistic $T = \sum_i T_i$ is compared against its expectation and variance conditional on the minimal sufficient statistics for the parental genotypes. For example, with $u(Y) = 1$ for cases and -1 for controls, and with $v(M) = M$, the number of M alleles, the test becomes a simple comparison of the proportion of M alleles in cases versus controls within sibships, as in the SDT described earlier. However, the phenotype scores can be very general functions, say for quantitative traits or residuals from a survival analysis; likewise, the genotype scores can incorporate assumptions about dominance. The approach is also applicable to arbitrary family structures with arbitrary patterns of missing data and to dense sets of multiple markers. Applications of their approach to data on *SDR5A2* and prostate cancer by Tu et al. (2000) and by Shih and Whittemore (2002) indicate that their method can be substantially more powerful when there are any untyped parents. Clayton and Jones (1999) use a similar approach for multilocus haplotype associations, but limited to a dichotomous disease trait. Lunetta et al. (2000) describe an alternative score test that allows for unaffected siblings, covariates, and interaction effects and is also robust to population stratification. Their method is also applicable to quantitative traits, as described in the following section. Their approach is similar in spirit to one by Bourgain et al. (2003), who use a robust quasi-likelihood score function to allow for the known genealogical relationships, even in large inbred pedigrees for which exact likelihood calculations would be intractable.

Quantitative Traits

Association of quantitative traits with candidate genes (or markers in LD with them) usually relies on standard t-tests, F-tests for multilevel genotypes or multiple genes, and the corresponding regression analog. All these procedures based on unrelated individuals are subject to the same problems of confounding by population stratification as the corresponding approaches for disease traits, and similar genomic control approaches could be applied (Bacanu et al., 2002). Hence, family-based designs are preferred for testing candidate gene associations for quantitative traits as well. For example, the genotype decomposition method for sibship data discussed earlier can be applied to continuous outcomes (Abecasis et al., 2000; Fulker et al., 1999); one would use a regression model of the form

$$E(Y_{ij}) = \alpha + \beta[Z(G_{ij}) - \bar{Z}_i] + \gamma \bar{Z}_i$$

where $Z(G)$ is a covariate coding of the genotype to reflect the assumed dominance model, and $\bar{Z}_i$ is the mean of $Z(G_{ij})$ in family i. Inference about the association of Y with G is based on β, providing a stratification-resistant within-family test known as the *quantitative TDT (QTDT)*.

By analogy with the TDT, one can also use parental genotypes to adjust a regression of Y_i on G_i without using any phenotype data on the parents (Allison, 1997; Rabinowitz, 1997). Lunetta et al. (2000) showed that this test can be formulated as a regression

$$E(Y_i) = \alpha + \beta[Z(G_i) - \gamma_{MT_i}]$$

where $\gamma_{MT_i} = E[Z(G_i) \mid G_m, G_f]$, the expected value of $Z(G)$ for offspring of parental mating type MT_i. However, this approach assumes that the intercept term α is independent of parental mating type. If we allow α to depend on mating type, the expression can be rewritten as

$$E(Y_i) = \alpha_{MT_i} + \beta Z(G_i)$$

without the need to subtract the γ_{MT} terms. Gauderman (2003) has shown that this version of the test can be substantially more powerful than the standard QTDT.

As formulated above, these two versions of the QTDT are based on a prospective model $\Pr(Y_i \mid G_i, G_m, G_f)$. As with binary disease traits, one can also consider a retrospective model of the form $\Pr(G_i \mid Y_i, G_m, G_f)$ (Liu et al., 2002). Applying Bayes' formula yields

$$\Pr(G_i \mid Y_i, G_m, G_f) = \frac{\Pr(Y_i \mid G_i, G_m, G_f) \Pr(G_i \mid G_m, G_f)}{\Pr(Y_i \mid G_m, G_f)}$$

If one were then to assume that $Y_i \sim \mathcal{N}(\alpha_{MT_i} + \beta Z(G_i), \sigma^2)$, one would obtain a likelihood of the form

$$\mathcal{L}(\alpha, \beta) = \prod_i \frac{\exp\left(-\frac{[Y_i - \alpha_{MT_i} - \beta Z(G_i)]^2}{2\sigma^2}\right)}{\sum_{G_* \mid G_m, G_f} \exp\left(-\frac{[Y_i - \alpha_{MT_i} - \beta Z(G_*)]^2}{2\sigma^2}\right)}$$

For further discussion, see Sun et al. (2000) and Zhu et al. (2001). Allison et al. (1999) provide a comparable approach for sibship data, not requiring any parental genotypes. Gauderman et al. (2003) review various extensions of the QTDT to longitudinal family data.

Conclusions

A gene can be associated with a trait either because it has a directly causal effect or because its alleles are associated in the population with another gene that is the truly causal factor. Some allelic associations are purely spurious, due to chance, drift, or population stratification, and are of no particular use in studying the etiology of disease. Noncausal associations due to LD, however, can be very useful for fine mapping of disease genes, or one might have a causal hypothesis for a candidate gene, based on prior knowledge of its biological function. Association studies alone, of course, cannot determine whether a population association is causal or not. However, appropriate design of such studies can eliminate those that are simply due to population stratification. Well-designed traditional case-control or cohort studies using unrelated individuals can be a very efficient way to test hypotheses about candidate genes or for LD mapping, but it is essential that ethnic origin be carefully controlled by matching or stratification. Family-based designs—case-sibling or case-parent trio designs, for example—are attractive alternatives because they are completely robust to the problem of population stratification, although they tend to be somewhat less efficient because of overmatching on genotype. Both approaches are currently being used to investigate the possible role in breast cancer of polymorphisms in various genes other than *BRCA1* and *BRCA2*, such as those on hormone synthesis or DNA repair pathways.

10

Linkage Disequilibrium Mapping

Chapter 8 dealt with the origins and evolution of LD and Chapter 9 with cohort and case-control designs for testing associations between a disease and a genetic marker, which could be applied to proposed causal (candidate) genes or to markers not thought to be causal themselves but perhaps in LD with a causal gene being sought. We now turn our attention to the latter use of association studies as a means of further localizing the region containing a still undiscovered mutation.

As we have seen, several mechanisms can produce LD between a marker and a disease gene. Two are of particular interest for the purpose of LD mapping: (*1*) recent admixture and (*2*) founder effects in isolated populations. After considering them, we turn to analytic approaches. So far, we have concentrated on methods for looking at associations between disease and a single marker at a time. Now we must face the problem of having many markers within a region where we think the disease gene lies. After describing some relatively simple curve-fitting approaches to estimating the location of the disease gene given this set of LD estimates, the chapter moves on to more sophisticated methods that rely on associations with entire haplotypes rather than one marker at a time.

Recently Admixed Populations

As demonstrated in Table 8.4, the mixture of two populations with differing allele frequencies at two loci tends to induce an allelic association between the loci in the combined populations, even if the loci are independently distributed within each subpopulation separately. This is simply a reflection of *Simpson's paradox* (noncollapsibility) in statistical parlance or *confounding* by ethnicity in epidemiologic parlance. Such an association can arise between any two loci that have differing allele frequencies between the two populations, *whether or not they are linked*. However, as such admixed populations interbreed, such spurious associations tend to disappear, following the rule $\delta(t) = \delta(0)(1 - \theta)^t$, where t is measured in generations (Eq. 8.3). Hence, after the passage of 20–50 generations, there are few such spurious associations, except between loci that are relatively tightly linked: after 20 generations, δ will have declined to 1% of its initial value at $\theta = 0.2$ but will still be 82% of its initial value at $\theta = 0.01$ (Table 8.6).

This is the basis of the localization technique known as *mapping by admixture linkage disequilibrium* (*MALD*) (Briscoe et al., 1994; McKeigue, 1997; Stephens et al., 1994). In particular, Dean et al. (1994) have described a panel of 257 RFLP markers, spaced at roughly 20 cM intervals on average, that were selected on the basis of having quite heterogeneous allele frequencies between Caucasian, African-American, Asian (Chinese), and American Indian (Cheyenne) populations, whose use they have advocated for this approach. The critical consideration is the selection of a population that was admixed long enough ago for most long-range disequilibrium to have disappeared, while short-range disequilibrium will have remained.

The other major consideration is the selection of a panel of markers within the region of interest that shows quite different allele frequencies between the two (or more) founding populations. Recently, several panels of markers have been described that have been selected on the basis of large δ differences between the founding populations for African-Americans, Hispanics, and other admixed groups (Bamshad et al., 2003; Collins-Schramm et al., 2002; Rosenberg et al., 2002; Smith et al., 2001; Williams et al., 2000). And of course, the founding populations would have had to have different frequencies of the disease gene; thus, the technique is likely to be most useful for diseases that show quite different incidence rates between populations. In any event, this technique is generally believed to be most useful for coarse mapping of genes, as the expected peaks in disequilibrium tend to be fairly broad, while still showing considerable local variation from one marker to the next due to differences in the initial disequilibrium (a function of their initial allele frequency differences). Sillanpaa et al. (2001) have described a Bayesian approach to LD mapping in admixed populations that exploits a panel of unlinked markers using the genomic control techniques described in Chapter 9 to infer subpopulation membership.

It is important to appreciate the extreme variability in δ from marker to marker that would normally be expected. Figure 10.1 illustrates this phenomenon from a simulation of admixture of two large populations with disease allele frequencies of $q = 0.1$ and 0.2, each initially in complete linkage equilibrium with each of a set of SNP markers spaced at 1 cM intervals. Each of the marker allele frequencies was assumed to be uniformly

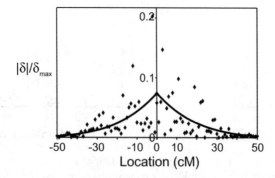

Figure 10.1 Simulated LD coefficients in a large admixed population after five generations of random mating. The solid line gives the theoretical curve $\bar{\delta}_0'(1-\theta)^5$, but note the considerable scatter about the line due to random variation in initial allele frequency differences from marker to marker, assuming perfect equilibrium in the founding populations and no random drift.

distributed in the two populations, with a correlation of 0.5 between the two populations. These values produce an average value of $\delta' = |\delta_0|/\delta_{max}$ of 0.07 in the combined population, a value that depends on the difference in disease allele frequencies between the two populations and the joint distribution of marker allele frequencies. However, the distribution of δ' is highly skewed, with a standard deviation of about 0.07. After five generations, the values of δ' have decayed as shown in the figure, together with the predicted curve $\bar{\delta}_0'(1-\theta)^5$. Although the LD coefficients are generally highest near the location of the disease gene, there are many markers with very small δ' values immediately adjacent to the gene, and others with relatively large values as much as 20 cM away.

The situation portrayed in Figure 10.1 represents a large population in which (*1*) there is no random drift and perfect equilibrium in the founding populations, (*2*) the disease genotype is in fact observed, rather than a phenotype with incomplete penetrance, and (*3*) the estimated δ' is based on an infinitely large sample. In short, the *only* component of variation simulated is in the allele frequency differences between the founding populations from marker to marker. In practice, the extent of LD that can be expected to result from admixture will be both smaller and more variable for all these reasons. In finite populations, we would expect there to be some disequilibrium between various markers and the disease locus simply due to drift, selection, founder effects, and so on, which tend to add to the variability in initial LD. As shown in Table 9.4, incomplete penetrance leads to considerable attenuation of the magnitude of the association between markers and a disease *phenotype* that might be expected, compared with what might be

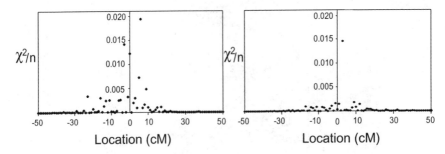

Figure 10.2 Simulated 1 *df* chi square noncentrality parameters for the simulations shown in Figure 10.1 under a fully penetrant recessive model (left) and a fully penetrant dominant model (right).

expected if the *genotypes* could be directly observed. And of course, having a modest-sized epidemiologic sample will add additional sampling variability to the observed associations.

To get a feeling for the expected association with a disease phenotype, Figure 10.2 shows the noncentrality parameters (λ) for a correctly specified chi-square test corresponding to the same simulated parameters as Figure 10.1 under fully penetrant recessive and dominant models. Under the recessive model, the mean of λ in generation zero is 0.0067, and under the dominant model it is 0.0022. Thus, to attain a chi square of $(1.96 + 1.28)^2 = 11.5$ (for 80% power at a nominal significance level of 5%, ignoring multiple comparisons), a sample size of $11.5/0.0022 = 1567$ cases and 1567 controls would be needed under the recessive model or 4773 each under the dominant model. Of course, these sample size requirements depend in a complicated way on the various model parameters, and the values shown here may be a best-case scenario: although they appear to be relatively insensitive to f_2, even slight increases in the sporadic case rate (f_0) greatly increase the sample size requirements; lower marker allele frequencies or smaller differences in allele frequencies between populations at either locus also lead to larger sample size requirements.

Isolated Populations

In contrast, the situation of an isolated population is likely to generate extremely localized peaks (but still showing substantial variability from one marker to the next). A population that has been isolated for 500 generations, for example, would have less than 0.01 of its initial disequilibrium at $\theta > 0.01$. Here the prevailing model is for a single mutation that was introduced by one of the founder members of the population (or by new mutation relatively soon after founding) and that has expanded by random drift to attain a substantial prevalence today. Diseases that tend to occur with unusually high prevalence in such an isolate would be good candidates for mapping by LD. The causal mutation in the founding individual must have occurred on a specific haplotype of surrounding markers. Over time, this haplotype would gradually have become whittled away by recombination, but most carriers of the founding mutation would tend to share some portion of the original haplotype. The closer to the disease locus, the stronger the disequilibrium would be.

However, the variability in LD from marker to marker again tends to be very high for many of the same reasons discussed in the previous section. A hotly debated question is whether the range of LD in most human populations is wide enough or large enough in magnitude to be useful for mapping purposes. Theoretical calculations based on coalescent theory (Kruglyak, 1999) indicated that significant LD was unlikely to extend much beyond 10–40 kb, but subsequent empiric studies (Dunning et al., 2000) provided evidence of significant LD extending to 100 kb ($\sim$0.1 cM) or more. In any event, it is clear that LD in population isolates is generally so narrow as to be useful only for fine mapping after the gene has been localized to a quite small region, in contrast to the situation in admixed populations, where it could potentially be used for genome-wide scans if the founding populations are different enough genetically to produce LD that is sufficiently large in magnitude.

A wide variety of techniques have been proposed to detect such patterns. These can be broadly classified into (*1*) parametric methods that attempt to model the dynamics of the genes over the history of the population and (*2*) empiric methods that simply aim to detect a pattern of decay of LD across the marker map. Parametric methods are highly complex and involve maximum likelihood or MCMC methods for fitting population genetics models, incorporating some knowledge of the history of the population (its age and rate of growth, for example) (Graham and Thompson, 1998; Hastbacka et al., 1992; Hill and Weir, 1994; Kaplan et al., 1995; Rannala and Statkin, 1998; Xiong and Guo, 1997). The central technique underlying all these methods is the *coalescent* (Chapter 8), a mathematical representation of the evolution of alleles in a population leading back to a common ancestor in the form of a distribution of tree structures showing the possible ancestral relationships between the members of a sample of the present-day population (Griffiths and Tavaré, 1994a, 1994b) and extensions of this approach to multilocus problems with recombination (Griffiths and Marjoram, 1996). These parametric models could in principle also be applied to admixed populations (Bahlo and Griffiths, 2000, 2001; Herbots, 1997), but so far, most of the applications of these methods have been to population isolates.

Because of their complexity, we defer further discussion of these approaches to the end of this chapter and begin by describing empiric methods that might be applicable to either type of population. Peltonen et al. (2000) provide an excellent review of the advantages and disadvantages of using isolated populations for gene mapping and the various statistical approaches that have been used.

Empiric Methods for Estimating the Location of a Disease Gene or Mutation

Lazzeroni (1998) and Cordell and Elston (1999) have described relatively simple methods to fit smooth curves to the estimated disequilibrium values $\hat{\delta}_m$ across a series of markers $m = 1, \ldots, M$, allowing for their interdependency, and thereby estimate the location of the peak of the curve and a valid confidence interval for that location. Lazzeroni approximates the theoretical $\delta \propto (1 - \theta)^T$ relationship by a Taylor series of the form

$$y(\delta_m) = \sum_{j=0}^{J} \beta_j |x_m - x_0|^j$$

for some normalizing transformation $y(.)$ of the δ_m, where x_m are the observed marker locations and β and x_0 are parameters to be estimated, x_0 being the location of the disease gene that is of primary interest. For additional flexibility, different slope coefficients β can be estimated proximal and distal to x_0. A bootstrap method is used to estimate the confidence interval around $\hat{x}_0$, allowing for the LD between markers.

Cordell and Elston use similar methods, but based instead on a quadratic approximation for the relationship between some transformation of LD, $y(\delta_m)$, and some transformation of distance, $X(|x_m - x_0|)$, of the form

$$y(\delta_m) = \beta_0 + \beta_1 X(|x_m - x_0|) + \beta_2 [X(|x_m - x_0|)]^2$$

The observed $\mathbf{y} = (y_1, \ldots, y_M)$ is treated as a single multivariate normal vector so that β can be estimated as $\hat{\beta} = (\mathbf{X}^T \mathbf{V}^{-1} \mathbf{X})^{-1} \mathbf{X}^T \mathbf{V}^{-1} \mathbf{y}$. However, since there is only a single realization of the $\mathbf{y}$ vector, the covariance matrix V is estimated by a bootstrap procedure similar to that of Lazzeroni. Given this estimate of β, a new estimate of x_0 is given by $x_0' = x_0 - \hat{\beta}_1 / 2\hat{\beta}_2$ and a confidence limit on $\hat{x}_0$ is obtained by the delta method.

Zhao et al. (1998a, 1999) have described GEE approaches to combining the highly localized by highly unstable LD information with the smoother long-range information from linkage using family data. Thus, Zhao et al. (1999) propose considering a joint parameter of the form $\delta(\theta - 0.5)$ and plotting this index for each marker separately. Zhao et al. (1998a) focus instead on multipoint LD analysis of associations with SNPs, exploiting the correlations between markers using an empirical covariance matrix without explicitly forming haplotypes.

All these methods are essentially based on separate estimates of $\hat{\delta}_m$ for each marker. Although the correlations between markers are allowed for in various ways, such approaches fail to exploit the full information content of tightly linked markers. To accomplish this, it is essential to consider how they are arranged into haplotypes. The difficulty is that without family data, it is not generally possible to determine with certainty how the observable multilocus genotypes are arranged into two haplotypes each. In addition, with each additional marker locus, the number of possible haplotypes that could exist becomes larger and larger, raising the related problems of multiple comparisons and sparse data: with many possible haplotypes, the frequency of false positive associations increases, and the amount of data to estimate any particular haplotype association becomes more limited. A number of methods have been proposed to address some of these problems. Several authors (Chiano and Clayton, 1998; Schaid et al., 2002; Stram et al., 2003b; Zaykin et al., 2002) have described E-M algorithm approaches to the problem of haplotype assignment. Letting $\mathbf{H}_i = (H_{i1}, H_{i2})$ denote the pair of haplotypes for individual i and $\mathbf{G}_i$ the corresponding genotypes, the likelihood is formed by summing over all possible haplotype assignments

$$\mathcal{L}(\boldsymbol{\beta}, \mathbf{q}) = \prod_i \sum_{\mathbf{h}} \Pr(Y_i \mid \mathbf{H}_i = \mathbf{h}; \beta) \Pr(\mathbf{H}_i = \mathbf{h} \mid \mathbf{G}_i; \mathbf{Q})$$

where $\boldsymbol{\beta}$ are the relative risk parameters for a logistic model for the penetrance associated with each haplotype and $\mathbf{Q}$ is a vector of the population frequencies of each of the possible haplotypes. The expression given above is a form of "prospective" likelihood that would be strictly valid only for cohort studies. When applied to case-control data, it would tend to overestimate the Q_h of high-risk haplotypes (that would be overrepresented in a case-control sample) and lead to some bias in the β_h as well. Stram et al. (2003) describe an ascertainment-corrected prospective likelihood and Epstein and Satten (2003) describe an alternative parameterization for the retrospective likelihood; see Thomas et al. (2003) for a comparison of the two approaches. Zhao et al. (2003) provide a robust GEE approach to fitting essentially the same model.

To address the problems of multiple comparisons and sparse data, Thomas et al. (2001) proposed a Bayesian smoothing of the βs using either an independence model, $\beta_h \sim \mathcal{N}(0, \sigma^2)$, *iid* or an intrinsic autoregressive model, $\beta_h \sim \mathcal{N}(\bar{\beta}_{-h}, \tau^2 / \sum_{k \sim h} w_{hk})$, where $\bar{\beta}_{-h} = \sum_{k \sim h} w_{hk} \beta_k / \sum_{k \sim h} w_{hk}$ and the weights w_{hk} are some measure of the *prior similarity* of any two haplotypes, say the number of markers at which they agree or the length of the longest shared segment. In order to estimate the location of a mutation, x, these weights might be taken as the length $L_{hk}(x)$ of the segment surrounding x that is shared by haplotypes h and k, which is then allowed to vary over the MCMC fitting process (Molitor et al., 2003a).

An attractive alternative, in the spirit of the coalescent methods described below, is to assume that haplotypes are clustered into a smaller number of clusters $c = 1, \ldots, C$, conceptualized as the descendants of common ancestral haplotypes. One could then assume that $\beta_h \sim \mathcal{N}(\gamma_{c_h}, \sigma^2)$, $\gamma_c \sim \mathcal{N}(0, \tau^2)$, and $\Pr(\mathbf{c} \mid \mathbf{H})$ exploit the spatial similarities of the haplotypes using a Bayesian spatial clustering model (Molitor et al., 2003b). Thomas et al. (2003) provide a comprehensive review of haplotype association methods.

Haplotype Sharing Methods

Sharing of haplotypes among family members has been used as a fine mapping technique for years, as described in Chapter 8. Among closely related individuals, however, shared segments tend to be very long, so only a handful of critical recombinants might be observed within the region of interest. Among apparently unrelated individuals who in fact carry a common ancestral mutation, the expected length of the shared ancestral segment surrounding that mutation will be much smaller, as described in Chapter 8. Such information has been used informally by various investigators in an attempt to map genes by LD (Houwen et al., 1994). Recently, a variety of approaches have been developed to provide a statistical basis for such comparisons (Boon et al., 2001; Bourgain et al., 2000, 2001a, 2001b; Devlin et al., 2000; Fischer et al., 2003; Nolte, 2002; Qian and Thomas, 2001; Schork et al., 1999; Te Meerman and Van Der Meulen, 1997; Tzeng et al., 2003; Van Der Meulen and Meerman, 1997; Zhang et al., 2003; Zhang and Zhao, 2000). Here the basic idea is that such pairs may descend from a common ancestor who transmitted the same mutant disease allele to them, together with some segment of the surrounding haplotype. Such pairs should thus share a common haplotype *in the neighborhood of the disease locus* more than randomly selected pairs of individuals.

Te Meerman and Van Der Meulen proposed a *haplotype sharing statistic (HSS)* based on the variance of the shared lengths $L_{hk}(x)$ of haplotypes surrounding a possible location x across all possible pairs (h, k) of case haplotypes. A randomization test (based on randomly reassigning case or control status) is used to evaluate the significance of the observed statistic. Qian and Thomas's procedure is similar in spirit but relies on family data to assign haplotypes and to assign to each founder haplotype a *disease score* d_h based on the number of transmissions and/or nontransmissions to affected and/or unaffected members of the family. Their *haplotype sharing correlation (HSC)* statistic is then based on the correlation between $D_{hk} = (d_h - \bar{d})(d_k - \bar{d})$ and their corresponding shared lengths $L_{hk}(x)$ across all pairs of haplotypes for apparently unrelated individuals. A randomization test is again used to assess the significance of this correlation. The maximum identity length contrast (MILC) method (Bourgain et al., 2000, 2001a, 2001b) also uses family data (specifically case–parent trios) to compare the maximum difference of mean sharing between transmitted and nontransmitted haplotypes over an entire region, again tested against its permutation distribution obtained by random reassignment of transmitted and nontransmitted alleles for each parent; this method does not provide an estimate of the location of the causal mutation, only a test of region-wide significance. It has been shown to have better power than using unrelated individuals. Zhang et al. (2003) describe a TDT based on haplotype sharing, which appears to have better power than standard single-marker or haplotype TDTs, essentially because of it's reduced df. Various transformations of $L_{hk}(x)$ might be helpful, such as replacing them by the conditional expectation of time to a common ancestor $E(T \mid L) = 3/[2L + 1/(2N)]$ (see page 246), but the properties of such transformations do not appear to have been systematically investigated. Tzeng et al. (2003) provide a unified framework for many of these haplotype sharing statistics in terms of a quadratic form, for which a general expression for its asymptotic variance can be derived. They show by simulation that haplotype sharing tests can be more powerful than haplotype association tests for common disease haplotypes, but for rare haplotypes, association methods are more powerful.

Parametric Methods Based on the Coalescent

The full probability distribution for all the unknowns in a coalescent model, including the location of a disease gene x, given a set of genotype data on cases and controls, might be written as

$$[\mathbf{Y} \mid \mathbf{H}, x, \beta] \cdot [\mathbf{G} \mid \mathbf{H}] \cdot [\mathbf{H} \mid H_{\text{anc}}, \Lambda, \mathbf{m}, \mathbf{r}] \cdot [\mathbf{m} \mid \Lambda, \mathbf{T}, \mu]$$
$$\cdot [\mathbf{T} \mid \Lambda] \cdot [\mathbf{r} \mid \Lambda] \cdot [\Lambda] \cdot [H_{\text{anc}}]$$

$$(10.1)$$

where for notational simplicity $[\cdot|\cdot]$ indicates a conditional probability distribution. Here Λ ranges over the space of all possible ancestral recombination graphs, $\mathbf{T}$ over coalescence or recombination times, $\mathbf{m}$ over mutations, $\mathbf{r}$ over recombination locations, $\mathbf{H}$ over haplotype assignments for the observed multilocus genotypes $\mathbf{G}$, and H_{anc} over possible haplotypes of the MRCA. From this, a likelihood for the observable data $\mathbf{Y}$ and $\mathbf{G}$ could in principle be computed by summing (or integrating) over all the unobservable variables $(\mathbf{H}, \mathbf{T}, \Lambda, \mathbf{m}, \mathbf{r})$ as a function of x, the penetrance parameters β, and mutation rate μ. Needless to say, the size of these summations is far too vast to allow direct calculation and maximization of this likelihood. Hence most implementations of parametric LD mapping methods have relied on approximations to this likelihood and/or MCMC methods.

While methods relying on the full treatment of ancestral recombination graphs are prohibitively complex, some progress has been made by considering one locus at a time, using similar likelihood formulations based on coalescent trees. For example, Graham and Thompson (1998) have described an MCMC approach to fitting the likelihood for a given mutation location. Others (Hill and Weir, 1994; Kaplan et al., 1995; Rannala and Statkin, 1998; Xiong and Guo, 1997; Zollner and von-Haeseler, 2000) have proposed a *composite likelihood* approach to estimating the likelihood by combining such *marginal* likelihoods for each possible mutation location in ways that allow for the dependency in coalescent structures from one location to the next.

McPeek and Strahs (1999) considered a likelihood-based approach that does not rely explictly on coalescent theory but exploits the theoretical results discussed in Chapter 8. They infer the ancestral mutation-bearing haplotype h_{anc} from which present-day mutant haplotypes h_i are derived using a likelihood of the form

$$\mathcal{L}(x, h_{\text{anc}}, T) = \prod_i \sum_{\ell < x < r} I[h_i(\ell, \dots, r) \sim h_{\text{anc}}(\ell, \dots, r)]\, g(T, \ell, r)$$
$$\times P_{\text{null}}[h_i(1, 2, \dots, \ell - 1)]\, P_{\text{null}}[h_i(r + 1, \dots, M)]$$

where $g(T, \ell, r)$ is given by Eq. (8.6), the notation $I(h_i \sim h_{\text{anc}})$ is an indicator of whether h_i and h_{anc} are identical over the indicated range of markers, and $P_{\text{null}}(h_i)$ is the probability of the observed sequence of markers by chance, given their allele frequencies and any LD between them. In this approach, h_{anc} is treated as a *parameter* to be estimated by maximum likelihood (together with T and x), rather than as a latent variable to be summed over as in the full likelihood, Eq. (10.1).

There are several additional simplifying assumptions implicit in this formula. First, the present-day haplotypes h_i are assumed to be known with certainty, without the complications of having to be inferred from observed genotypes; this would generally require the existence of some family data to make this assignment. Likewise, the set of haplotypes included in the analysis are all assumed to carry a disease mutation, as might be the case for a fully penetrant recessive gene for which *both* haplotypes carried by cases could be assumed to carry the mutation. For notational simplification, this expression assumes that there is only a single disease mutation, although McPeek and Strahs also allow for the possibility of a second common mutation and an indistinguishable set of additional rare mutations. The expression given above also does not allow for mutations at the marker loci, although again, their paper includes an extension to allow for that situation. Finally, each of the present-day haplotypes is assumed to be independently descended from the ancestral haplotype (a *star-shaped* genealogy) rather than to have the hierarchical structure of relationships that might be expected from a coalescent model. A similar approach to *ancestral haplotype reconstruction* has also been described by Service (1999). Ophoff et al. (2002) describe an application of this approach to LD mapping of bipolar disorder in a Costa Rican isolate.

Some of these limitations are relaxed in a subsequent paper by Morris et al. (2000), who describe an MCMC implementation of this basic approach. The most important difference between their two approaches is that Morris et al. treat the ancestral haplotypes h_{anc} and their associated ages as random variables rather than as parameters and sample them using MCMC methods to derive a marginal distribution for x that reflects the uncertainty in the assignment of h_{anc} and T's. They also generalize the approach in several other ways, such as allowing for phenocopies and non-independent ancestral histories. Morris et al. (2002) further extend their approach to relax the assumption of a star-shaped genealogy using what they call a *shattered coalescent*. Additional generality could be obtained by using reversible jump MCMC methods (Green, 1995) to allow for uncertainty in the number of ancestral haplotypes by including moves to add and delete ancestral haplotypes from the model. Recent developments along these lines have been described by Lin et al. (2002), Liu et al. (2001), Niu et al. (2002), Stephens et al. (2001b), and Zhang et al. (2002b).

Kuhner and Felsenstein (2000; Kuhner et al., 1995) describe a more ambitions MCMC sampler that does directly entail sampling from the space of possible ancestral recombination graphs Λ for an observed sample of haplotypes. Although this work is described as preliminary, in principle a full implementation of such an approach would entail a number of different MCMC moves, each entailing sampling from one of the distributions being summed over in Eq. (10.1): for example, sampling topologies Λ, coalescence/recombination times $\mathbf{T}$, haplotypes $\mathbf{H}$, mutation locations x, and the various model parameters μ, β, while summing over **m** using a peeling-like recursion algorithm.

How Much Linkage Disequilibrium Is There in the Human Genome?

These techniques are undergoing rapid development. At this point, the key unknown issue is how useful such techniques will turn out to be in practice. Despite some limited success in identifying genes for such conditions as cystic fibrosis (Kerem et al., 1989), Huntington's disease (MacDonald et al., 1991, 1992), and diastrophic dysplasia (Hastbacka et al., 1992), it is still not clear whether these are unique situations or whether similar methods will be useful in other situations.

Crucial to resolution of this question will be how much LD actually exists in different populations. In an influential paper, Kruglyak (1999) described theoretical predictions, based on coalescent simulations, of the decay of LD with physical distance and concluded that "a useful level of LD is unlikely to extend beyond an average distance of roughly 3 kb in the general population," where "useful LD" corresponds to roughly an r^2 of at least 0.1. Thus, he concluded that a panel of approximately 500,000 SNPs would be required for genome-wide association studies. He also predicted that the extent of LD would be similar in isolated populations unless the founding bottleneck was very narrow or the mutation was rare ($<5\%$). Ott (2000), however, pointed out that Kruglyak's simulations were conducted assuming a continuously expanding population, and argued that bottlenecks and cycles of expansion and contraction would be expected to produce more LD. He cited the article by Collins et al. (1999) as indicating that the calculations were "clearly contradicted by observed data" and concluded that perhaps only 30,000 SNPs might be required.

Numerous empirical studies have been reported, showing highly discrepant patterns in different populations and different regions of the genome (Abecasis et al., 2001; Dunning et al., 2000; Goldstein, 2001; Mohlke et al., 2001; Przeworski and Wall, 2001; Reich et al., 2001; Stephens et al., 2001a; Taillon-Miller et al., 2000). For example, Reich et al. (2001) examined 19 randomly selected genomic regions in a sample of 44 unrelated individuals from Utah and found that LD typically extends 60 kb from common alleles. A similar pattern was found in a sample of 48 southern Swedes. In contrast, in a sample of 96 Yorubans (from Nigeria), the half-length of LD was less than 5 kb. Stephens et al. (2001a) described pairwise LD and haplotype variation in 313 genes in 82 individuals from four populations and found a highly variable pattern of LD, with 30% of pairs that were separated by >20 kb having a $\Delta' = 1$.

Caution is needed in interpreting patterns of LD from small samples such as these: since the average value of the *estimated* LD coefficients, $E(\hat{r}^2)$, will be $r^2 + \text{var}(r)/N$, small samples tend to exaggerate the amount of LD actually present in a population. In a much larger sample of 837 NIDDM cases and 386 controls from the Finnish population, Mohlke et al. (2001) found quite substantial LD among a panel of microsatellite markers on chromosome 20 at distances as great as 3–4 cM. On the other hand, in an analysis of 38 SNPs from three chromosomal regions in a sample of 1600 individuals of European descent (Afrikaners, Ashkenazim, Finns, and East Anglian British), Dunning et al. (2000) found mean D' of 0.68 for marker pairs less than 5 kb apart, 0.24 for pairs 10–20 kb apart, and no significant LD for pairs greater than 500 kb apart. Pritchard and Przeworski (2001) provide an excellent review of both the theory and empirical data. Figure 10.3 illustrates some of the variability in LD that has been observed in various populations.

The first genome-wide survey of SNP variation was reported by Reich et al. (2002), who characterized data from 1.42 million SNPs from the SNP Consortium (Sachidanandam et al., 2001) and the BAC overlap project. They found considerable local variation in the rate of heterozygosity across the genome, with a correlation between segments that declined from about 0.97 at distances of 100 bp to about half that at 8 kb and remained significant as far as 100 kb (Fig. 10.4). This correlation could be due either to shared ancestry or to autocorrelation in the true mutation rate along the chromosomes. Using coalescent simulation, Reich et al. showed that the former accounted for about 75% of the variation in rates of sequence variation. Much has been written recently on the characteristics of human genetic diversity (e.g., Cargill et al., 1999; Pritchard and Cox, 2002; Reich and Lander, 2001; Tishkoff and Verrilli, 2003). We revisit this literature in terms of its implications for genome wide association studies in Chapter 13 (p. 358).

Haplotype block structure

A flood of papers (Ardlie et al., 2002; Cardon and Abecasis, 2003; Clark et al., 1998; Conti and Witte, 2003; Daly et al., 2001; Gabriel et al., 2002; Goldstein, 2001; Jeffreys et al., 2001; Patil et al., 2001; Phillips et al., 2003; Stephens et al., 2001a; Stumpf and Goldstein, 2003; Zhang et al., 2002a) has pointed out that the pattern of LD in the human genome appears to be highly nonrandom, with well-defined *blocks* in which only a very small proportion of all possible haplotypes account for most of the variation actually seen, separated by regions of relatively low LD. Jeffreys et al. (2001) provide a typical picture, shown in Figure 10.5, for the 216 kb long class II region of

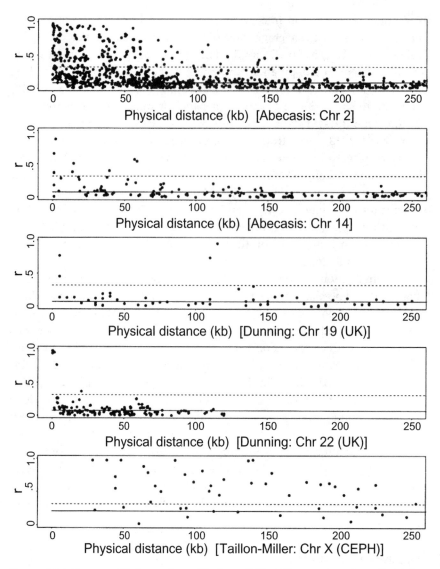

Figure 10.3 Decay of linkage disequilibrium (LD) (r^2) as a function of physical distance (in kb) for single nucleotide polymorphism data from five regions. Points above the solid line represent significant LD at the 0.05 level and points above the dotted line correspond to what Kruglyak (2000) called *useful* LD. (Reproduced with permission from Pritchard and Przeworski, 2001)

the MHC region (from *HLA-DNA* to *TAP2*). The degree of shading below the diagonal indicates the strength of LD (measured by the $|D'|$ statistic), and that above the diagonal indicates the degree of statistical significance (measured by the LR statistic) for each pair of loci. For common SNPs (minor allele frequency >15%, panel B), the entire region appears to be

(A)

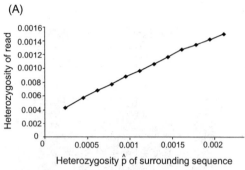

Figure 10.4 Correlation in single nucleotide polymorphism heterozygosity. (A) Heterozygosity of individual sequence reads in relation to the heterozygosity of the flanking sequences 2.5 kb on either side of the read. (B) Correlation in heterozygosity between pairs of reads (corrected for stochastic variance) as a function of the distance between them. (Reproduced with permission from Reich et al., 2002)

(B)

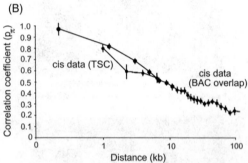

broken up into three major blocks (indicated by lighter shading), with generally low degrees of LD between blocks (the off-diagonal blocks). Panel C provides the comparable picture for rare SNPs, showing a finer block structure. Panels D and E provide expansions of two of the blocks shown in panel B (the *HLA-DNA* and *HLA-DMB* regions, respectively). These data are based on genotyping sperm samples from 50 British donors. Because sperm are haploid, it is easy to estimate LD directly without having to use the E-M approach described in Chapter 8 to resolve haplotypes in double heterozygotes. Recall, however, that estimates of $|D'|$ are upwardly biased in small samples.

Daly et al. (2001) have investigated this phenomenon further by examining extended haplotypes rather than just pairwise LD in a 500 kb region of chromosome 5q31. The data derived from a study of Crohn's disease in 256 case-parent trios from Toronto, primarily Caucasians of Western European descent (Rioux et al., 2001). The analysis first examined the haplotype diversity in the entire region in overlapping five-marker haplotypes, comparing the observed to expected heterozygosity. On this basis, regions with locally low heterozygosity were identified and expanded or contracted to define haplotype blocks. The frequency of the major haplotypes within each block and the patterns of LD between haplotypes in adjacent blocks were then estimated using a hidden Markov models approach. The resulting

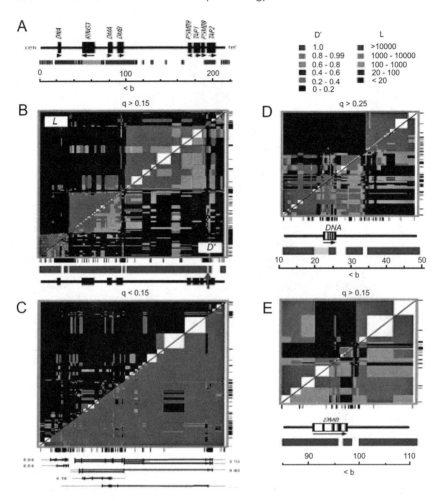

Figure 10.5 Pairwise linkage disequilibrium measured in the class II major histocompatibility complex region; see text for explanation. (Reprinted with permission from Jeffreys et al., 2001)

pattern is shown in Figure 10.6. In panel a, the first block comprises eight SNPs, with only two haplotypes accounting for 96% of the total frequency (panels b and c). Even the longest block (number 7, 92 kb with 31 SNPs) has only four haplotypes accounting for 93% of the total frequency. The LD between blocks is summarized in panel d, with the most common associations indicated by dotted lines between pairs of adjacent haplotypes in panel a.

Daly et al. (2001) and Gabriel et al. (2002) interpret these block boundaries as hot spots of recombination, which is certainly a possible interpretation, although they could also simply represent old recombination events

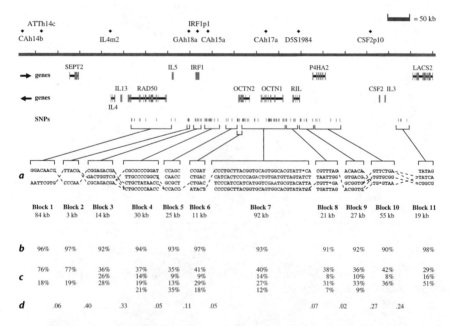

Figure 10.6 Block-like haplotype diversity at 5q31 : *a*) common haplotype patterns in each block of low diversity. *b*) Percentage of observed chromosomes that match one of the common patterns exactly. *c*) Percentage of each of the common patterns among untransmitted chromosomes. *d*) Rate of haplotype exchange between blocks. (Reprinted with permission from Daly et al., 2001)

in the coalescent process, where the recombinant haplotypes have since expanded to high prevalence today. Wang et al. (2002), Wall and Pritchard (2003a,b); and Phillips et al. (2003) have described coalescent simulations that demonstrate that block structure can arise purely from drift under constant recombination rates, although their distribution does not fit the observed patterns well without allowing for some variation in recombination rates. Certainly there is evidence of substantial variation in recombination rates across the genome. Kong et al. (2001) typed 869 individuals from 149 Icelandic sibships, representing a total of 628 paternal and 629 maternal meioses, at 5136 microsatellite markers across the human genome. Figure 10.7 illustrates the variation in recombination rates (male and female combined) across chromosome 3. Note the extremely local variability in these recombination rates. Whether the haplotype block structure found by Daly et al. actually correlates with variation in recombination rates remains to be seen. Again, sperm typing provides a direct measurement of recombination rates, based on very large sample sizes, without the need to assemble families (Arnheim et al., 2003; Boehnke et al., 1989; Hubert et al., 1994; Lazzeroni et al., 1994). In the study of LD in the MHC region discussed

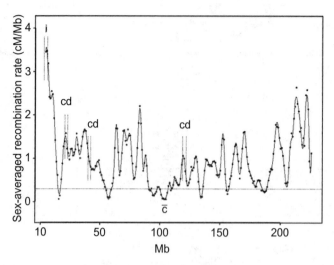

Figure 10.7 Sex-averaged recombination rate for chromosome 3. (Reprinted with permission from Kong et al., 2001)

above, Jeffreys et al. (2001) found five narrow (1–2 kb) recombination hot spots (three around *HLA-DNA* and two around *HLA-DMB*) corresponding to intervals of low LD. Further research on methods of estimating haplotype block structure, testing whether it corresponds to variation in recombination rates, allowing for the dependency in the coalescent process, and using this information in haplotype-based LD mapping methods would be very useful.

Patil et al. (2001) were the first to describe the haplotype block structure of an entire chromosome (chromosome 21) by genotyping 24,047 SNPs in a sample of 20 rodent-human somatic cell hybrids. Their algorithm identified a total of 4135 haplotype blocks, averaging 7.83 kb in length with an average of 2.72 common haplotypes per block. These common haplotypes required a total of 4563 *haplotype tagging SNPs (htSNPs)* to distinguish them, obviously many fewer than the total number tested to identify these haplotypes originally. Zhang et al. (2002b) have applied an alternative *dynamic programming* algorithm to these data that appears to be computationally more efficient. Their solution was somewhat more parsimonious, yielding only 2575 blocks that could be characterized by 3582 htSNPs. Variants of this approach provide methods for quantifying the significance of block boundaries (Mannila et al., 2003) and for finding the optimal partition yielding a given maximum number of htSNPs (Zhang et al., 2003). These applications were all applied to phase-known haplotype data. A variety of alternative methods have recently been proposed for selecting subsets of SNPs for subsequent use in case-control studies, where the haplotypes are not directly observed but must be reconstructed from unphased genotype data. Broadly, these fall into two types: htSNP selection algorithms (Huang et al., 2003; Stram et al., 2003b; Meng et al., 2003) aim to find a parsimonious subset of SNPs for predicting common haplotypes; Johnson et al. (2001), Thompson et al. (2003), and Weale et al. (2003) aim instead to predict each SNP's genotype based on a subset of the remaining ones, on the theory that any one of the SNPs in the data set could be a causal SNP. An application of Stram et al.'s method to data on *CYP19* (Haiman et al., 2003) revealed a significant global association of breast cancer risk with common haplotypes in one block of the gene; they also identified one long-range haplotype composed of haplotypes from two adjacent blocks that conferred a significant *RR* of 1.3.

A massive resequencing project known as the HapMap Project (Couzin, 2002) is currently underway, aimed at characterizing haplotype blocks across the entire genome and identifying a minimal subset of SNPs that would be sufficient to characterize the most common haplotypes. The hope is that this will reduce the number of SNPs that would be required for genome-wide association studies (as suggested by Risch and Merikangas, 1996) from several million by at least an order of magnitude. Of course, it remains to be seen whether such common variants are really the cause of common complex diseases (Pritchard, 2001). The computational challenges posed by trying to identify haplotype blocks and haplotypes from genome-wide diploid genotype data are formidable and deserve further attention.

Despite the considerable attention that is currently being devoted to describing haplotype block structure and searching for htSNPs, it remains an open question whether associations with disease genes can be detected with greater power using haplotypes or genotypes. As of this writing, there is only a very small literature on this question (Akey et al., 2001; Bader, 2001; Judson et al., 2000; Kirk and Cardon, 2002; Long and Langley, 1999; Morris and Kaplan, 2002; Schaid, 2002a; Schaid et al., 2002). Although it is generally held that haplotypes have greater potential than analyses of one SNP at a time when the causal variant is not included in the set of available SNPs or when there is a complex pattern of association with multiple SNPs, nevertheless there are several factors militating against their use. First, the number of possible haplotypes can become very large when many loci are under consideration, leading to the problems of sparse data and multiple comparisons. Second, the effect of a single causal variant may be spread out across a whole set of haplotypes that contain the same variant. Third, when one is analyzing case-control data on unrelated individuals, the uncertainty in the resolution of multilocus genotypes into haplotypes must be taken into account in the test. Most investigations of this question have compared haplotype associations with multiple single-SNP associations, using some form of correction for multiple comparisons for the latter. An exception is Conti and Witte (2003), who describe a hierarchical spatial models approach to simultaneously modeling the effects of all SNPs together, an approach that could potentially be extended to allow for SNP × SNP interactions. Further research comparing appropriate multivariate models for haplotype and genotype associations would be helpful.

Conclusions

With the growing recognition of the limited power of family-based linkage analysis for detecting genes for complex diseases, there has been an explosion of interest in the use of LD for fine mapping or even for future genome-wide association scans. Relatively simple curve-fitting approaches can be used to model the pattern of pairwise LD between a disease and markers one at a time in order to smooth out the highly variable associations from marker to marker and thereby estimate the possible location of the causal mutation. More powerful techniques exploit multiple tightly linked markers, using such techniques as the multilocus TDT test, haplotype sharing between pairs of unrelated cases, and formal coalescent modeling. These techniques have had some success with the identification of rare major genes in isolated populations, where the disease is caused by a single founder mutation, but their utility for mapping complex diseases is still uncertain. A great deal of interest is currently directed at understanding the phenomenon of haplotype block structure and its potential utility for reducing the number of SNPs that might need to be tested in either a candidate gene association study or a genome-wide association scan by using only a subset of htSNPs. The next generation of the Human Genome Project, known as the HapMap Project, may generate valuable data on the potential of these methods for future gene-mapping efforts.

11

Gene Characterization

Suppose that we have identified a locus as a likely causal gene for the disease under study, a *candidate gene*. There are now a number of things we might wish to learn about that gene, including:

- whether in fact it is associated with the disease, after controlling for other risk factors such as ethnicity (see Chapter 9)
- the spectrum of mutations that occur among cases, as well as any *neutral polymorphisms* that occur no more commonly among cases than among the general population
- the biological effect of each mutation
- the genetic relative risks and dominance associated with each polymorphism
- the absolute age-specific penetrance function for each polymorphism
- the population allele frequencies for the different polymorphisms
- the molecular function of the gene

Depending on the specific aims of the study, how much is already known about the gene, and the anticipated frequency of mutations, one might adopt any of a number of different study designs. This chapter covers approaches to characterizing genes that are thought to be causally related to the disease.

Estimation of Genetic Risks

In principle, any of the designs for testing candidate gene associations discussed in Chapter 9 could also be used to characterize cloned genes, but some of them would not be very efficient for this purpose. In particular, for characterizing rare major susceptibility genes, a cohort study or a case-control study with unrelated controls would likely yield only a very small proportion of carriers, so that much of the genotyping burden would be essentially wasted. In most sections of this chapter, we will therefore focus on more efficient family-based designs that provide a means of obtaining samples that are enriched for gene carriers. For characterizing more common, low-penetrance genes, however, standard case-control and cohort designs using unrelated individuals are likely to be the design of choice. In the next section, following a brief review of epidemiologic designs using independent individuals, we discuss familial cohort study designs, including those based on anecdotal samples of heavily loaded families and various forms of multistage sampling to improve efficiency. We begin by focusing on genetic main effects and then turn to testing $G \times E$ and $G \times G$ interactions. The chapter concludes with a discussion of approaches to estimating carrier probabilities and searching for additional genes.

Cohort and case-control designs using unrelated subjects

Chapter 4 provided a general introduction to the design and analysis of cohort and case-control studies using unrelated individuals. The application of these designs to testing familial aggregation and to genetic associations was further elaborated in Chapters 5 and 9. The basic approach entails estimation of standardized incidence ratios (for a cohort study) or odds ratios (for a case-control study). To make a simple categorical exposure classification, contingency table methods for Poisson or binomial data can be used; for analyses of multiple or continuous covariates, Cox regression models (Eq. 4.5) or logistic regression models (Eq. 4.4) would be appropriate. We will discuss some extensions of these models to incorporate $G \times G$ and $G \times E$ interactions.

Although most epidemiologic studies focus primarily on the estimation of relative risk, absolute risk as a function of genotype (i.e., penetrance) is also of interest to the geneticist. Cohort studies allow direct estimation of this quantity, while case-control studies require incorporation of ancillary information on the population rate. For a cohort study, a traditional person-time analysis yields a grouped-time estimator of the age-specific incidence rates $\hat{\lambda}_{gs} = D_{gs}/T_{gs}$ for genotype g and age stratum s, where D_{gs} are the number of incident cases and T_{gs} is the total person-time in the corresponding cell (see Chapter 9 for details). (Obviously, s could include other stratifying factors like gender and race.) Cox regression yields an estimate of both the relative risk parameter(s) $\hat{\beta}$ and the baseline hazard function $\hat{\lambda}_0(t)$, so the modeled absolute incidence rate is $\hat{\lambda}_0(t) \exp(\mathbf{Z}'\hat{\beta})$. Of course, this assumes that the hazard ratio is constant over time, which is clearly not the case for breast cancer and *BRCA1,* so in this case one would either have to include an age interaction term in the model (as a time-dependent covariate) or stratify the analysis by genotype. For case-control data, an *OR* or a logistic regression model provides an estimator of the *RRs* $\hat{r}_g$ but no direct estimate of absolute risk. However, if the population risk $\bar{f}$ is known and, among controls, proportion $\hat{p}_g$ has genotype g, then the absolute penetrances f_g can be estimated by solving the equation $\bar{f} = \sum_g \hat{p}_g f_g = f_0 \sum_g \hat{p}_g \hat{r}_g$ for f_0 to obtain

$$\hat{f}_g = \frac{\hat{r}_g \bar{f}}{\sum_g \hat{p}_g \hat{r}_g}$$

As with the cohort method, this calculation could be applied to age-specific population rates $\bar{f}_t$ by assuming constant RRs [adjusting the genotype prevalences for differential survival if the penetrances are high via $p_g(t) = p_g S_g(t) / \sum_g S_g(t)$] or by including age interaction terms. Whether cohort or case-control data are used, the estimated incidence rates can then be combined in a life table approach to estimate the cumulative risk to any given age, as described in Chapter 4 (Table 4.1).

Familial cohort study designs

Population-based studies. As discussed in Chapter 5, one can also view family data as a cohort study, and this design has been popularized as an approach to characterization of measured genes as well, particularly in the context of efforts to characterize *BRCA1/2*. There are several variants of this idea. In its conceptually (but not operationally) simplest form, one might simply genotype everyone in a set of families (or all available members) and then analyze them as if they were a cohort of independent individuals under the assumption that the major dependencies between family members would be accounted for by the measured genes. In any event, residual familial dependencies would not bias the estimate of the candidate gene association, but it would lead to underestimation of its variance; some adjustment in the analysis, such as use of a robust sandwich variance estimator or bootstrap methods, could be used to allow for this dependency (Chapter 4).

This also assumes that families were not enrolled because of their disease status. Under single ascertainment, for example, one could simply exclude the probands from the analysis; under complete or multiple ascertainment, it is less clear how to proceed. We revisit this question below.

However, the major problem with this design is the need to genotype all the other family members. This could be quite expensive and could lead to bias if availability was related to phenotype, for example if mutation-carrying cases were more likely to have died. We therefore turn our attention to the simplest of the alternative designs, which has come to be known as the *kin cohort* design (Wacholder et al., 1998). Here one genotypes only the proband in each family (who could be either affected or unaffected) and then computes the age-specific incidence rates in the first-degree relatives of carriers and noncarriers separately using a standard Kaplan-Meier survival curve estimator (Chapter 4). If the gene is a rare dominant, then roughly 50% of the first-degree relatives of carriers will be carriers and most of the first-degree relatives of noncarriers will be noncarriers. More precisely, the probability distribution for a mother's genotype given her daughter's is computed by summing over the possible genotypes of the father:

$$\Pr(G_m \mid G_o) = \frac{\sum_{G_f} \Pr(G_o \mid G_m, G_f)\Pr(G_m)\Pr(G_f)}{\Pr(G_o)}$$

For example,

$$\pi_0 = \Pr(G_m = dd \mid G_o = dd) = \frac{(1)(1-q)^2(1-q)^2 + \frac{1}{2}2q(1-q)(1-q)^2}{(1-q)^2}$$

$$= 1 - q$$

$$\pi_1 = \Pr(G_m = dd \mid G_o = dD) = \frac{\frac{1}{2}(1-q)^2 2q(1-q) + (1)(1-q)^2 q^2}{2q(1-q)}$$

$$= \frac{1-q}{2}$$

Hence, the mother of a noncarrier has probability $1 - \pi_0 = q$ of being a carrier, while the mother of a carrier has probability $1 - \pi_1 = (1+q)/2$ of being a carrier. Although sisters have the same expected number of alleles as mothers, their distribution is more complex, owing to the possibility that they could share two alleles. Table 11.1 provides the exact distributions.

Thus, the survival function $S_1(t)$ in carrier relatives is roughly a 50-50 mixture of the survival functions for carriers ($\tilde{S}_1(t)$) and noncarriers $\tilde{S}_0(t)$

Table 11.1 Genotype Probabilities for First-Degree Relatives of a Proband, Given the Proband's Genotype

Proband's Genotype	Relative's Genotype		
	dd	dD	DD
PARENTS OR OFFSPRING			
dd	$1-q$	q	0
dD	$\frac{1-q}{2}$	$\frac{1}{2}$	$\frac{q}{2}$
DD	0	$1-q$	q
SIBLINGS			
dd	$1-q+\frac{q^2}{4}$	$q-\frac{q^2}{2}$	$\frac{q^2}{4}$
dD	$\frac{1}{2}-\frac{3q}{4}+\frac{q^2}{4}$	$\frac{1}{2}+\frac{q}{2}-\frac{q^2}{2}$	$\frac{q}{4}+\frac{q^2}{4}$
DD	$\frac{(1-q)^2}{4}$	$\frac{1}{2}-\frac{q^2}{2}$	$\frac{1}{4}+\frac{q}{2}+\frac{q^2}{4}$

and likewise for noncarrier relatives:

$$(1 - \pi_1)\tilde{S}_1(t) + \pi_1\tilde{S}_0(t) = S_1(t)$$

$$(1 - \pi_0)\tilde{S}_1(t) + \pi_0\tilde{S}_0(t) = S_0(t)$$

The carrier and noncarrier survival functions (and hence the penetrances) can therefore be derived by solving this system of linear equations from the observed carrier-relative and noncarrier-relative survival functions (Wacholder et al., 1998). Saunders and Begg (2003) compared the kin-cohort and standard case-control approaches; they concluded that the kin-cohort design could be substantially more efficient either for relatively common diseases or for rare mutations with a large GRR.

The first application of this approach was to a study of penetrance of *BRCA1/2* in Ashkenazi Jews in the Washington, D.C., area (Struewing et al., 1997). (This population was chosen because it was already known that Ashkenazi Jews have a high prevalence of three specific mutations in *BRCA1* or *BRCA2*; thus, genotyping costs could be minimized by testing only for these three mutations rather than having to sequence the entire gene.) A sample of 5318 volunteers, not selected by a personal or family history of disease, was genotyped, yielding 133 carriers of mutations in *BRCA1* or *BRCA2*. The estimated cumulative incidence rates of breast cancer in relatives of carriers and noncarriers are shown in Figure 11.1A, and the estimated penetrances are shown in Figure 11.1B. The cumulative risk to age 70 was estimated to be 56% for breast cancer (95% CI 40%–73%) and 16% for ovarian cancer (6%–28%) (not shown), both significantly lower than previous estimates from the Breast Cancer Linkage Consortium (Easton et al., 1993).

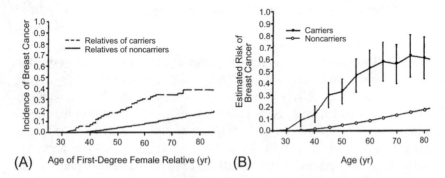

(A) Age of First-Degree Female Relative (yr)   (B)   Age (yr)

Figure 11.1 Kaplan-Meier estimates of the risk of breast cancer in Ashkenazi Jews: (A) Cumulative incidence in first-degree relatives of carriers (dashed line) and non-carriers (solid line). (B) Estimated penetrance (cumulative incidence) in carriers and noncarriers. (Adapted with permission from Struewing et al., 1997)

This approach does not make full use of all the available information. First, it is restricted to first-degree relatives. Second, it may be possible to genotype other family members as well, using an allele-specific oligonucleotide assay for the specific mutation carried by the proband. Third, the analysis is not fully efficient because it does not exploit the relationships of the relatives to each other, only their relationships to the proband. Finally, there is no requirement that the estimated penetrances be monotonic. These considerations led Gail et al. (1999a, 1999b) to propose several variants of this basic design that would exploit this information. In what they called the *genotyped-proband-genotyped-family-member (GPGF) design,* one would include all members of the family and use a likelihood-based analysis similar to segregation analysis, but conditional on the available genotypes. Letting $\mathbf{g} = (\mathbf{g}_{obs}, \mathbf{g}_{unk})$ denote the observed and the unobserved genotypes, respectively, the likelihood is then a modified form of the standard segregation analysis, now summing only over the genotypes of the untyped individuals,

$$\mathcal{L}(\lambda_g(.), q) = \sum_{\mathbf{g}_{unk}} \Pr(\mathbf{y} \mid \mathbf{g}; \lambda_g(.)) \Pr(\mathbf{g} \mid q) \qquad (11.1)$$

excluding the proband from the penetrance term to allow for ascertainment correction. This likelihood also extends the approach to other dominance and allele frequency models, as these parameters can be estimated jointly with the penetrances.

This approach was used by Hopper et al. (1999b) in the analysis of a population-based case-control family study of breast cancer under age 40. This analysis was restricted to first- and second-degree relatives of probands who had themselves been found to be carriers of a protein truncating mutation in exons 2, 11, or 20 of *BRCA1* or in exons 10 or 11 of *BRCA2* by the protein truncation test. The modified segregation analysis yielded an estimate of cumulative risk to age 70 in cases of only 40% (95% CL 15%–65%), smaller even than that from the study of Ashkenazi Jews and considerably smaller than that from the Breast Cancer Linkage Consortium. Other population-based studies (Anglian-Breast-Cancer-Study-Group, 2000; Risch et al., 2001; Thorlacius et al., 1998) have yielded similarly low penetrance estimates. A meta-analysis of 22 studies of families unselected by FH (Antoniou et al., 2003) obtained penetrance estimates (to age 70) for *BRCA1* of 65% (95% CI 44%–78%) for breast cancer and 39% (18%–54%) for ovarian cancer; for *BRCA2* the corresponding penetrances were 45% (31%–56%) and 11% (2%–19%).

The reasons for this discrepancy are still being debated (see, e.g., Begg, 2002, and the correspondence following), but it is possible, on the one hand, that the kinds of mutations found in high-risk families have a more deleterious effect than other mutations in these genes (such as the three ancestral mutations in Ashkenazi Jews). For example, it has been suggested that there is an *ovarian cancer cluster region* in *BRCA2,* where mutations are associated with a higher risk of ovarian cancer and a lower risk of breast cancer (Gayther et al., 1997; Thompson et al., 2001). On the other hand, high-risk families are probably more likely to have other breast cancer risk factors (genetic or environmental) that may modify the penetrance of *BRCA1/2,* so that the risk in such families is indeed higher than in the general population of carriers. Yet another possible explanation is that, despite the use of a mod score approach in the analysis of the Breast Cancer Linkage Consortium that ostensibly corrects for ascertainment bias (Eq. 7.6) and later in this chapter, there could be some bias in this approach if families are sampled not just on the basis of their disease phenotypes but also on the basis of the marker data. This could happen if the analysis was limited to families that show evidence of linkage. Siegmund et al. (1999a) have shown that either restriction to linked families (as in the analyses of the Breast Cancer Linkage Consortium [Easton et al., 1993, 1995; Ford et al., 1994, 1998]) or omission of a modifying factor that is correlated within families could lead to an overestimation of the penetrance in carriers. Hopper (2001) provides an excellent discussion of this controversy.

An important study design consideration is deciding whom to genotype. Unlike the kin cohort design, in which only the proband is genotyped, use of the full likelihood (Eq. 11.1) allows the genotypes of as many family members as are available to be included in the analysis without requiring everyone in the pedigree to be genotyped. Is the improvement in precision from having additional family members genotyped worth the cost? If so, does it make more sense to concentrate on affected family members, near or distant relatives of the proband, relatives of carrier probands, and so on? Such questions have been investigated by Siegmund et al. (2001), who found that the cost effectiveness of various strategies depended on the genetic model and the particular parameters of interest. For example, there was little to be gained by testing unaffected family members for a rare gene, but testing unaffected relatives greatly improved the estimation of the genetic *relative* risk for a common low-penetrance gene.

Recently, King et al. (2003) estimated the penetrance of the three ancestral *BRCA1/2* mutations among Ashkenazi Jews using the GPGF design, genotyping all available family members of carrier probands. Their analysis was restricted to family members (excluding probands) whose genotypes could be unambiguously determined, either by direct sequencing of blood samples of living relatives, by extracting DNA from surgical specimens for deceased cases, or by reconstructing genotypes from those of surviving children, thereby allowing direct estimation of penetrance using simple Kaplan-Meier survival functions rather than requiring the maximum likelihood method discussed above (Eq. 11.1). The resulting penetrance estimates—70% for breast cancer by age 70 for carriers of mutations in either gene, 54% or 12% for ovarian cancer in *BRCA1* and *BRCA2* carriers respectively—are substantially higher than those from other population-based series discussed above. Inconsistent with this, the overall prevalence of mutations among the affected probands—10.3%—was similar to that estimated from other studies of Ashkenazi Jews from which the lower penetrances referred to above were estimated. The reasons for these discrepancies are not clear but could be due to bias in the earlier likelihood-based estimates if the model was misspecified (e.g., by failing to allow for other causes of familial aggregation, genetic or environmental), ascertainment bias in families identified through affected probands (Begg, 2002), or real differences between populations or specific mutations (King et al.'s analysis is strictly generalizable only to ancestral mutations among Ashkenazi Jews). The most likely explanation, however, is selection bias in King et al.'s analysis due to unaffected individuals (particularly deceased ones) being preferentially unavailable for genotyping. The advantage of the likelihood-based approach is that it incorporates the phenotypes of *all* subjects, irrespective of whether their genotypes are known, properly allowing for the uncertainty about the genotypes of the untyped pedigree members.

Later on, we will review the risk of breast cancer in relation to another gene, *ATM*, which in homozygotes causes the recessive neurological disease ataxia-telangiectasia (A-T). It has also been suggested that *ATM* heterozygotes are at elevated risk of cancer, particularly breast cancer. This hypothesis is easily tested by studying the incidence of cancer in parents of A-T patients, who are obligatory heterozygotes, and comparing them with population rates using standard cohort analysis methods. In this case, no adjustment for residual familial aggregation is needed because the parents are genetically unrelated (although one might want to allow for the possibility of shared unmeasured environmental influences). Siblings, grandparents, aunts, and uncles of *ATM* cases are independently at a 50% risk of being *ATM* heterozygotes and could be included in such an analysis using methods like the kin cohort design described above. Since the gene is very large and, as with *BRCA1/2*, many mutations and polymorphisms have been identified, it is natural to wonder whether they all have the same penetrance. For example, Gatti et al. (1999) have suggested that missense mutations, which in their homozygous state do not cause A-T, may be more important than truncating mutations than in causing cancer in heterozygotes. Since the parents of A-T cases are unlikely to carry the same mutation or polymorphism, comparison of risks in the two sides of a family in relation to the alleles each carries will be a powerful approach to resolving this question. A study along these lines is currently underway (R. Haile, P.I.).

Use of high-risk families. If the gene is thought to be responsible for only a small proportion of the cases in the population, it may not be very efficient to use a population-based case series to characterize its prevalence and penetrance. This situation can arise either because the mutant allele(s) have very low population frequency or because the penetrance is low. In this case, there is a natural inclination to want to focus resources on families that are likely to carry the mutation. Thus, one might want to use families with many cases or restrict the study to the subset of these families that has already been shown by linkage to be likely carriers (*linked* families). It should be obvious that without correction for ascertainment, no valid estimates of population parameters could be obtained from such series. They would produce spuriously high estimates of mutation frequency as well as penetrance. Since they must have many cases to get into the sample, it would appear that disease rates (among carriers and noncarriers both) must be very high.

Nevertheless, there is a role for such studies. First, in the early stages of the characterization of a new gene, it is important to identify all the mutations, and if mutations are thought to be rare in the general population, any mutations among cases are likely to be causal. For this purpose, use of heavily loaded families is quite reasonable since no population parameters are being estimated.

Second, if the families have been sampled according to a simple and well-defined ascertainment scheme, it may be possible to correct for this to estimate population parameters. To illustrate this point, consider the following thought experiment. Suppose that one had only a population-based series of cases, with no controls. Obviously, one could not estimate penetrance from such a series, since all subjects had to have the disease to get into the sample. Likewise, the disease allele would also tend to be overrepresented in cases, so a naive estimate of that fraction would grossly exaggerate the population allele frequency. But if one knew the penetrances, then one could compute the ascertainment-corrected allele frequency by maximizing the likelihood

$$\mathcal{L}(q) = \left(\frac{f_0 (1-q)^2}{\Sigma(q)} \right)^{C_0} + \left(\frac{2 f_1 q (1-q)}{\Sigma(q)} \right)^{C_1} + \left(\frac{f_2 q^2}{\Sigma(q)} \right)^{C_2} \tag{11.2}$$

where $\Sigma(q)$ denotes the sum of the numerators and C_g are the number of cases with genotype g. This would require numerical solution, since there is no closed form expression for the MLE. In practice, of course, one probably would not know the penetrances either, and it would not be possible to use this likelihood to jointly estimate both penetrances and allele frequency from only a series of cases. Furthermore, for the highly selected families that are typically used for linkage analysis, there is generally no way to characterize mathematically how they were selected and hence no feasible ascertainment correction. Even for relatively simple multiplex ascertainment schemes, correction methods may still be intractable.

Pursuing this thought experiment further, since population controls are likely to have so few carriers that estimates of carrier risk using them would be highly unstable, how might one estimate the penetrances without obtaining population controls? The family members of the proband provide the solution. Some of these carry the same mutation as the proband and some do not. Since they were not involved in the sampling of probands, their outcomes should be representative of carriers and noncarriers in the general population, conditional on their genotypes, assuming no familial aggregation of other genetic or environmental risk factors. (Of course, their genotype prevalences tend to be higher than the general population.) Hence, penetrances can be estimated simply as disease rates in the usual way, with no further correction for ascertainment needed, say, using the standard person-years estimator. Alternatively, one might select matched controls from within the families, as described in Chapter 9, to estimate the relative risk. This can be a relatively cost-efficient design when no screening test for all mutations is available, since family members would need to be screened only for the particular mutation carried by the proband. Family members of probands with no mutation might also be assumed to be phenocopies if the mutation rate is very low. Be warned, however, that for more common mutations, this approach is potentially biased. In a matched case-control study, the only discordant pairs identified by such a design would be of the case-carrier/control-noncarrier type; the converse type would never be identified because controls for noncarrier cases would never get tested. Hence such a study would be expected to estimate an infinite genetic *RR*, even if the true *RR* was 1.0.

Finally, although absolute penetrances cannot be estimated from selected samples without ascertainment correction, estimates of *relative* risks are fairly insensitive to ascertainment bias because both the carrier and noncarrier rates are upwardly biased by comparable amounts. (Proof of this claim is somewhat technical, so the reader who is primarily interested in design issues can skip the following section.)

Proof: The likelihood contribution for family i under complete ascertainment is

$$L_i(f_0, f_1) = \frac{\prod_g \binom{N_{ig}}{C_{ig}} f_g^{C_{ig}} (1 - f_g)^{N_{ig} - C_{ig}}}{1 - \prod_g (1 - f_g)^{N_{ig}}}$$

where N_{ig} is the total number of individuals with genotype g of family i and C_{ig} is the number of family i cases with genotype g. Letting $N_g = \sum_i N_{ig}$, $C_g = \sum_i C_{ig}$, and $A_i = 1 - \prod_g (1 - f_g)^{N_{ig}}$, the total loglikelihood becomes

$$\ell(f_0, f_1) = \sum_g [C_g \ln f_g + (N_g - C_g) \ln(1 - f_g)] - \sum_i \ln A_i$$

The score function with respect to f_g is therefore

$$
\begin{aligned}
U_g &= \frac{C_g}{f_g} - \frac{N_g - C_g}{1 - f_g} - \frac{1}{1 - f_g} \sum_i N_{ig} \frac{(1 - A_i)}{A_i} \\
&= \frac{1}{f_g(1 - f_g)} [C_g - f_g(N_g + N'_g)] \\
&= \frac{1}{f_g(1 - f_g)} [(C_g - f_g N'_g) - f_g N_g]
\end{aligned}
$$

where $N'_g = \sum_i N_{ig}(1 - A_i)/A_i$. This suggests two possible iterative schemes for estimating the penetrances by replacing the current estimates by either of the following expressions:

$$
f'_g = \frac{C_g}{N_g + N'_g}
$$

$$
f'_g = \frac{C_g - f_g N'_g}{N_g}
$$

Obviously, without ascertainment correction, the crude penetrance estimators C_g/N_g would be seriously biased upward, but it is instructive to consider the corresponding crude estimators of relative risk $(C_g/N_g)/(C_0/N_0)$ or the odds ratio $C_g(N_0 - C_0)/(C_0(N_g - C_g))$. At convergence of the above iterative processes, the risk ratio would be given by the following expressions:

$$
\frac{f_g}{f_0} = \left(\frac{C_g/N_g}{C_0/N_0} \right) \left(\frac{1 + N'_0/N_0}{1 + N'_g/N_g} \right) = \left(\frac{C_g/N_g}{C_0/N_0} \right) \left(\frac{1 - f_g N'_g/C_g}{1 - f_0 N'_0/C_0} \right)
$$

The right-hand factors are generally very close to 1, so the crude risk ratio (the left-hand factor) is a close approximation to the true penetrance ratio f_g/f_0.

A possible use of this design might be to test the hypothesis the certain childhood cancers are caused by the *BRCA1* gene. Since *BRCA1* mutants are extremely rare in the general population and are therefore likely to be rare in childhood cancers, taking a random sample of childhood cancer cases would be highly inefficient. Instead, one might sample childhood cancers (probands) with a family history of breast cancer at an early age. Perhaps about 25% of these affected family members will be *BRCA1* carriers, and a subset of the probands of these will share the same gene IBD with the proband. One would first type the parent of the proband who could have transmitted that gene and, among those who test positive for *BRCA1*, then type the proband. The observed frequency of *BRCA1* mutations among these probands could then be compared to the null expectation of 50%.

Mod score approach to gene characterization. Given the complexity of ascertainment correction for high-risk families, an attractive alternative is to apply the mod score approach (Eq. 7.6) to the modified segregation analysis likelihood for the genotyped-proband design (Eq. 11.1). Kraft and Thomas (2000) compare four general approaches to likelihood construction for gene characterization studies:

$$\Pr\!\left(\mathbf{Y}_i \mid \mathbf{G}_i, \sum_j Y_{ij}\right) \quad \text{Conditional likelihood}$$
$$\Pr(\mathbf{Y}_i \mid \mathbf{G}_i, Asc_i) \quad \text{Prospective likelihood}$$
$$\Pr(\mathbf{G}_i \mid \mathbf{Y}_i) \quad \text{Retrospective likelihood}$$
$$\Pr(\mathbf{Y}_i, \mathbf{G}_i \mid Asc_i) \quad \text{Joint likelihood}$$

where Asc_i represents the ascertainment of family i, assumed to depend only on $\mathbf{Y}_i$, not on $\mathbf{G}_i$. Using a logistic function for $\Pr(Y_{ij} \mid G_{ij})$ in the conditional likelihood leads to the standard conditional logistic regression for matched data

$$\mathcal{L}_i^{(C)}(\beta) = \frac{\exp\left[\sum_j Z(G_{ij}) Y_{ij}\right]}{\sum_P \exp\left[\sum_j Z(G_{ij}) Y_{ip_j}\right]}$$

where $\mathcal{P}$ represents a set of all permutations $\mathbf{p} = (p_j)$ of the family members. The prospective and joint likelihoods require families to have been ascertained in some manner that can be described by a probability distribution for $\Pr(Asc_i \mid \mathbf{y}_i)$, which effectively limits their use to relatively simple random sampling schemes (e.g., single or complete ascertainment). The retrospective likelihood

$$\mathcal{L}_i^{(R)}(\beta, q) = \frac{\Pr(\mathbf{Y}_i \mid \mathbf{G}_i)\Pr(\mathbf{G}_i \mid q)}{\sum_{\mathbf{G}_i} \Pr(\mathbf{Y}_i \mid \mathbf{G}_i)\Pr(\mathbf{G}_i \mid q)}$$
$$= \frac{\prod_j \Pr(Y_{ij} \mid G_{ij})\Pr(G_{ij} \mid G_{ip_j}, q)}{\sum_{\mathbf{G}_i} \Pr(Y_{ij} \mid G_{ij})\Pr(G_{ij} \mid G_{ip_j}, q)}$$

(where p_j denotes the parents of subject j) has no such requirement and turns out to be remarkably efficient (in terms of the precision of estimates of penetrances and allele frequency), even where the other ascertainment schemes are possible—generally *more* efficient than the prospective likelihood. However, all these likelihoods assume no residual familial aggregation. Kraft and Thomas discuss the robustness of the various likelihood formulations to heterogeneity in penetrance parameters and/or allele frequencies and propose a mixed models approach to dealing with it. Gong and Whittemore (2003) compare the use of the retrospective likelihood for high-risk families with the joint likelihood for population-based families and conclude that the former gives more accurate penetrance estimates for rare mutations mainly because these families tend to include more mutation carriers.

These likelihoods can be applied to only the subset of family members for whom both phenotype and genotype information is available. However, phenotype information for other family members can be exploited by forming a likelihood similar to that used in segregation analysis by summing over the genotypes of all untyped family members conditional on the available genotype information.

Multistage sampling and countermatching

For characterizing rare mutations, a particular attraction of family designs is the opportunities they offer to improve efficiency by sampling in such a way as to increase the yield of mutation carriers in the sample. This can be done by some form of multistage sampling, with each successive stage of sampling being based on the accumulating information on genotypes, phenotypes, or other risk factors assembled from earlier stages. There are quite a few variants of this basic idea, depending on how the data are to be analyzed. In this section, we consider two such variants.

Whittemore and Halpern (1997) introduced the idea of multistage sampling of pedigrees and proposed a form of analysis based on *Horvitz-Thompson estimating equations* (Horvitz and Thompson, 1952). Their example of a genetic study of prostate cancer in African-Americans begins with a random sample of prostate cancer cases and unrelated population controls. These are stratified by family history (FH, the presence or absence of an affected first-degree relative based on a telephone interview) and a random sample of each of the four groups defined by case/control status, and FH is used in the second stage of sampling. These subjects then complete a more detailed interview, inquiring about family history in more distant relatives, and medical confirmation is sought for all reported familial cases. On this basis, a third-stage subsample comprised of families with three or more cases is selected to obtain blood samples for association and linkage studies.

The analysis of such designs using Horvitz-Thompson estimating equations would use only the data from the final stage and the sampling fractions that yielded these data. Consider a two-stage design with $s = 1, \ldots, S$ sampling strata, comprising N_s individuals in the original random sample S_1 and n_s in the second stage S_2. Let $U_i(\theta)$ denote the score contribution of the ith subject for estimating some parameter θ. Then the Horvitz-Thompson estimating equation is of the form

$$U(\theta) = \sum_{i \in S_2} \left(\frac{N_{s_i}}{n_{s_i}} \right) U_i(\theta) = 0$$

Table 11.2 Results for the Second Stage of Sampling in the Prostate Cancer Study of African-Americans

	Cases		Controls	
	FH+	FH−	FH+	FH−
EXPECTED NUMBERS OF SUBJECTS				
Probands, stage I	209	1291	92	1408
Mutation carriers	133.1	52.3	5.8	2.3
OPTIMAL SAMPLING FRACTIONS (NUMBER IN STAGE II)				
To minimize variance of:				
A. carrier penetrance	100% (209)	20% (258)	50% (46)	4% (56)
B. noncarrier penetrance	100% (209)	12% (155)	34% (31)	13% (183)
C. disease allele frequency	100% (209)	20% (258)	64% (59)	3% (42)
To maximize mutation yield	100% (209)	21% (271)	100% (92)	0% (0)

Source: Whittemore and Halpern (1997).

the solution to which, $\hat{\theta}$, has an asymptotic variance in the form of the familiar sandwich estimator for GEEs, Eq. (4.9).

With this form of analysis in mind, it is possible to decide what the optimal weights would be to minimize the variance of the parameter estimates. The form of weights requires that there be at least some representatives of all sampling strata, and the optimal weights depend on which parameter is of particular interest in a multiparameter model. Table 11.2 illustrates the results of such calculations for the second stage of sampling in the prostate cancer study described above, based on 1500 cases and 1500 controls in the initial sample and a budget sufficient to genotype a total of 570 subjects in the second stage.

Thus, for any parameter, the optimal design entails taking a 100% sample of FH+ cases, a somewhat smaller percentage of FH+ controls, a still smaller percentage of FH− cases, and the smallest percentage of FH− controls. (For different genetic models, the optimal design might be different.) For further discussion, including the implementation of these ideas in a family registry of colorectal cancer, see Siegmund et al. (1999b).

In some circumstances, it may be possible to consider sampling strategies that use genotype or exposure information collected on the proband before deciding whether to enroll other family members. For example, in an ongoing study of colorectal cancer, investigators are interested in pursuing the phenomenon of *microsatellite instability (MSI)* in relation to the *mismatch repair (MMR)* genes, *hMLH1* and *hMSH2* (Chapter 12), using the resources of an existing international Collaborative Family Registry. Probands have been enrolled from various centers, some registries using multistage sampling designs based on age and/or FH. All these probands will be initially assessed for MSI status, and 100% of MSI-high or -low cases and 10% of MSI-stable cases will then be genotyped for mutations in the MMR genes. For those found to carry mutations, all their available family members will then also be genotyped for the same mutation. Such studies must be designed with great care so that a valid analysis for the resulting data will be possible. Designs of such complexity are not generally amenable to optimization by analytical methods such as those described by Whittemore and Halpern, so simulation is commonly used to assess the statistical power of alternative sampling schemes.

A somewhat different approach might be taken for case-control studies, in which multistage sampling of subjects might be based on some easily measured surrogate for one or more of the risk factors under study. This could be done using either unmatched or matched designs. The idea was first introduced by White (1982) in the context of unmatched case-control studies, where cases and controls are initially stratified on the basis of a surrogate for exposure and different sampling fractions are taken in each of the cells of the resulting 2×2 table. The logarithm of these sampling fractions is then included as an *offset* term (a covariate with a coefficient fixed at unity) in a standard unconditional logistic regression of the more precise data that were collected on the second-stage subjects:

$$\text{logit } \Pr(Y_i = 1 \mid \mathbf{Z}_i) = \beta_0 + \mathbf{Z}_i'\boldsymbol{\beta} - \ln\left(\frac{N_{s_i}}{n_{s_i}}\right)$$

Breslow and Cain (1988), Cain and Breslow (1988), and Fears and Brown (1986) provide additional details.

For matched studies, Langholz and Borgan (1995) introduced the idea of *countermatching* on a surrogate for exposure. In a $1:1$ matched case-control study involving a dichotomous surrogate variable, for example, each surrogate-exposed case is paired with a surrogate-unexposed control and vice versa. The rationale for this procedure is to maximize the discordance in true exposure within the matched sets, as only discordant pairs are informative. Of course, this would be a biased design were the sampling fractions not taken into account in the analysis. This is easily done by including the log of the control sampling fractions for each case as an offset term in the standard conditional logistic regression

$$\mathcal{L}_i(\beta) = \frac{\exp[\mathbf{z}_i'\boldsymbol{\beta}]}{\sum_{j \in \tilde{R}_i} \exp[\mathbf{z}_j'\boldsymbol{\beta} - \ln(N_j)]}$$

where N_j is the number of potential countermatched controls that could have sampled for subject j had that person been the case. The case-control pairs could still be matched on other confounding factors the investigator wished to control.

Andrieu et al. (2001) extended this idea to studies of gene–environment interactions for which surrogates for exposure, genotype (e.g., FH), or both might be available. Specifically, they compared a standard $1:3$ matched design with $2:2$ countermatched designs based on surrogates for genotype or surrogates for exposure, or with a $1:1:1:1$ countermatched design using surrogates for both—that is, each set containing one case and three controls, representing one of each of the four possible surrogate–variable combinations.

This idea is currently being used in a study of the interaction between the *ATM* gene and radiation exposure in the etiology of second breast cancers in a cohort of survivors of a first breast cancer (Bernstein et al., under review). In this design, cases of second breast cancer are being countermatched to two controls each (those with first cancers who were diagnosed at the same age as the case and survived at least as long) on the surrogate variable of radiotherapy (yes or no) for treatment of the first breast cancer, requiring that each matched set contain two radiotherapy and one nonradiotherapy patient. Exposure assessment then requires abstraction of the details of the treatment protocols and dose reconstruction using phantoms. In all, 2700 women (900 cases and 1800 controls) will be included in this stage of sampling for dose reconstruction, genotyping, and interviewing for other risk factors. In a substudy of *BRCA1/2* interactions, the FH information will be used to estimate the probability that each case and each control is a mutation carrier for either of these genes using the BRCAPRO program (Parmigiani et al., 1998). Matched triplets from the main study will then be subsampled based on the probability that at least one member is a carrier.

Relative efficiency of the alternative designs

To compare the alternative designs, we introduce the concept of *asymptotic relative efficiency (ARE)*, defined as the ratio of the large-sample variances for estimators from alternative study designs and/or methods of analysis. Equivalently, it can be interpreted as the ratio of sample sizes that would be required to attain the same degree of statistical precision. Recall that the asymptotic variance of a parameter is given by the inverse of the expected Fisher information (Eq. 4.6), the second derivative of the loglikelihood,

$$\text{var}(\hat{\beta}) = \{E[\imath(\hat{\beta})]\}^{-1} = -\left\{E\left[\frac{\partial^2 \ell(\beta)}{\partial \beta^2}\right]_{\beta=\hat{\beta}}\right\}^{-1}$$

This expected information is computed by summing over all possible combinations of the observed data, in this case the genotypes and phenotypes, conditional on the ascertainment scheme of the data. For the simple logistic model, the information contribution from a family with genotype vector **g** is given by

$$\imath(\boldsymbol{\beta}, \mathbf{g}) = p_g(1 - p_g)\mathbf{Z}(g)'\mathbf{Z}(g)$$

where p_g is the predicted logistic probability of disease for genotype g and $\mathbf{Z} = (1, Z(g))$. Hence, the expected information is

$$E[\imath(\boldsymbol{\beta})] = \sum_{\mathbf{y}} \sum_{\mathbf{g}} \Pr(\mathbf{y}, \mathbf{g} \,|\, Asc) \, \imath(\boldsymbol{\beta}, \mathbf{g})$$

The relative efficiency of two design/analysis combinations is then given by

$$ARE(1:2) = \frac{\mathrm{var}(\hat{\beta}^{(2)})}{\mathrm{var}(\hat{\beta}^{(1)})} = \frac{E[\imath(\hat{\beta}^{(1)})]}{E[\imath(\hat{\beta}^{(2)})]}$$

For multiparameter models [e.g., $\boldsymbol{\beta} = (\beta_0, \beta_1)$], the variance of β_1 is given by the (β_1, β_1) element of the inverse matrix of $\imath(\boldsymbol{\beta})$, not by $1/i(\beta_1)$.

Figure 11.2 illustrates these calculations for a comparison of four alternative case-control designs for estimating the relative risk of a binary disease for a rare major susceptibility locus. For a dominant gene, the most efficient design uses unrelated controls (the reference for this comparison, i.e., $ARE = 100\%$), although the case-parent design provides virtually the same efficiency per case-control set. However, since the latter design requires three genotypes per set, compared with only two for the standard case-control design, its relative efficiency *per genotype* (i.e., the cost efficiency

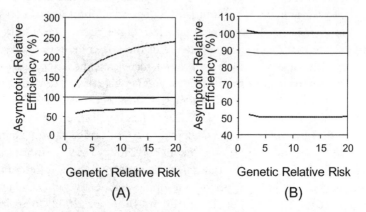

Figure 11.2 Asymptotic relative efficiency for estimating the main effect of a gene under (A) a recessive model or (B) a dominant model as a function of the genetic relative risk (e^β), holding the population attributable risk fixed at 20%. Asymptotic relative efficiencies are expressed relative to a case-control design with unrelated controls: dotted line, case–sibling; solid line, case–cousin; dashed line, case–parent trios, all expressed relative to the case-control design using unrelated individuals (100%). (Adapted with permission from Gauderman et al., 1999)

if the major cost is for genotyping rather than subject recruitment) is only about 67%. For a recessive model, the case-parent design becomes much more efficient—even on a per-genotype basis—than any of the other designs. The relative efficiency of a case-sibling design is only about 50% under this model, whereas that of the case-cousin design is about 88%. These reductions reflect the greater similarity of genotypes within matched pairs that would be expected using unrelated controls (overmatching). Witte et al. (1999) and Gauderman et al. (1999) provide further comparisons of alternative case-control designs. As emphasized in Chapter 9, there are a variety of other nonstatistical considerations in choosing between study designs, such as representativeness, freedom from bias, and so on.

Gene–Environment and Gene–Gene Interactions

The term "interaction" is used loosely in both the genetic and epidemiologic literature in many different senses, so before discussing study designs and statistical methods, it is worth beginning by clarifying its meaning. In general, one could think of $G \times E$ interaction equivalently as either as increased (or decreased) vulnerability to environmental exposures in carriers of a certain genotype relative to noncarriers, or as increased (or decreased) genetic expression in exposed subjects compared to unexposed subjects. On p. 74, "interaction" or "effect modification" was defined as a variation in some measure of the effect of one variable across levels of another variable. Thus, the precise meaning of interaction depends upon the scale on which effect size is measured—constancy of the relative risk corresponding to a multiplicative model whereas constancy of the risk difference corresponding to an additive model—so *statistical interaction* means a departure of the observed risks from some model for the main effects of two or more factors. As mentioned before, statistical interaction does not necessarily imply biological interaction and vice versa. Nevertheless, such interactions are often interpreted as having biological significance about underlying mechanisms. For example, Ottman (1990) and Yang and Khoury (1997) outline various patterns of $G \times E$ interaction that might be expected under different causal models, and Cordell (2002) provides a similar perspective on $G \times G$ interactions (epistasis). Rothman et al. (2001) and Brennan (2002) focus instead on the ways in which study of $G \times E$ interactions can help clarify the effects of environmental carcinogens. On the other hand, Clayton and McKeigue (2001) highlight some of the difficulties in interpretation of interaction effects and argue for greater emphasis on the study of main effects.

Biological systems are frequently very complex, perhaps involving a pathway with multiple genes and substrates, and even multiple interrelated pathways. A variety of exploratory and mechanistic modeling approaches have been proposed to synthesis patterns across a potentially large number of interactions. These approaches will be discussed in Chapter 12, but for now we will focus on interactions involving only two factors at a time.

Case-control designs

Case-control studies, whether with related or unrelated controls, can be used in a very natural way to investigate interaction effects. The basic descriptive analysis for an unmatched case control study is illustrated in Table 11.3A. Epidemiologic papers often present ORs conditional either on genotype (Table 11.3B) or on exposure (Table 11.3C), depending on the scientific question. Also, depending on the rarity of the A or a allele and the assumed dominance model, it might be appropriate to combine one of the genotype categories with the heterozygotes. The ORs given in panel A provide the most complete summary of the results (together with confidence limits and tests of interaction).

However, a significant OR for a single exposure/genotype category does not necessarily constitute significant *interaction*. A multiplicative interaction means that the odds ratios in the first column, OR_{ge} (where g denotes

Table 11.3 Basic Descriptive Analysis of $G \times E$ Interactions in an Unmatched Case Control Study

(A) UNCONDITIONAL ODDS RATIOS (ORs)

Genotype	Exposure	Cases	Controls	Joint OR	Interaction IOR^{mult}
aa	$-$	c_{00}	d_{00}	1	
aa	$+$	c_{01}	d_{01}	$OR_{01} = c_{01}d_{00}/c_{00}d_{01}$	
Aa	$-$	c_{10}	d_{10}	$OR_{10} = c_{10}d_{00}/c_{00}d_{10}$	
Aa	$+$	c_{11}	d_{11}	$OR_{11} = c_{11}d_{00}/c_{00}d_{11}$	$IOR_{11} = \dfrac{OR_{11}}{OR_{10}OR_{01}}$
AA	$-$	c_{20}	d_{20}	$OR_{20} = c_{20}d_{00}/c_{00}d_{20}$	
AA	$+$	c_{21}	d_{21}	$OR_{21} = c_{21}d_{00}/c_{00}d_{21}$	$IOR_{21} = \dfrac{OR_{21}}{OR_{20}OR_{01}}$

(B) ORs FOR GENOTYPE CONDITIONAL ON EXPOSURE

Genotype		Not Exposed			Exposed	
	Cases	Controls	$OR_{G\mid\bar{E}}$	Cases	Controls	$OR_{G\mid E}$
aa	c_{00}	d_{00}	1	c_{01}	d_{01}	1
aA	c_{10}	d_{10}	OR_{10}	c_{11}	d_{11}	OR_{11}/OR_{01}
AA	c_{20}	d_{20}	OR_{20}	c_{21}	d_{21}	OR_{21}/OR_{01}

(C) ORs FOR EXPOSURE CONDITIONAL ON GENOTYPE

Genotype		Not Exposed			Exposed	
	Cases	Controls	$OR_{\bar{E}\mid G}$	Cases	Controls	$OR_{E\mid G}$
aa	c_{00}	d_{00}	1	c_{01}	d_{01}	OR_{01}
aA	c_{10}	d_{10}	1	c_{11}	d_{11}	OR_{11}/OR_{10}
AA	c_{20}	d_{20}	1	c_{21}	d_{21}	OR_{21}/OR_{20}

genotype and e environment), differ from what would be expected under a multiplicative model, that is, $OR_{g1} \neq OR_{g0} \times OR_{01}$ or, equivalently, that the ORs in the last two columns differ from each other, $OR_{g|E=1} \neq OR_{g|E=0}$ and $OR_{E|G=g} \neq OR_{E|G=aa}$. We can define the multiplicative *interaction odds ratio* in terms of any of the following ratios of ORs:

$$IOR_g^{\text{mult}} = \frac{OR_{g1}}{OR_{g0}OR_{01}} = \frac{OR_{g|E=1}}{OR_{g|E=0}} = \frac{OR_{E|G=g}}{OR_{E|G=aa}}$$

with the null value of no multiplicative interaction being $H_0 : IOR^{\text{mult}} = 1$. Alternatively, one might wish to test for a departure from an additive model of the form $OR_{g1} \neq 1 + (OR_{g0} - 1) + (OR_{01} - 1)$. In a similar way, we can define the additive $IOR_g^{\text{add}} = OR_{g1} - OR_{g0} - OR_{01} + 1$, with null value $H_0 : IOR_g^{\text{add}} = 0$. Chapter 4 and Rothman and Greenland (1998) provide further discussion of the epidemiologic principles underlying additive versus multiplicative models as null hypotheses for synergistic effects and methods for testing interaction effects; in particular, they argue for an additive model as the natural null hypothesis for the public health concept of absence of *synergy*, in the sense of a joint effect that is greater than the sum of the effects of each factor separately. Siemiatycki and Thomas (1981) make a useful distinction between *biological* and *statistical* interaction, arguing that biological independence, in the sense of the action of two factors by unrelated mechanisms, could yield either a multiplicative or an additive statistical model, or neither, whereas an adequate fit to a statistical main effects model without interaction terms does not necessarily imply biological independence. In the remainder of this section, we will focus on testing for multiplicative statistical interactions.

Standard conditional or unconditional logistic regression methods can be used to test for interaction effects in matched or unmatched case-control studies, respectively, by including as covariates the various main effects and interactions. In a logistic model of the form

$$\text{logit } \Pr(Y = 1 \mid G, E) = \alpha + \beta_1 Z(G) + \beta_2 E + \beta_3 Z(G) \times E$$

the parameter β_3 is an estimator of $\ln(IOR_g^{\text{mult}})$. For testing $G \times G$ interactions, the data would be laid out in a manner similar to that in Table 11.3, with the entries for environment being replaced by the second gene. Logistic regression would again be used, with a variety of possible codings of the interaction effect $Z(G_1, G_2)$; Table 11.4 provides some typical alternatives. Needless to say, more complex models incorporating both $G \times E$ and $G \times G$ interactions, perhaps with multiple genes or environmental exposures, or even including higher-order interactions (e.g., $G \times G \times E$), could be analyzed in this framework, although in reality, the sparseness of the data and the multiplicity of hypothesis tests will seldom support too elaborate models,

Table 11.4 Some Possible Codings of Gene–Gene Interaction Effects: Upper Left, a Multiplicative Coding of Two Additive Loci; Upper Right, a Sufficient Effect of Any Three Alleles; Lower Left, Dominant Effect of G_1 Interacting with a Recessive Effect of G_2; Lower Right, Fully Saturated Model for Two Codominant Genes

| | G_2 | | | G_2 | | |
G_1	bb	bB	BB	bb	bB	BB
aa	0	0	0	0	0	1
aA	0	1	2	0	1	1
AA	0	2	4	1	1	1
aa	0	0	0	0	0	0
aA	0	0	1	0	Z_{31}	Z_{32}
AA	0	0	1	0	Z_{33}	Z_{34}

unless guided by strong prior understanding of the relevant biological pathways. Cortessis and Thomas (2002) discuss the use of physiologically based pharmacokinetic models for complex metabolic pathways.

Case-only studies

Another design that can be used to examine $G \times E$ interactions is the *case-only* or *case-case* design. Piegorsch et al. (1994) pointed out that if one was prepared to assume that the gene and an environmental risk factor were independently distributed in the population at risk, then one could detect $G \times E$ interactions (in the sense of departures from a multiplicative model) simply by looking for association between the two factors among cases. Table 11.5 illustrates a dominant gene with high-risk genotype probability P and prevalence of the environmental factor Q. By construction, we have assumed that the two risk factors are independent in the population. Then it can easily be seen that the two risk factors will be independent among cases if and only if $R_{GE} = R_E R_G$: the expected odd ratio among cases is

$$OR_{GE}(\text{cases}) = \frac{C_{11}C_{00}}{C_{01}C_{10}} = \frac{PQR_{GE} \times (1-P)(1-Q)}{(1-P)QR_E \times P(1-Q)R_G} = \frac{R_{GE}}{R_E \times R_G} \equiv R_I$$

Thus, the interaction relative risk R_I can be estimated under this assumption simply by the OR for association between G and E among cases.

Table 11.5 Expected Distribution of Genotypes and an Environmental Factor Among Cases

Genotype	Environment	Population	RR	Cases
aa	−	$(1-P)(1-Q)$	1	$E(C_{00}) = (1-P)(1-Q)/\Sigma$
aa	+	$(1-P)Q$	R_E	$E(C_{01}) = (1-P)QR_E/\Sigma$
aA or AA	−	$P(1-Q)$	R_G	$E(C_{10}) = P(1-Q)R_G/\Sigma$
aA or AA	+	PQ	R_{GE}	$E(C_{11}) = PQR_{GE}/\Sigma$

where Σ denotes the sum of the numerators

What may be less obvious is that this estimator of the interaction effect is more efficient than the corresponding one from a case-control comparison, essentially because the estimate of association among controls (with its inherent variability) is replaced by an assumed value. Of course, this method is entirely dependent on the assumption of independence of G and E in the source population. In many circumstances this might be reasonable, for example if there is no plausible mechanism by which one's genotype would affect one's environment. In other circumstances, however, this may not be obvious, for example if the environmental factor is a biological characteristic such as a hormone level or if the genotype might influence one's appetite or tolerance for the factor. Furthermore, even if E and G were independent at birth, differential survival can produce such an association at later ages (Gauderman and Millstein, 2002). In fact, for high enough penetrances, it is possible for a greater-than-multiplicative interaction at baseline to turn into a less-than-multiplicative interaction as the exposed-carrier group becomes depleted of cases preferentially. Gauderman and Millstein describe how to correct for this bias by including an age interaction term in a logistic model for E given G (or vice versa).

Case-parent trios

The case-parent trio design was introduced in Chapter 9 as a means of testing candidate-gene associations. This design can also be used for testing $G \times E$ or $G \times G$ interactions, under somewhat weaker assumptions of $G - E$ independence than required by the case-only design. Used in this way, the design utilizes the genotypes on all three members of the trio, but the exposure information only on the case. (In any event, age, gender, or generational differences would make a case-control comparison between the case's and the parent's exposures meaningless.) Hence, the basic idea is to stratify the genetic RRs estimated from the case-parent trio design by the exposure status of the case: in the absence of a $G \times E$ interaction, the two genetic RRs should be the same; in the presence of an interaction, their ratio will estimate the interaction relative risk. To see this, consider the likelihood for the genetic main effect given in Eq. (9.1) and add the environmental factor E:

$$\mathcal{L}(\beta) = \prod_i \Pr\big(G_i \mid Y_i = 1, G_{f_i}, G_{m_i}, E_i\big)$$

$$= \prod_i \frac{\Pr(Y_i = 1 \mid G_i, E_i) \Pr\big(G_i \mid G_{f_i}, G_{m_i}, E_i\big)}{\sum_{G_*} \Pr(Y_i = 1 \mid G_*, E_i) \Pr\big(G_* \mid G_{f_i}, G_{m_i}, E_i\big)}$$

The first factor in the numerator follows from the assumption that the case's disease status is conditionally independent of the parents' genotypes, given the case's own genotype; this factor would generally take the form $\exp[\beta_1 Z(G_i) + \beta_2 E_i + \beta_3 Z(G_i) E_i]$. Under the assumption that the case's genotype and environment are independent *conditional on the parents' genotypes*, the second factor can be simplified to $\Pr(G_* \mid G_{f_i}, G_{m_i})$, the same as would appear in the standard likelihood for the case-parent trio design. Now the terms involving $\beta_2 E_i$ cancel out from the numerator and denominator, as might be expected since there is no comparison that would permit the main effect of environment to be estimated in this design, leaving a likelihood than can be written as

$$\mathcal{L}(\beta) = \prod_{i \mid E_i = 0} \frac{e^{\beta_1 Z(G_i)} \Pr(G_i \mid G_{f_i}, G_{m_i})}{\sum_{G_*} e^{\beta_1 Z(G_i)} \Pr(G_* \mid G_{f_i}, G_{m_i})}$$

$$\times \prod_{i \mid E_i = 1} \frac{e^{(\beta_1 + \beta_3) Z(G_i)} \Pr(G_i \mid G_{f_i}, G_{m_i})}{\sum_{G_*} e^{(\beta_1 + \beta_3) Z(G_i)} \Pr(G_* \mid G_{f_i}, G_{m_i})}$$

Each of the two parts of the likelihood can be maximized separately to obtain estimates of the lnRR in unexposed subjects (β_1) and in exposed subjects ($\beta_1 + \beta_3$), so the test of $H_0 : \beta_3 = 0$ is thus a test of no $G \times E$ interaction. Schaid (1999), Thomas (2000b), and Weinberg and Umbach (2000) provide further discussion.

The case-parent design is thus an appealing way to examine $G \times E$ interactions, both because of its conceptual simplicity—one simply compares the genetic relative risks estimated from exposed and unexposed cases—and because the assumption of $G - E$ independence that is required is somewhat weaker than that required for the case-only design. A stratified analysis can be used to control for potential within-family dependencies induced by measured confounding variables.

Essentially the same approach could be used for testing for interactions between unlinked genes; one simply stratifies the RRs for one gene by the genotype of the proband at the other locus. Unfortunately, this approach does not have the desirable symmetry in the handling of the two genes, since the ratio of estimated RRs for locus 1 between genotypes at locus 2 will not generally be the same as the ratio of estimated RRs for locus 2 between genotypes at locus 1, since the genotypes at only one locus for the parents contribute to this comparison. A better approach would be to use the genotype information at both loci for the entire trio. Letting $\mathbf{G} = (G_1, G_2)$ denote the joint genotype, the likelihood becomes

$$\mathcal{L}(\beta) = \prod_i \Pr(\mathbf{G}_i \mid Y_i = 1, \mathbf{G}_{f_i}, \mathbf{G}_{m_i})$$

$$= \prod_i \frac{\Pr(Y_i = 1 \mid \mathbf{G}_i) \Pr(\mathbf{G}_i \mid \mathbf{G}_{f_i}, \mathbf{G}_{m_i})}{\sum_{\mathbf{G}_*} \Pr(Y_i = 1 \mid \mathbf{G}_*) \Pr(\mathbf{G}_* \mid \mathbf{G}_{f_i}, \mathbf{G}_{m_i})}$$

where the sum in the denominator is now over the 16 possible joint genotypes that could have been transmitted, given the joint genotypes of the parents (Gauderman, 2002b). If the two loci are unlinked, these 16 possibilities are equally likely, so the resulting likelihood reduces to

$$\mathcal{L}(\boldsymbol{\beta}) = \prod_i \frac{\exp[\beta_1 Z_1(G_{i1}) + \beta_2 Z_2(G_{i2}) + \beta_3 Z_3(G_{i1}, G_{i2})]}{\sum_{\mathbf{G}_*} \exp[\beta_1 Z_1(G_{*1}) + \beta_2 Z_2(G_{*2}) + \beta_3 Z_3(G_{*1}, G_{*2})]}$$

where the covariates Z_1, Z_2, Z_3 encapsulate whatever assumptions one wishes to test about dominance relationships for the two genes jointly. If $\beta_3 = 0$, the likelihood factors into the product of two likelihoods, one for each gene separately with four terms in the denominator of each, but this test of interaction still requires the full expression involving all 16 possible joint genotypes. If the genes are linked, the 16 terms in the denominator have probabilities that depend on the recombination fraction θ between them. With only case-parent trios, this recombination fraction cannot be estimated, but if their locations were already known, θ could be treated as fixed. In particular, for two polymorphisms in the same gene, it would be reasonable to set $\theta = 0$, yielding a relatively simple likelihood that entails $\boldsymbol{\beta}$ as well as the haplotype frequencies. In this situation, one might consider reparameterizing $\mathbf{Z}$ in terms of haplotype RRs rather than main effects and interactions. Generalization of the test to sibships would allow joint estimation of θ and $\boldsymbol{\beta}$.

Gene–environment interactions for breast cancer

As an example, consider the possible interactions between *BRCA1* and OC use, as suggested for breast cancer by Ursin et al. (1997) and for ovarian cancer by Narod et al. (1998), using case-only and case-sib designs, respectively. The relevant data are shown in Tables 11.6 and 11.7, respectively. The case-only analysis in young Ashkenazi breast cancer cases found that a higher proportion of carrier cases were long-term OC users than were noncarrier cases, leading to an interaction *OR* estimate of 7.8 (with wide confidence limits due to the small number of cases); that is, the effect of long-term OC use is estimated to be 7.8 times higher in carriers than in noncarriers, or equivalently, the effect of being a mutation carrier is 7.8 times higher in

Table 11.6 Interaction Between *BRCA1/2* Mutations and Oral Contraceptive (OC) Use Before First Full-Term Pregnancy (Months) for Breast Cancer Using a Case-Only Design

OC use	Carriers	Noncarriers	Adjusted *OR*	95% CI
0–11	3	15	1.0	
12–48	4	11	1.8	0.3–13
49+	7	7	7.8	1.1–55

Source: Ursin et al. (1997).

Table 11.7 Interaction Between *BRCA1/2* Mutations and Oral Contraceptive (OC) Use (Months) for Ovarian Cancer Using a Case-Sibling Design

	Mutation Carriers		
	Cases (N = 207)	Sisters (N = 53)	
Users Mean	50%	77%	General
Duration (yr)	4	5	Population*
OC Use (mo)	OR (95% CI)		OR
0	1.0		1.0
Any	0.4 (0.2–0.7)		0.66
1–35	0.4 (0.3–0.9)		—
32–71	0.4 (0.1–1.0)		—
72+	0.3 (0.1–0.7)		0.30

*From Collaborative-Group-on-Hormonal-Factors-in-Breast-Cancer (1996).

Source: Narod et al. (1998).

long-term users than in nonusers. This positive interaction for breast cancer could be due to $G - E$ association, perhaps because of population stratification (although this study was limited to Ashkenazi Jews), or more likely by confounding by FH or hormonal/reproductive factors.

Narod et al. identified 207 ovarian cancer cases who were carriers of a mutation in *BRCA1* or *BRCA2*. Among their 161 sisters, 53 were found to be carriers, 42 to be noncarriers, and 66 were not tested; these three subgroups of sisters had similar OC histories and were combined for most analyses, but Table 11.7 shows the results using only the carrier sisters. Carrier cases were less likely to have used OCs and to have used them for shorter periods than their sisters, leading to estimates of the protective effect that increase with duration of use, comparable to that seen in a meta-analysis of studies in the general population (Collaborative-Group-on-Hormonal-Factors-in-Breast-Cancer, 1996). Thus, OCs appear to have essentially the same protective effect (in a multiplicative sense) in carriers and noncarriers rather being a true interaction. Because the authors used sibling controls, no assumption of $G - E$ independence is required, as such an association would be estimated from the controls. The protective effect thus cannot be explained on this basis (although because only a small number of cases had an eligible sib control, an unmatched analysis was used, leading to other potential problems).

To date, no study of this interaction has been reported using the case-parent design, in part because parents would be difficult to obtain unless the study was restricted to young breast cancer cases. However, we can speculate on the credibility of the $G - E$ independence assumption in such a hypothetical study. Perhaps the most important source of potential dependence would be confounding by FH: women with a positive FH might be more or less inclined to use OCs, and FH would also be associated with the likelihood of being a *BRCA1* carrier. This would induce a population association between *BRCA1* carrier status and OC use that could bias the case-only design, but it could not bias the case-parent design because within a family all cases would have the same FH. This argument would not apply to individual-specific risk factors, like age at menarche or first pregnancy. However, as with the case-only design, such confounders could be controlled in the analysis by stratification.

If the source of $G - E$ dependence was the FH, F, then one must determine which family members are involved. The relevant dependence can be written as $\Pr(E_i \mid G_i, G_{f_i}, G_{m_i}) = \sum_F \Pr(E_i \mid F) \Pr(F \mid G_i, G_{f_i}, G_{m_i})$. If F includes the descendants of the proband, then the second factor will certainly depend on G_i and will induce such a dependence. Otherwise, the second factor will depend only on G_f, G_m and $G - E$ independence will hold, conditional on G_f, G_m. For example, if a woman's use of OCs was influenced only by the disease status of her sisters, parents, grandparents, aunts, or cousins, but not that of her daughters, this would not bias the case-parent approach to $G \times E$ interactions.

Narod (2002) and Narod and Boyd (2002) have reviewed the literature on modifying factors for *BRCA1/2* mutations in breast and ovarian cancers and have discussed their implications for prevention. Other genes that have been studied as potential modifiers include those involved in the metabolism of sex hormones (the androgen receptor (*AR*) gene and *NCOA3*) and those involved in DNA repair (*RAD51, HRAS*). In terms of environmental factors, the strongest evidence of modifying effects is for oophorectomy (protective against breast cancer), pregnancy (increasing the risk of early-onset breast cancer; also associated with an increased risk of ovarian cancer in *BRCA1* carriers while being protective in noncarriers [Narod et al., 1995]), breastfeeding (protective against breast cancer in *BRCA1* but not *BRCA2* carriers), tubal ligation (equally protective against ovarian cancer in *BRCA1* carriers and noncarriers but apparently not in *BRCA2* carriers), and tamoxifen (protective against breast cancer in *BRCA2* carriers, conflicting results for *BRCA1* carriers). The data on OC use and hormone replacement therapy (HRT) is less clear. Oral contraceptives appear to have at most a small effect on breast cancer risk in the general population, but there may be a stronger risk factor in mutation carriers, as indicated by the case-only analysis described above and by a significant association with OC use (*OR* 3.3, CI 1.6–9.7) among sisters and daughters of cases (Grabrick et al., 2000), although this study did not test for mutations. A large case-control study (Narod et al., 2002) of 1311 breast cancer cases with known *BRCA1* or *BRCA2* mutations, each matched with one unrelated control carrying the same mutation, found a significant positive association with OC use in *BRCA1* (but not *BRCA2*) carriers, particularly among cases diagnosed before age 40 or those who used OCs before age 30, before 1975, or for more than five years. Subsequent studies of the protective effect of OC use for ovarian cancer have been conflicting (Modan et al., 2001; Narod et al., 2001). Results for HRT are similarly ambiguous, with an apparently positive interaction between HRT and FH (Steinberg et al., 1991) but a reduced risk in women with a history of HRT in two tamoxifen prevention trials for women with a positive FH (Powles et al., 1998; Veronesi et al., 1998); to date, however, there have been no studies of HRT use specifically in mutation carriers. Finally, there is evidence that *BRCA1/2* carriers with ovarian cancer have better survival than those without a mutation (Narod and Boyd, 2002), although it is not clear whether this is because of differences in natural history or response to treatment.

Relative efficiency of alternative designs for interaction effects

The relative efficiency for estimating $\beta_3 = \ln IOR$ is shown in Figure 11.3 for two hypothetical situations: an interaction between a rare major gene and an environmental exposure that is only weakly correlated within families (e.g., *BRCA1* and OC use) and a common low-penetrance gene and an environmental factors that is strongly correlated within families (e.g., *GSTM1* and environmental tobacco smoking). In contrast with Figure 11.2, here we see that siblings can be more efficient than unrelated controls for testing an

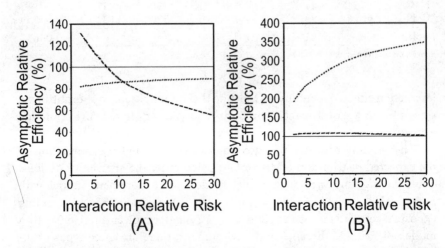

Figure 11.3 (A) Asymptotic relative efficiency for estimating the $G \times E$ effect for an interaction between *GSTM1* and environmental tobacco smoke as a function of R_I ($p_E = 0.4$, $\psi = 10$, $q = 0.25$ (recessive) and $R_E = 2$, $R_G = 2$). (B) Asymptotic relative efficiency for estimating the $G \times E$ effect for an interaction between *BRCA1* and oral contraceptive use as a function of R_I ($p_E = 0.3$, $\psi = 2$, $q = 0.01$) (dominant) and $R_E = 1$, $R_G = 5$). Dotted line, siblings; dashed line, case–parent trios, both expressed relative to the case-control design using unrelated individuals (100%). (Based on data from Gauderman, 2002c)

Table 11.8 Expected Distribution of Discordant Pairs for a Dominant Model: N = Noncarrier, C = Carrier, U = Unexposed, E = Exposed ($P_E = 0.25$, $Q = 0.1$, $\psi = 2$, $R_G = 10$, $R_E = 2$, $R_I = 2$)

(A) JOINT DISTRIBUTION OF ALL CASE-CONTROL PAIRS

Cases	Population Controls				Sibling Controls			
	N,U	N,E	C,U	C,E	N,U	N,E	C,U	C,E
N,U	285	285	67	66	991	278	107	30
N,E	190	190	44	44	525	321	57	34
C,U	667	667	156	155	1067	300	1499	418
C,E	883	883	207	205	1124	688	1578	959

(B) DISTRIBUTIONS OF INFORMATIVE PAIRS BY DISCORDANCE ON EXPOSURE, GENOTYPE, OR BOTH

	Population Controls			Sibling Controls		
Genotype Concordant, Exposure Discordant						
	U–E	E–U	var(ln OR)	U–E	E–U	var(ln OR)
N–N	285	190	—	278	525	—
C–C	155	207	0.0201	418	1578	0.0085
Genotype Concordant, Exposure Discordant						
	U–U	E–E		U–U	E–E	
N–C	67	44	—	107	34	—
C–N	667	883	0.0403	1067	688	0.0408
Discordant on Both Factors						
	U–E	E–U		U–E	E–U	
N–C	66	44	—	30	57	—
C–N	667	883	0.0402	300	1124	0.0555
Pooled			0.0101			0.0063

Source: Gauderman et al. (1999).

interaction effect, depending on the model. This may seem counterintuitive, since siblings are overmatched on both genotype and shared environmental exposures.

The resolution of this paradox comes from a detailed examination of the expected distribution of discordant pairs under the alternative designs. Table 11.8A illustrates such a distribution for a dominant model with $\beta_1 = \ln(10)$, $\beta_2 = \ln(2)$, $\beta_3 = \ln(2)$, $q = 0.1$, $p_E = 0.25$, and a sibling exposure concordance odds ratio $\psi = 2$ (Gauderman et al., 1999). In a model involving both genes and environment, there are three types of informative pairs: (1) those discordant for exposure with the same genotype; (2) those discordant for genotype with the same exposure; and (3) and those discordant for both. These three comparisons are separated in panel B. The interaction OR parameter β_3 is approximately a weighted average of the three pairs of ratios of ORs from the three types of discordant pairs (it is easy to see that these IORs are 2 for all three comparisons). The precision of these OR estimates is driven most by the size of the smallest cells in each 2×2 table. In this example, it turns out that the most informative contrast is between the genotype-concordant, exposure-discordant pairs. The over-matching on genotype in sib pairs has had the effect of greatly increasing the number of such sets, yielding a variance for this comparison that is less than half that using population controls. Even though the variances for the other two comparisons are somewhat smaller for population controls, when a weighted average of the three contributions is taken, the pooled variance using population controls is 1.6-fold larger than that for sibling controls. Of course, this conclusion is influenced by the amount of exposure concordance among siblings. Here we have assumed moderate sharing of the environment ($\psi = 2$), but as this increases, the advantage of using sibs for $G \times E$ studies decreases, eventually becoming less than for unrelated controls.

Garcia-Closas and Lubin (1999), Gauderman (2002c), and Selinger-Leneman et al. (2003) provide further comparisons of case-control, case-sibling, and case-parent-trio designs for testing $G \times E$ interactions. Similar comparisons for $G \times G$ interactions are discussed in (Gauderman, 2002b). The procedures for estimating power and sample size requirements have been implemented in two computer programs available on the Internet: POWER (http://dceg.cancer.gov/power/) and QUANTO (http://hydra.usc.edu/gxe/).

Estimation of Gene Frequencies and Carrier Probabilities

Another major aim of gene characterization studies is to estimate the population allele frequencies q of mutation(s) in a gene and their variation between ethnic groups. These data can then be used to assess how much of the differences in disease rates between groups might be attributable to differences in allele frequencies and, in a genetic counseling setting, to estimate the probability that an individual carries a mutation given FH information.

Conceptually, estimation of a population allele frequency is a trivial undertaking. All that needs to be done is to take a random sample of unrelated individuals from a population (unselected by disease status), genotype them, and estimate the allele frequency from the observed fractions of carriers C and homozygotes, H, that is, $\hat{q} = C/2 + H$. Of course, the difficulty is that if mutations are rare, as in $BRCA1/2$, this would require an enormous sample size. The current estimate of $q = 0.0006$ for $BRCA1$, for example, would lead to only about 1 carrier expected in a sample of 1000 individuals from the general population! Hence, most efforts to estimate the gene frequency are based on cases, using estimates of penetrance derived from the family-based designs described earlier in this chapter; see,

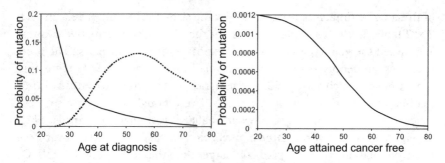

Figure 11.4 Estimates of the *BRCA1* carrier probabilities. Left: for individuals with breast cancer (solid line) or ovarian cancer (dotted line) as a function of age at diagnosis; right: for individuals free of either disease as a function of their attained age. (Adapted from Berry et al., 1997)

for example, the likelihood (Eq. 11.2) of a case series under single ascertainment. More elaborate segregation analysis-like likelihood methods can be used for family-based designs with some individuals genotyped, such as the kin cohort or genotyped-proband design, yielding a likelihood for joint estimation of penetrances and allele frequencies (Eq. 11.1). Thus, estimates of carrier frequencies in unselected series of breast cancer cases are typically about 1% and in high-risk families about 5%, although these numbers depend heavily on age at diagnosis and FH (Fig. 11.4). Peto et al. (1999) estimate that about 6% of unselected cases under age 50, 1.3% of cases over age 50, and 0.2% of the general population are carriers of mutations in one of these genes; similar estimates have been found in a population-based Australian series (Dite et al. 2003).

Given a set of allele frequency estimates q_e for different ethnic groups e, one might inquire whether the differences in population rates $\bar{P}_e$ can be explained by differences in allele frequencies. To keep things simple, suppose that we ignore the dependence of risk (and perhaps even the GRR) on age and consider a simple logistic model for penetrance of the form logit $P_e(g) = \alpha_e + \beta Z(g)$, assuming a constant *RR* parameter β across ethnic groups. Then the population average risk would be of the form $\bar{P}_e = \sum_g Q_g(q_e) P_e(g)$, where Q_g denotes the Hardy-Weinberg probabilities corresponding to allele frequency q. For example, for a low-penetrance, rare dominant gene, this is approximately $\bar{P}_e = e^{\alpha_e}[1 + 2q_e(e^{\beta} - 1)]$. The factor in square brackets is thus the portion of risk attributable to the gene, and the first factor is the variation in risk attributable to other factors. Table 11.9 illustrates the calculations.

Notice how, despite a large GRR $e^3 \approx 20$, the population attributable risk $ARG_G = Q_{aA}[P_e(aA) - P_e(aa)]/\bar{P}_e$ is only about 4% in the low-allele-frequency populations and about 17%–21% in the high-frequency populations. Also, the *RR*s comparing populations with low and high allele

Table 11.9 Relative Risks and Population Attributable Risks Corresponding for Different Allele Frequencies

α_e	q_e	β	$P_e(aa)$	$P_e(aA)$	$\bar{P}_e$	RR	AR_G
−4.0	0.001	3.0	0.0180	0.2689	0.0185	1.00	3.8%
−4.0	0.005	3.0	0.0180	0.2689	0.0205	1.11	17.0%
−2.0	0.001	3.0	0.1192	0.7311	0.1204	6.51	4.3%
−2.0	0.005	3.0	0.1192	0.7311	0.1253	6.78	20.6%

frequencies are much smaller than those comparing populations with low and high background rates.

Once estimates of age-specific penetrance and allele frequency are available, it is possible to estimate carrier probabilities for individuals based on their personal and family histories. This entails a straightforward application of Bayes' formula:

$$\Pr(G \mid Y) = \frac{\Pr(Y \mid G; \mathbf{f}) \Pr(G \mid q)}{\sum_G \Pr(Y \mid G; \mathbf{f}) \Pr(G \mid q)}$$

For example, consider the parameters in the first line of Table 11.9. The carrier probability for an unselected case would then be $(0.2689 \times 0.002)/(0.2689 \times 0.002 + 0.0180 \times 0.0998) = 2.9\%$. To incorporate FH into this calculation would entail replacing G and Y for the individual in this formula by vectors of genotypes and phenotypes for the entire family and summing over all possible combinations of $\mathbf{G}$. For breast and ovarian cancers in relation to *BRCA1/2*, these calculations have been implemented in the BRCAPRO program (Berry et al., 1997; Parmigiani et al., 1998), which can also include any available mutation testing information on relatives. These calculations are complex, in part because they allow for the uncertainties in the assumed penetrance and allele frequency parameters, as well as incomplete sensitivity and specificity of the genetic tests, using Monte Carlo methods. Figure 11.5 illustrates the joint distribution of *BRCA1* and *BRCA2* carrier probabilities estimated from a series of 4849 individuals from an international consortium of population-based family registries for breast cancer (A.S. Whittemore, personal communication), based on their age and reported FH in first-degree relatives.

These results are summarized in Table 11.10 in relation to their personal disease status. Using logistic regression on a sample of 424 Australian Ashkenazi Jewish women who either had had breast or ovarian cancer themselves or had a first- or second-degree relative with breast or ovarian cancer, Apicella et al. (2003) developed a logistic regression model for the carrier probability of the form

$$\text{logit } \Pr(G_i = 1 \mid Y_i, T_i, \mathbf{Y}) \approx -4 + \sum_j Score_j$$

where the scores for the proband and her relatives are given in Table 11.11.

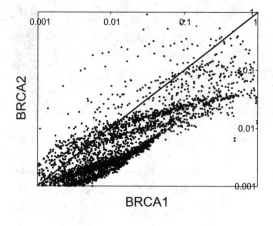

Figure 11.5 Estimates of the *BRCA1* and *BRCA2* carrier probabilities for individuals in a population-based family registry for breast cancer. (AS Whittemore, personal communication)

Table 11.10 Carrier Probabilities in Relation to Disease Status

Breast Cancer Status	Carrier Probability	
	BRCA1	*BRCA2*
Unaffected	0.020	0.005
Affected	0.052	0.016
Unilateral	0.042	0.014
Bilateral	0.247	0.054

Table 11.11 Scores Used in the Logistic Regression Model Developed by Apicella et al. (2003) for the Carrier Probability

Phenotype	Age T_i	Score		
		Proband	First Degree	Second Degree
Breast cancer	0–39	+3.0	+1.5	+1.0
	40–49	+2.0	+1.0	—
	50–59	+1.0	+0.5	—
Bilateral breast cancer	Any	+1.0	—	—
Ovarian cancer	Any	+3.0	+1.5	+1.0
Unaffected	0–39	−0.5	—	—
	40–49	−1.0	—	—
	50–59	−1.5	—	—
	60+	−2.0	—	—

Searching for Additional Genes

Now that one or more major susceptibility genes for a disease have been identified and characterized, the next question is whether there are additional major genes yet to be found. If the already identified genes are rare, the obvious strategy is to exclude those families that are known to be segregating these genes and then repeat the cycle of segregation, linkage, and association studies on the remainder. Alternatively, one might leave them in the series and fit multilocus models on the entire series, conditioning on the available genotype information for those tested at the already identified loci. The latter strategy has the advantage that it would be possible (in principle) to allow for epistatic interactions between the known and unknown loci if the allele frequencies of both loci were high enough for there to be a substantial number of carriers of both mutations. These two approaches are illustrated by the search for additional breast cancer genes.

Cui et al. (2001) conducted one- and two-locus segregation analyses on first- and second-degree relatives of 858 Australian breast cancer probands under age 40, excluding 34 families known to carry mutations in *BRCA1* or *BRCA2*. Their analyses strongly rejected any models with no additional genetic effect in favor of either a dominant major gene with $q = 0.0008$ and a relative risk declining with age from 180 to 12 or a recessive major gene with $q = 0.065$ and a constant risk of 132. Two-locus models with a multiplicative effect of both a dominant and a recessive component ($q = 0.001$ and 0.063 with constant $RR = 13$ and 142, respectively) or a mixed model with a recessive and polygenic component ($q = 0.072$, $RR = 123$, and polygenic $SD = 0.73$) fit significantly better than either one-locus model.

Antoniou et al. (2001) also fitted segregation analysis models to first-degree relatives of a series of 1484 U.K. breast cancer cases under age 55. Rather than excluding *BRCA1/2* carriers, these investigators fitted two-locus models, including a polygenic background, where one locus was a composite of the two measured genes (a three-allele system: *BRCA1* positive, *BRCA2* positive, neither). The second locus (designated *BRCA3* but unmeasured) was also assumed to be rare, so that no subject would be a carrier of mutations at both loci. The authors' best-fitting model involved a recessive effect of *BRCA3* with an allele frequency of 24% and a penetrance of 42% by age 70. A purely recessive model gave a similarly good fit, and a dominant model fitted only slightly worse. In the mixed models, the polygenic component did not add significantly to a recessive genetic effect, while the dominant genetic effect did not add significantly to the polygenic effect. After adjusting for parity, a polygenic model fitted best. A further segregation analysis (Antoniou et al., 2002), exploiting in addition a series of high-risk families (using the mod score approach to adjust for ascertainment), yielded similar results.

The suggestion of a recessive effect for non-*BRCA1/2* familial breast cancer is supported by a subsequent descriptive cohort analysis (Dite et al., 2003) of the same Australian case-control family study described above. Standard SMR and proportional hazards regression models (with robust variance estimators) were used to describe the penetrance and relative risk of breast cancer in relatives of cases by the age and *BRCA1/2* carrier status of the proband. As in previous analyses of familial aggregation, relative risks declined with the age of the proband. In general, these relative risks were reduced only slightly when carrier families were removed. In noncarrier families, sisters of 40-year-old cases had a 10.7-fold excess risk and aunts a 4.2-fold excess, while mothers were not at excess risk, as might be expected under a recessive model. The authors point out that the Breast Cancer Linkage Consortium families were selected in part with the expectation that a dominant gene was being sought, so unlinked families in that series would be less likely than this population-based series to show evidence of a residual recessive component. Claus et al. (1998) reanalyzed the CASH study data, stratifying on the proband's predicted *BRCA1/2* carrier probability, and found a 2.0-fold increase in mothers and a 1.7-fold increase in sisters of cases who were unlikely to carry a mutation in these genes. In relatives of predicted carrier cases, the familial aggregation appeared to be explained by their carrier status.

To estimate the proportion of breast cancer families due to *BRCA1/2* mutations, Serova et al. (1997) performed mutation testing in 31 multiple-case families. They estimated that 8–10 of these families carried mutations in genes other than *BRCA1* or *BRCA2*. A study of 37 families with no mutations in either gene (Kainu et al., 2000) has suggested a linkage to a marker at 13q21 (a multipoint lod score under heterogeneity of 3.46, with $\theta = 0.10$ from marker D13S1308). A genomic map of this region revealed eight known genes and many other predicted genes; sequencing of five of these in 19 breast cancer families revealed numerous polymorphisms but no deleterious mutations (Rozenblum et al., 2002). However, this region was not confirmed in a linkage analysis of 128 families from the Breast Cancer Linkage Consortium who were not segregating mutations in *BRCA1* or *BRCA2* (Thompson et al., 2002).

Other genes are under investigation for their effects on breast cancer. Swift et al. (1991) suggested that relatives of patients with A-T were at elevated risk of cancer, particularly breast cancer. Ataxia-telangiectasia is a recessive disease caused by a mutation in the *ATM* gene, which among other features causes extreme sensitivity to ionizing radiation. Thus parents of A-T patients are obligatory heterozygotes, and half of all siblings and second-degree relatives are also heterozygotes. Swift (1994) later provided preliminary data suggesting a $G \times E$ interaction between the gene and ionizing radiation, a hypothesis currently under investigation in the study described

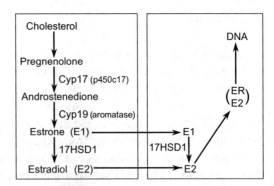

Figure 11.6 Genes on the estrogen synthesis pathway. (Adapted from Feigelson and Henderson, 1998)

earlier in this chapter. In a meta-analysis of the available data, Easton (1994) estimated a relative risk in *ATM* heterozygotes of 3.9 (95% CI 2.1–7.2) for breast cancer [3.2 (2.4–4.2) after correction for the use of spouse controls] and 1.9 (1.5–2.5) for all other cancers combined. Watts et al. (2002) showed that *ATM* carriers had distinct patterns of expression of many genes in lymphoblastoid cells, both at baseline and over time following ionizing radiation exposure, suggesting a possible mechanism for their increased cancer risk and radiosensitivity.

Because of the strong epidemiologic evidence implicating hormones, particularly estrogens, in breast and ovarian cancer, it is also natural to consider genes on the estrogen synthesis pathway (Fig. 11.6). All of these genes—*CYP17*, *CYP19*, *17HSD1*, and *ER*—are known to be polymorphic and appear to be weakly associated with a breast and/or ovarian cancer risk. Although their genetic relative risks are small compared with those of *BRCA1/2*, their population attributable risks could be substantial because polymorphisms in these genes are much more common, and the plausibility of their interactions with other reproductive risk factors or exogenous hormone use makes them particularly interesting targets for the study of $G \times E$ interactions. Feigelson et al. (2001) conducted a nested case-control study of *CYP17* and *HSD17B1* and found that risk increased in a dose-related fashion with the number of *A2* alleles of the former and *A1* alleles of the latter. The risk among women carrying four high-risk alleles was 2.21 (95% CI 0.98–5.00; p for trend = 0.03) compared with those who carried none. This risk was largely limited to women who were not using HRT (*RR*-2.60; 95% CI, 0.95–7.14) and was most pronounced among those weighing 170 pounds or less (*RR*-3.05; 95% CI, 1.29–7.25). Cui et al. (2003b) applied regressive logistic and proportional hazards familial models to population-based family data from Australia and found that a recessive model yielded an *RR* of 1.47 (95% CI 1.28–1.68) for the *CC* genotype of the 5′ UTR $T \to C$ MspA1 polymorphism in *CYP17* relative to the *CT* and *TT* genotypes.

Conclusions

The identification of a causal gene—whether by traditional positional cloning or by candidate gene association methods—is far from the end of a genetic epidemiologist's work. Some of the most interesting questions can then be attacked, such as how the gene affects the risk of disease, how it functions biologically, how it is distributed across populations, and how it interacts with other genes or other environmental factors. Both population-based and family-based study designs can be useful for answering these questions. Even collections of highly selected families can be used, with appropriate techniques of analysis that adjust appropriately for the way the families were ascertained. However, the generalizability of the results from such families may depend on untestable assumptions, such as the absence of heterogeneity in unmeasured risk factors. The family-based kin cohort design provided one of the first population-based estimates of the penetrance of the three common mutations in *BRCA1* and *BRCA2* among Ashkenazi Jews, indicating that in the general population, the lifetime risk appeared to be substantially lower than in the highly selected families used for linkage analysis. More sophisticated likelihood-based analyses, allowing more distant relatives and measured genotypes of other family members to be exploited, have led to similar or even lower penetrance estimates. Multistage and countermatched sampling designs have the potential to greatly improve the efficiency of these studies. A particularly simple approach to study $G \times E$ interaction is the case-only design, which requires an assumption of $G - E$ independence in the source population, although case-control, case-sibling, or case-parent trio designs have the advantage of not requiring this assumption. Both case-only and case-sibling designs have been used to investigate the interaction of *BRCA1/2* with OC use in breast and ovarian cancers, and a countermatched case-control study of the interaction of *ATM* and ionizing radiation in second breast cancers is currently underway.

Even after one or more genes have been identified, the possibility of residual familial aggregation that could be caused by yet undiscovered genes remains to be considered, leading back through the cycle of familial aggregation, segregation, linkage, and association studies in families not segregating the already known genes. This is the point at which we currently find ourselves with breast cancer, where there is mounting evidence that other genes remain to be discovered. The years to come are likely to be exciting ones in this field as we continue to pursue such questions.

12

Tying It All Together: The Genetic Epidemiology of Colorectal Cancer

This concluding chapter will illustrate the entire process of genetic epidemiology with the colorectal cancer story and show how the study of familial cancer sheds light on fundamental mechanistic processes. We begin with a historical perspective and insights from the descriptive epidemiology of familial and sporadic cancers and the role of nongenetic risk factors. We then explore the role of germline and somatic mutations in cancer, the two-hit hypothesis, and the different types of cancer genes that are involved. The two major forms of familial colorectal cancer—familial adenomatous polyposis coli (FAP) and hereditary nonpolyposis colorectal cancer (HNPCC)—are then discussed separately, showing the role that familial aggregation, segregation, linkage, and association studies have played and discussing ongoing efforts to characterize the relevant genes. This section concludes with a discussion of apparently sporadic cancers and the role that other genes and complex pathways might play in some of them. Finally, we look ahead to the future and speculate on the potential impact of high-volume genotyping methods, gene expression arrays, DNA methylation, imprinting, and proteomics.

History, Descriptive Epidemiology, and Familiality

Colorectal cancer is the second leading cause of cancer mortality in the United States, with a crude annual incidence rate of about 39/100,000 (U.S. SEER whites, 1988–92, both sexes) and a mortality rate of 21/100,000 (United States, 1999, all races, both sexes). The relative accessibility of the colon by means of sigmoidoscopy is a definite advantage in studying the genetics and pathophysiology of the disease. Colorectal cancer was first recognized as a familial syndrome late in the nineteenth century by Warthin (1913), who described a cluster of cases in his seamstress's family. This family initially had primarily gastric and uterine cancers, but as it has been followed in four additional publications, more recent generations have had a high incidence of colorectal cancers (Lynch and Krush, 1971). Lynch et al. (1966) defined two classes of familial cancer syndromes—Type I, limited to colorectal cancer, and Type II involving other cancers such as those of the female genital tract—although it now appears that these may not have a distinct genetic basis.

Familial risk of colorectal polyps and colorectal cancer has been described in a number of publications (Bale et al., 1984; Carstensen et al., 1996; Lovett, 1976; Lynch et al., 1973; Macklin, 1960; Woolf, 1958). For example, Fuchs et al. (1994) conducted a cohort study of 32,085 men and 87,031 women who had not previously been examined by endoscopy. Each provided baseline data on first-degree relatives with colorectal cancer, diet, and other risk factors for the disease. During the follow-up period, colorectal cancer was diagnosed in 148 men and 315 women. The familial relative risk in first-degree relatives of colorectal cancer patients was found to be about 1.7, rising to 2.8 if two or more first-degree relatives were affected or and to 5.4 if both relatives were less than 45 years old at diagnosis. Studies of familial coaggregation of different cancers have also suggested that a family history of breast, ovarian, and endometrial cancers may be associated with an increased risk of colorectal cancer (Andrieu et al., 1991; Cramer et al., 1983; Schildkraut and Thompson, 1988). In contrast, Winawer et al. (1996) examined familial aggregation in relation to colorectal polyps using a case-control family design. A random sample of 1199 patients found to have polyps identified by the National Polyps Study were enrolled as cases and 1411 unaffected spouses served as controls, and the incidence of colorectal cancer in their first-degree relatives was compared. Polyps were found to be associated with a 1.8-fold risk of colorectal cancer in first-degree relatives and a 2.6-fold risk in first-degree relatives of polyps cases affected below age 60. The relative risk to a sibling of a polyps case who also had a parent with colorectal cancer was 3.3. The tendency for polyps and colorectal cancer to coaggregate in families has been replicated in numerous other studies (Ahsan et al., 1998; Aste et al., 1984; Nakama et al., 2000; Novis and Naftali, 1999; Ponz de Leon et al., 1987).

Given the evidence discussed below for environmental factors like diet that are likely to be highly shared by family members, it is not at all obvious whether the consistent but modest familial risks for polyps and cancer are due to genetic influences or shared environment. In an attempt to answer this question, several authors have conducted segregation analyses of the pattern of familial aggregation, but without using specific information on environmental covariates. Burt et al. (1985) conducted a segregation analysis of colorectal cancer and polyps in a single six-generation kindred of 5000 Utah Mormons ascertained on the basis of a brother, sister, and nephew affected with colorectal cancer. Using sigmoidoscopy, 21% of kindred members and 9% of their spouses were found to have polyps. In addition, 15 pedigree members and 3 spouses were found to have had colorectal cancer; these showed no obvious pattern of inheritance, either by inspection or by formal segregation analysis of this trait alone. When combined with the polyps data, however, segregation analysis rejected the sporadic and autosomal recessive models in favor of a dominant model for the joint phenotype (either polyps or cancer). Cannon-Albright et al. (1988) followed up these results in the same population with a segregation analysis of 670 individuals from 34 kindreds identified through either a polyp or a cluster of colorectal cancers, with an ascertainment correction that depended on how the family was identified; they also concluded that a dominant model fitted best (with an allele frequency of $q = 0.19$) and that polyps and cancer occurred only in carriers. In both of these studies, polyp and cancer cases were both treated as affected, leaving open the questions of whether they share a common genetic etiology and how their penetrances might differ.

It is now recognized that there are two distinct forms of familial colorectal cancer syndromes, those characterized by large numbers of polyps and those without them. In FAP, at-risk individuals develop thousands of such polyps over the course of their lives, typically beginning in their 20s. While polyps are a precursor lesion for carcinoma, those that occur in FAP appear individually to be at no higher risk of progression than those occurring in nonfamilial cases (Kinzler and Vogelstein, 2002a). However, the sheer number of such polyps puts the individual at very high risk of cancer. Unless the colon is removed prophylactically, virtually all patients with FAP will develop colorectal cancer at a median age of about 40. (In addition to FAP, there are several other rare syndromes involving polyps that are now known to have different genetic origins [e.g., Puetz-Jaeger syndrome, juvenile polyposis, Cowden syndrome]; in the remainder of this chapter, we will focus on FAP.)

In contrast, HNPCC cases have no such recognizable precursor and, prior to the recognition of the specific genetic defect, could only be defined in terms of the pattern of familial aggregation. By consensus, HNPCC is now defined by the *Amsterdam criteria* (Vasen et al., 1991): at least three verified cases in two or more generations, with at least one of them being a first-degree relative of the other two and at least one cancer having occurred before age 50; FAP must also be excluded. A subsequent NCI Workshop extended this definition to include certain other cancers that commonly cosegregate with colorectal cancer, such as endometrial, ovarian, and gastric cancers (Rodriguez-Bigas et al., 1997). Testing for familial aggregation or segregation for this type of cancer is complicated by the need to allow for this highly restrictive ascertainment criterion.

In the aggregate, these familial forms still account for only about 3%–5% of all colorectal cancers (Kinzler and Vogelstein, 2002a). Nevertheless, genetics may play a role in the remainder (which we will call *sporadic*, although some may have an FH not meeting the criteria for FAP or HNPCC). Nongenetic factors also clearly play a role in sporadic cancers and may also be modifiers of the genetic effect in the familial forms. Hypotheses about other risk factors are suggested by the 20-fold international variation in incidence rates (high in North America, Europe, and, recently, Japan; low in Africa, India, and South America). Migrant studies suggest that migrants tend to adopt the disease rates of the country to which they move (at a rate depending in part on their age at migration) to a greater extent than their descendants. For example, although Japan had a low rate of colorectal cancer until recently, the rate among Japanese in Hawaii is among the highest in the world. Similarly, African-Americans have even higher rates than whites in the United States (Haenszel, 1961; Haenszel and Kurihara, 1968; McMichael and Giles, 1988). These patterns have been interpreted as suggesting that acculturation may play a role, most likely through dietary factors.

A large number of epidemiologic studies, using both ecologic correlation and analytic (cohort and case-control) designs, have been done to investigate specific hypotheses, particularly for diet (see Potter, 1999; Potter et al., 1993, for comprehensive reviews). The dietary hypotheses that have the greatest support relate to three interrelated groups of foods and nutrients: fruits/vegetables/fiber/folate, meat/fat, and calcium. Unscrambling these effects is beyond the scope of this brief review, but we will return to two of them later as we examine the role of $G \times E$ interactions, specifically those of folate with the *MTHFR* gene and red meat with a series of metabolic genes. Other established risk factors include physical activity and obesity, HRT, tobacco smoking, alcohol, and nonsteroidal anti-inflammatory drugs, but the remainder of this chapter will focus on genetic factors.

Polyps in particular must be noted as a risk factor for colorectal cancer in the general population. Although the familial coaggregation of polyps and cancer is well established and there are good mechanistic reasons to believe that most cancers develop out of an adenomatous polyp (Hill et al., 1978) (as discussed in the following section), there are limited data the risk of cancer following polyps in individuals, if only because the current standard of treatment for polyps consists of searching the entire colon by colonoscopy and removing all polyps before they can turn into cancers (Winawer et al., 1990). From 30% to 50% of individuals with one polyp will be found to have one or more additional polyps at the same time, and 30% will develop additional ones later. Levi et al. (1993) conducted a cohort study of 2496 individuals with intestinal polyps followed for an average of 4 years each. A 2.1-fold excess of colorectal cancer was found (35 cases compared with 17 expected). No excess of other cancers was seen, except for 2 cases of small intestine cancer compared with 0.4 expected.

Mechanistic Hypotheses

Models of carcinogenesis

It is generally accepted that both germline and sporadic mutations are involved in most cancers, including colorectal cancers. In a study of retinoblastoma, Knudson (1971) advanced the hypothesis that the same gene is involved in both familial and sporadic forms. Specifically, he proposed that two hits to the same gene in the same cell are required to produce a cancer. In sporadic cancers, both of these events occur somatically; since these are rare events, the probability of two of them occurring at the same locus in the same cell is small. In familial cancers, however, one of the two mutations is transmitted in the germline and thus is carried in every somatic cell; thus, a single additional somatic mutation in any cell of target tissue is sufficient, thereby accounting for the much higher risk in familial cases. In order to account for the steep rise in incidence with age, Knudson also proposed that cells with a single mutation undergo clonal expansion. A mathematical representation of this process was developed by Moolgavkar, known as the *two-mutation clonal-expansion model* (Moolgavkar and Knudson, 1981), that has now been applied to a wide range of cancers and environmental agents.

Long before the Moolgavkar-Knudson model was developed, Armitage and Doll (1954) proposed that a series of mutational events was required, leading to what has become known as the *multistage model of cancer*. Specifically, if k such events are required, they showed that the age-specific incidence rate would be proportional to age^{k-1}, where for most solid cancers, the best fit for k is about 5–7. From studies of the molecular changes in the progression from normal mucosa, to polyps, to increasing grades of dysplasia and carcinoma (Fearon, 1995), it has become evident that more than two mutations are required to cause colorectal cancer. Moolgavkar and Luebeck (1992) have extended the two-event model to incorporate these additional stages.

According to the multistage theory of carcinogenesis, colorectal cancers are thought to derive from a single cell having undergone a sequence of mutations and clonal expansions (Nowell, 1976). A first mutation confers a

competitive growth advantage over normal cells. Among this clone of intermediate cells, one cell acquires a second mutation, leading to further clonal
expansion and/or an increased risk of a further mutation, and so on. The first
empiric evidence for this single-cell origin of colorectal cancers came from
studies of X inactivation. In females, only one of the two copies of the X
chromosome is expressed, the particular copy being randomly selected early
in embryonal development by DNA methylation, which is then transmitted
to all successive daughter cells. Thus, normal colonic mucosa comprises
a random distribution of cells with the maternal or paternal copy inactivated. In contrast, colorectal tumor cells invariably have the same copy inactivated, indicating that all cells of the tumor are descended from a single
cell (Fearon et al., 1987).

The normal architecture of the colonic mucosa consists of tiny crypts
that are approximately 50 cells deep, containing the stem cells from which
the epithelial cells differentiate and migrate to the surface of the gut. A
possible evolutionary basis for this structure is to protect the stem cells
from the highly mutagenic environment of fecal material. Thus, it has been
suggested that the first hit in the Knudson model is more likely to be from
blood-borne rather than fecal-borne mutagens (Potter, 1999). Once cells
with a mutation have migrated to the surface, they tend to form a lesion
known as an *aberrant-crypt focus (ACF)* or microadenoma. After further
exposure to the contents of the colon, these foci are then thought to develop
into polyps and cancers. Nevertheless, although ACFs occur frequently and
polyps are premalignant, they rarely develop into cancers even in FAP.

Cancer genes

We now recognize two broad classes of major susceptibility genes for cancer.
Oncogenes are altered forms of genes called *proto-oncogenes* that are involved
in normal regulation of the cell cycle, cell division, and differentiation. When
activated, these oncogenes experience a gain of function, for example rescu-
ing cells from apoptosis (programmed cell death), or immortalizing genes
that block cell differentiation, or reducing growth factor dependence leading
to loss of contact inhibition. Mutation of *tumor-suppressor genes,* in contrast,
leads to a loss of function. There are two main categories of tumor suppressor genes—*gatekeepers* and *caretakers* (Kinzler and Vogelstein, 2002b,
pp. 209–210):

> Gatekeepers are genes that directly regulate the growth of tumors by inhibit-
> ing their growth or by promoting their death. The functions of these genes
> are rate-limiting for tumor growth, and as a result, both the maternal and
> paternal copies of these genes must be inactivated for a tumor to develop....
> In contrast, inactivation of caretakers does not directly promote growth of

tumors. Rather, inactivation of caretakers leads to a genetic instability that only indirectly promotes growth by causing an increased mutation rate. Because numerous mutations are required for the full development of a cancer, inactivation of caretakers, with the consequent increase in genetic instability, can greatly accelerate the development of cancers.

Genes involved in DNA repair, including the MMR genes *hMSH2* and *hMLH1* involved in HNPCC, are subject to loss-of-function mutations and are thus examples of caretaker tumor-suppressor genes. Other DNA repair pathways could also be relevant, such as those involved in repair of double-strand breaks that are caused, for example, by ionizing radiation (a complex involving, among others, the *ATM*, *BRCA1*, and *p53* genes interacting with Rad50/Mre11/Nbs1) and the nucleotide excision repair pathway. In contrast, the *APC* gene responsible for FAP is a gatekeeper, whose disruption is a very early event on the pathway leading to colorectal polyps by increased transcription of growth-promoting genes like *c-MYC* (Kinzler and Vogelstein, 2002a).

Genomic instability

This is not to say that colorectal tumors are genetically homogeneous. Indeed, HNPCC tumors with microsatellite instability are highly heterogeneous, as demonstrated by experiments in which colorectal tumors have been microdissected and the spectrum of mutations in different regions used to infer the age of the tumor (Tsao et al., 2000). In this experiment, the initial event is assumed to be loss of MMR capability (e.g., mutation or loss of *hMLH1* or *hMSH2* leading to accumulation of further mutations at a much accelerated rate). The data for these analyses were obtained from the distribution of microsatellite alleles in noncoding regions. The numbers of generations from loss of MMR to the start of the terminal expansion period and from there to diagnosis were estimated using the variance in allele lengths within loci across a tumor and the differences between the most common alleles and the germline, using coalescent methods similar to those discussed in Chapter 10.

Most colorectal cancers have some form of genetic instability. In HNPCC, it is MSI due to MMR mutations. But in the majority of sporadic cancers a different form of genomic instability, known as *chromosomal instability*, is seen, in which whole chromosomes or at least large chromosomal regions are lost or duplicated. In a small fraction of these cases, the mechanism for this appears to be mutation in the mitotic checkpoint gene *BUB1* (Cahill et al., 1998), but in most cases the genetic basis of chromosomal instability remains to be discovered.

Familial Cancer Syndromes

Familial adenomatous polyposis

Familial adenomatous polyposis has been known for decades to be inherited in a dominant fashion (Veale, 1965). The first clue that the *APC* gene was responsible for FAP was the observation of a germline deletion of the entire 5q chromosome in a single patient with Garner syndrome (one of the rare polyposis conditions associated with colorectal cancer) (Herrera et al., 1986), suggesting that a tumor-suppressor gene might be located somewhere in this region. Subsequent linkage analyses (Bodmer et al., 1987; Leppert et al., 1987; Nakamura et al., 1988) further localized the region to 5q21. Figure 12.1 summarizes the lod scores with respect to marker C11p11 reported by all three studies, showing virtually identical results, each producing a 1-lod support interval of about 14 cM, the aggregate narrowing the interval to 5 cM. Multipoint analyses by Leppert et al. (1987) suggested that the gene was distal to C11p11, possibly on either side of the nearest marker, MC5.61, 12 cM away. Nakamura et al. (1988) then added additional markers to the region, including one (YN5.48) between the previous two, which yielded a two-point lod score of 8.25 at $\theta = 0$ (compared with 3.32 for C11p11 and 8.05 for MC5.61) and a strong peak near YN5.48 by multipoint analysis (Fig. 12.2). On this basis, the 1-lod support interval was reduced to about 3 cM on either side of YN5.48, still a relatively large region to search by brute force sequencing. These three analyses included a subtype of FAP known as *Gardner syndrome,* characterized by such extracolonic manifestations as multiple osteomas, fibrous cysts, and congenital hypertrophy of the retina, and found no evidence of heterogeneity between these two subtypes.

Additional evidence for a tumor-suppressor gene in this region came from the observation that 20%–50% of sporadic cancers had somatic chromosomal losses in 5q. These losses occurred with equal frequency in

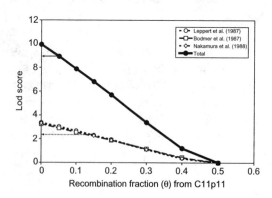

Figure 12.1 Summary of two-point linkage results for familial adenomatous polyposis coli and the C11p11 marker from Leppert et al. (1987) (open circles), Bodmer et al. (1987) (open squares), and Nakamura et al. (1988) (open diamonds), together with the combined lod score (solid circles); 1-lod confidence intervals are indicated by horizontal arrows.

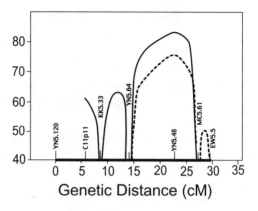

Figure 12.2 Multipoint lod scores for familial adenomatous polyposis coli using two overlapping panels of markers. Solid line: C11p11, KK5.33, YN5.64, YN5.48; dotted line: YN5.64, YN5.48, MC5.61, EW5.5. (Reprinted with permission from Nakamura et al., 1988)

small benign and larger malignant tumors, suggesting that this event was a very early one in the carcinogenic process (Vogelstein et al., 1988). Of the four genes found in the linked region, *APC* was the only one found to carry mutations in FAP and sporadic cancer patients (Groden et al., 1991; Nishisho et al., 1991). Mutations have been found in this gene in virtually all of the over 500 FAP kindreds studied so far (Laurent-Puig et al., 1998; Nagase and Nakamura, 1993), as well as in over 80% of sporadic colorectal cancers, including very early lesions affecting only a few crypts. The vast majority of these are truncating mutations, with some large deletions or mutations that lead to reduced expression. An important exception is the missense polymorphism I1307K, which occurs rarely in the general population but in about 6% of Ashkenazi Jews. It appears to be associated with an FH of colorectal cancer in that population and, in these families, to be carried by cases of colorectal polyps or cancer (Laken et al., 1997). Since these missense mutations do not have an obvious effect on function, the argument that they are the cause of these conditions relies on a Bayesian calculation of the ratio of the posterior probability that the mutation is causal to the probability that it is not, given the observed pedigree data (Peterson et al., 1998; Thompson et al., 2003). Molecular study of these individuals revealed that about half of them also carried a truncating mutation in the immediate vicinity, suggesting that the I1307K polymorphism leads to a *premutation* that is highly susceptible to somatic mutation in the adjacent region (Laken et al., 1997). This observation suggests that major mutations in both copies of *APC* are needed to produce *APC*, while minor mutations might lead to an increased risk of sporadic cancer but not the full-blown familial syndrome. About a third of sporadic cancers have been shown to have no functioning copy of *APC* (Powell et al., 1992), while in tumor cells from FAP patients, about 80% have no functioning copy (Smith et al., 1993). *APC* appears to act in a complex with β-catenin to activate growth-promoting genes such as c-MYC; thus, the initial hit in the Knudson model could be either an inactivating mutation in APC or an activating mutation in β-catenin. Kinzler and Vogelstein (2002a) provide further details on the FAP story and the function of APC.

Familial adenomatous polyposis is a very rare syndrome, accounting for only about 0.5% of all cases of colorectal cancer. Estimates of the population allele frequency q are less than $1/20,000$ (Fearon, 1995). Nevertheless, study of the genetics of the familial form is important in understanding the role of somatic mutations in APC in sporadic cancers.

Hereditary nonpolyposis colorectal cancer

Like FAP, HNPCC is inherited in an autosomal dominant fashion. Houlston et al. (1995) ascertained 305 pedigrees through an age-stratified sample of probands from the population-based registry for Northern Ireland, and, using the POINTER program for complex segregation analysis, concluded that the best-fitting model was a single dominant major gene with a population frequency of $q = 0.002$ and a lifetime penetrance of 85%, although the results depended on the particular likelihood method used. Bailey-Wilson et al. (1986) conducted segregation analysis on 11 large pedigrees comprising a total of 2762 individuals meeting the criteria for HNPCC and also concluded that a dominant model fitted best, with a lifetime penetrance of 71%–79% and a mean age of onset of 47. Scapoli et al. (1994) also limited their study to HNPCC kindreds from the Modena district of Italy, but their segregation analysis suggested instead a two-locus model in which the major locus acted in a codominant manner with an allele frequency of $q = 0.0044$ and a lifetime penetrance of 73% for heterozygotes.

Both of the latter two studies involved ascertainment of multicase families, raising questions about ascertainment correction. Scapoli et al. do not address how this was done, but Bailey-Wilson et al. provide an extensive comparison of their results without ascertainment correction, under single ascertainment for the original proband, also conditioning on the two cases most closely related to the proband. Because their pedigrees are large (252 on average), the two correction methods yielded fairly similar results, having somewhat greater influence on the allele frequency than on the penetrances. Additional analyses were conducted to assess whether other cancers were part of the syndrome: first, analyses of the phenotype *all cancer,* assuming a common age distribution but separate lifetime penetrances, yielded a poor fit under all models considered; second, separate analyses of colorectal cancer in families with only that cancer and those with other cancers yielded no evidence of heterogeneity between the two groups under any of the models considered.

The classic feature of HNPCC is microsatellite instability (MSI). In the 1980s, Loeb (1994) proposed that a *hypermutable phenotype* would be needed to account for the numerous somatic mutations found in most colorectal cancers. A mechanism was later shown to be the genome-wide instability in microsatellite sequences that was produced by mutations in the *MMR genes*, discovered independently by three groups using a variety of approaches (Ionov et al., 1993; Peltomaki et al., 1993; Thibodeau et al., 1993). Thibodeau et al., using sporadic colon cancer, found that the MSI was less likely to occur in patients with LOH on chromosomes 5q, 17p, and 18q. Peltomaki et al. applied linkage analysis to two large kindreds to map a locus to 2p15-16.

Elucidation of the mechanism of MSI came instead from studies of yeast genetics, which showed that mutations in several genes of the Mut HLS MMR pathway could lead to several-hundred-fold increases in the rates of mutation of poly(GT) sequences (Strand et al., 1993). This led to a search for the human homologues of these yeast MMR genes, the first of which to be discovered (*hMSH2*) was found in the region of 2p15-16 previously linked to HNPCC (Fishel et al., 1993; Leach et al., 1993). Soon thereafter, a second MMR gene (*hMLH1*) was mapped to 3p (Lindblom et al., 1993), a third (*hMLH6*) was found in the same region of 2p as the first (Miyaki et al., 1997), and two others (*hPMS1* on 2q and *hPMS2* on 7p) have also been identified, each based on linkage analysis in one or two large HNPCC kindreds. The MMR repair system involves a complex interaction among the protein products of all these genes (see Boland, 2002 for a description), the end result of which is to eliminate about 99.9% of the errors that occur spontaneously during DNA replication, reducing errors to a rate of about 1 per 10^{12} bp.

Efforts have now turned to the molecular characterization of these genes in terms of their spectrum and frequency of mutations in different populations, their effects on age-specific penetrance, and their interaction with other risk factors. Some data on prevalence of mutations are available from clinic-based families and even less from population-based cases unselected for family history.

In families meeting the Amsterdam criteria, estimates of carrier prevalence range from 25% (Weber et al., 1997) to 70% (Liu et al., 1996). A reanalysis (J. Hopper, unpublished) of data from five studies totaling 284 HNPCC clinic-based families yielded an estimate of the prevalence of deleterious mutations in either *hMLH1* or *hMSH2* of 47% with 95% confidence limits of 41%–53%. In clinic-based families not meeting the Amsterdam criteria, estimates range from 7% (Wijnen et al., 1998) to 16% (Moslein et al., 1996). Wijnen et al. (1998) provide a logistic model for estimating the probability of carrying an MMR mutation in families suspected of having HNPCC, similar to the LAMBDA model for *BRCAx* mutations described in Chapter 11.

There have been only two population-based studies of MMR mutations to date. Aaltonen et al. (1998) tested a consecutive series of 509 patients from nine hospitals in southeast Finland, first by MSI testing and then by sequencing of those found to be MSI+; 10% were found to have an MSI+ tumor and 2% to carry an MMR mutation. Farrington et al. (1998) studied 50 cases diagnosed before age 30 from the Scottish National Cancer Registry and reported an overall prevalence of 28%, varying with FH: 15% in those with no family history up to third-degree relatives, 46% in those with at least one affected family member but not meeting the Amsterdam criteria, and 50% in those that did meet the Amsterdam criteria.

Data on penetrance are even more limited. The largest clinic-based study to date is a retrospective cohort study of 360 carriers of mutations in *hMLH1* or *hMSH2* identified from 50 Finnish HNPCC families (Aarnio et al., 1999). The authors estimated a risk to age 70 of 100% in males and 54% in females, but it is not clear whether the index cases leading to ascertainment were excluded from the analysis. Two other studies based on HNPCC families (Lin et al., 1998; Vasen et al., 1996) yielding high estimates of penetrance appear to be similarly flawed by a failure to allow properly for ascertainment.

The only population-based study published to date (Dunlop et al., 1997) did MSI testing followed by sequencing of MMR genes in 27 cases ascertained between 1970 and 1993 from the Scottish National Cancer Registry, excluding those referred specifically because of a family history meeting the Amsterdam criteria. For the six probands found to carry a mutation in *hMLH1* or *hMSH2*, pedigrees were assembled, comprising a total of 156 individuals over age 18. Likelihood-based analyses using the techniques described in Chapter 11, based on computing carrier probabilities for each family member based on his or her own or other family members' genotypes, yielded an estimate of risk of all cancers to age 70 of 91% for males and 69% for females. In males, the majority of this risk (74%) was accounted for by colorectal cancer, while in females, the risk was dominated by uterine cancer (42%), followed by colorectal cancer (30%). Similar estimates of colorectal cancer risk (100% in males, 15% in females) were found by another population-based study from Australia (J. Hopper, unpublished data).

Because of the rarity of mutations in these genes, standard population-based case-control and cohort designs have limited utility, so family studies based on multiplex ascertainment schemes are attractive, as illustrated by the studies described above. To emphasize the subtleties of the design of such studies, we briefly describe ongoing efforts by a multinational consortium to characterize MMR mutations and their interactions with other factors. The National Cancer Institute has established a Cooperative Family Registry for Colorectal Cancer Studies (CFRCCS; see http://epi.grants.cancer.gov/CCFR/Q&A.html for details) that will comprise over 8000 pedigrees totaling over 250,000 individuals. Phenotypes, extensive questionnaire data on risk factors for surviving family members, and biological specimens for the probands and selected relatives (both affected and unaffected) are being collected. Families have been ascertained by six participating centers in the United States, Canada, and Australia using a variety of sampling schemes, some population-based (some using multistage sampling on such factors as age, race, or FH), some clinic-based.

Because of the cost of mutation screening, a multistage sampling design has been developed (see Chapter 11), first screening all probands for MSI status and then sequencing *hMSH2* and *hMLS1* in all MSI-high or MSI-low cases and a 10% sample of MSI-stable cases; all living relatives (out to the third degree) of mutation carriers will also be genotyped. Careful attention is needed to the statistical design of such studies to ensure that the results will not be subject to ascertainment bias and to estimate the power of the study. The analysis will use the likelihood-based approaches to gene characterization discussed in Chapter 11, including all individuals—whether genotyped or not—by summing over the genotypes of the untyped family members, conditional on the available genotype information. This analysis also needs to take account of the multistage sampling in the design, using techniques such as the Horwitz-Thompson estimating equations or weighted likelihood approaches described earlier.

The statistical power of the design was estimated by Monte Carlo simulation, in which data were simulated for typical pedigree structures under a given model for penetrance, allele frequency, and sensitivity/specificity of MSI testing using the proposed multistage sampling scheme. These simulated data were then analyzed using the proposed statistical methods, and the distribution of results across replicate simulations was used to estimate power.

These analyses will focus particularly on modifiers of the effects of MMR mutations—both environmental exposures and other genes—particularly in light of evidence of the sensitivity of MMR-deficient cell lines to environmental agents (Lopez et al., 2002), perhaps mediated through DNA methylation (see below) (Jirtle et al., 2000). Another aim will be to characterize the effects of different types of MMR mutations, which will require the use of hierarchical models to identify relevant mutation characteristics (Witte, 1997), because the rarity of any particular mutation and the multiple comparisons will preclude direct estimation of the effect of any particular mutation.

Sporadic Cancers

Genetic alterations in colorectal cancer

Returning to the theme introduced at the beginning of this chapter that the same genes might prove to be involved in the etiology of both hereditary and sporadic cancers—with the difference that in hereditary cancers one copy of a mutant allele was inherited in the germline and the other mutation occurred somatically, while in sporadic cancers both mutations are acquired somatically—we now consider a genetic model for colorectal carcinogenesis proposed by Vogelstein and colleagues (Fearon and Vogelstein, 1990; Kinzler and Vogelstein, 2002a). Figure 12.3 provides a schematic representation of the model, commonly referred to as a *Vogelgram*.

The process begins with inactivation of both copies of the *APC* gene. This event sets in motion an adenomatous process leading first to the creation of a single dysplastic cell, which then develops into a polyp by clonal expansion. (This first mutation could be the result of one of the metabolic processes described below.) Such a polyp could remain dormant indefinitely, but if one of its cells develops a further mutation (most often in *K-RAS*), it will acquire a proliferative advantage leading to a larger tumor. Subsequent waves of mutation and proliferation continue in a branching process, typically involving somatic mutations in such genes as *DCC, SMAD4, SMAD2,* and *p53,* each leading to the creation of more dysplastic, more unstable, and more aggressive cells that overtake the earlier clones. Once a cell has acquired a sufficient number of mutations, it becomes fully malignant, invading neighboring tissues and metastasizing.

This process has a high degree of randomness, so the actual sequence of mutations will vary from one tumor to another, and probably no gene in this sequence is either necessary or sufficient. Nevertheless, this model does essentially posit a minimum of seven genetic events (inherited or acquired)—the activation of one oncogene (*APC*) and the inactivation of

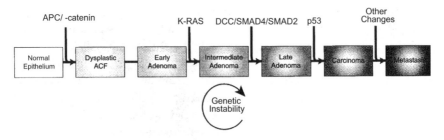

Figure 12.3 A genetic model for colorectal carcinogenesis. (Reprinted with permission from Kinzler and Vogelstein, 2002a)

three tumor-suppressor genes (two mutations each)—a considerably more complex model than the original Knudson hypothesis.

These various genes serve different purposes, so that the order in which mutations occur can have a major influence on the outcome. For example, *p53* mutations are extremely common in colorectal cancers. The *p53* gene appears to function as a tumor-suppressor gene by binding to the promoters of growth-inhibiting genes or by activating apoptosis-promoting genes. Those rare individuals who have inherited a mutant copy of *p53* (Li-Fraumeni syndrome) (Li et al., 1988) do not tend to develop polyposis, although they are at elevated risk of cancer. Thus, the *p53* gene cannot be an initiator of the carcinogenesis process (i.e., an oncogene), but rather acts as a gatekeeper.

Pathways: suppressor and mutator

The traditional view, described above, incorporates the basic notion that there are two main routes to colorectal cancer: the *suppressor pathway*, characterized by mutational inactivation of both alleles of a tumor-suppressor gene (such as *APC*) or by activation of oncogenes, and the *mutator pathway*, characterized by widespread genomic instability associated with defective MMR genes. However, the traditional view makes a closer identification between these two pathways and the FAP and HNPCC conditions than now appears warranted (Rodriguez-Bigas et al., 1997). First of all, MSI is manifest in 15%–30% of all colorectal cancers, including sporadic cancers (Aaltonen et al., 1993; Ionov et al., 1993; Thibodeau et al., 1993). Second, the term *hereditary nonpolyposis colorectal cancer* has commonly, but some say incorrectly, been used as synonymous with carrying a mutation in an MMR gene, although Aaltonen et al. (1998) found that in a consecutive series of 509 patients, germline MMR mutations were found in only 10 of 63 patients with MSI. More importantly, 20%–40% of HNPCC families (as defined by the Amsterdam criteria) do not carry germline mutations in known MMR genes or have tumors with MSI (S. Thibodeau, personal communication). For these reasons, the more restrictive term *hereditary mismatch repair deficiency syndrome (HMRDS)* has been proposed for cases carrying germline MMR mutations (Jass, 1998).

Three classes of MSI have been defined (Dietmaier et al., 1997; Thibodeau et al., 1998): MSS (microsatellite stable), MSI-L (fewer than 30%–40% of markers tested showing MSI), and MSI-H (high frequency of MSI); MSI-H tumors could have many mutations. Microsatellite instability high is characteristic of tumors with MMR mutations and distinguishes them from those caused by the suppressor pathway, but MMR mutations are not restricted to HNPCC; inactivation of both copies of an MMR gene can also occur somatically, leading to a sporadic case. Liu et al. (1995) found that the majority of cases under age 35 had MSI irrespective of their FH and most of these carry germline MMR mutations. Thus, the Amsterdam criteria are not sufficient to identify all MMR families (Lynch et al., 1996; Vasen et al., 1991).

There is also a growing body of evidence on biological differences between tumors caused by the two pathways (Thibodeau et al., 1998): the MSI-H tumors are more likely to have mutations in the TGF-β receptor gene and less likely to have loss of APC or mutations in $p53$ or K-RAS than MSS tumors; they are also more likely to be diploid, to have lower carcinoembryonic antigen (CEA) expression, to occur on the right side, to occur in females, and to have a better prognosis, as well as a host of histopathologic differences and differences in response to chemotherapeutic agents. In general, MSI-L tumors tend to be more similar to MSS than to MSI-H tumors, although frequent involvement of $MLH6$ has been reported in MSI-L HNPCC cases.

In contrast, there are few consistent molecular differences between sporadic and HNPCC cases with MSI-H tumors (Rodriguez-Bigas et al., 1997). The most important of these seems to be that the germline mutations found in HNPCC cases tend to be insertions, deletions, and point mutations, while most of the sporadic cancers tend to be caused by DNA methylation of the promoter region of $hMLH1$ (Thibodeau et al., 1998). (We will describe methylation in greater detail below.) Failure to distinguish between cancers caused by the two pathways (e.g., using the phenotypic definitions of FAP/HNPCC/sporadic rather than a molecular definition based on MSI) could well have obscured important differences in their etiology, prognosis, and response to treatment.

Metabolic pathways

This is probably not the only pathway that can lead to sporadic cancers, however. A number of environmental exposures are risk factors for colorectal cancer, and individual susceptibility to such factors is doubtless influenced by various metabolic pathways that involve polymorphic genes. Tobacco smoking and consumption of well-done red meat are two examples (Potter, 1999). Tobacco smoke contains literally hundreds of chemicals, many of which are known to be carcinogenic, including polycyclic aromatic hydrocarbons (PAHs). Cooking of red meats creates another class of carcinogens known as heterocyclic amines (HCA), the concentration of which increases with greater doneness. (In fact, both classes of chemicals can be found in both sources.)

These chemicals require metabolic activation to become fully carcinogenic via a sequence of biochemical reactions mediated by what are known as *phase I enzymes*. These reaction products can also be detoxified by another series of reactions catalyzed by *phase II enzymes*. For example, the PAH benzo(a)pyrene (BAP) is converted to its most carcinogenic form, BAP 7,8-dihydrodiol 9,10-epoxide, by a sequence of reactions involving any of several cytochrome p-450 enzymes, such as CYP1A1, and microsomal epoxide hydrolase (*mEH*, encoded by the gene *EPHX1*), and is detoxified by any of several glutothyione-S-hydrolases, such as GSTM3. Activation of HCAs is catalyzed by CYP1A2 and the *N*-acetyltransferases NAT1 or NAT2, and is detoxified by various UDP-glucuronosyltransferases. All these genes are polymorphic. Although the relative risks associated with the range of polymorphisms is relatively modest (typically less than 2 or 3), their high frequency in the general population means that they could perhaps account for a larger population attributable risk than the rare major genes responsible for the familial syndromes. Furthermore, since the function of these genes is to metabolize various environmental substrates, it is highly likely that $G \times E$ and $G \times G$ interactions are important. This could form a basis for prevention. Unscrambling such a complex network is challenging, since considering only one gene at a time or pairwise interactions of one gene with one exposure factor risks diluting an already weak signal with a large amount of misclassification or confounding. Cortessis and Thomas (2003) describe an approach to complex and competing metabolic pathways based on Bayesian pharmacokinetic modeling (Gelman et al., 1996; Wakefield, 1996) of the entire network. Conti et al. (2003) compare this approach with one using Bayesian model averaging. Sillanpää and Corander (2002) discuss similar techniques for linkage analysis in the presence of uncertainty about which loci to include in the model.

Other pathways that could be relevant to colorectal cancer include folate metabolism, involving the *MTHFR* gene (Chen et al., 1996; Ma et al., 1997) and calcium and vitamin D, involving the vitamin D receptor gene (Cross et al., 1996; Darwish and DeLuca, 1993). For example, the folate-*MTHFR* combination appears to have a real interaction effect, in that risk is increased only when both folate deficiency and a variant genotype are present, and may act by influencing the availability of the methyl donor *S*-adenosyl methionine (SAM), leading to DNA hypomethylation, as discussed further below (Potter, 1999). De Jong et al. (2002) conducted a pooled analysis of 30 polymorphisms that had been reported two or more times in colorectal cancer or polyps studies, and confirmed associations of seven of them—*GSTT1, NAT2, HRAS1, ALDH2, MTHFR, Tp53,* and *TNF-α*—with cancer but none with polyps.

The relationship between polyps and colorectal cancer

Relatively few studies have examined polyps and colorectal cancer jointly, and many of those that have combined them in uninformative ways, such as the segregation analyses discussed above. Polyps are an attractive endpoint because they are a more frequent event, requiring smaller sample sizes and shorter periods of observation to study, and because it is possible to intervene at a stage where the prognosis is greatly improved. Nevertheless, the utility of such interventions as a means of preventing cancer requires a better understanding of the relationship between the two endpoints and the way this relationship is modified by age, genotype, FH, environmental factors, and so on. This requires careful consideration of study design options as well as bivariate longitudinal analysis methods.

Discovery of novel colorectal cancer genes

The genes discussed in the previous section are examples of candidate genes suggested by functions that were already known and thought to be relevant in the light of established risk factors. What is the role for further gene discovery using genome-wide scans for linkage or association? Jenkins et al. (2002) conducted segregation analyses of 131 Australian families ascertained through a population-based series of young colorectal cancer cases. After excluding 6 found to carry MMR mutations, the best fitting model involved a recessive gene with 98% penetrance and $q = 0.0017$, accounting for 15% of all colorectal cancer under age 45. Efforts are currently underway to identify other genes in families that are not segregating any of the already known major genes. For example, combining the resources of the CFRCCS and another National Cancer Institute initiative, the Cancer Genetics Network, a sib-pair linkage study is currently attempting to enroll about 800 affected sib pairs (Kerber et al., under review) with the intention of performing nonparametric linkage analyses. In designing this study, the investigators recognized that additional information could be contributed by unaffected siblings and by the surviving spouse and offspring of affected cases who had died. In the standard affected-sib pair design, the mean IBD sharing of affected pairs is compared to its theoretical null value of 1/2; in this extended design, greater power or robustness may be obtained by comparing affected to discordant pairs, using GEE methods to allow for the dependence on IBD probabilities among multiple pairs within a sibship (Guo and Elston, 2000; Thomas et al., 1999). Also, the inclusion of additional relatives allows greater precision in the estimation of IBD probabilities, as well as recovery of some of the information that would otherwise be lost if dead cases had to be excluded. The first genome-wide linkage scan for colorectal neoplasia genes that excluded families with FAP or HNPCC used this approach (Wiesner et al., 2003). Kindreds containing at least one full-sib pair with either colorectal cancer or a large (≥ 1 cm) polyp before age 65 were identified and all available members of the sibship and their parents were genotyped. Six regions showed elevated allele sharing (lods $\geq$ 1) using the affected pairs; of these, only one—on chromosome 9q22.2-31.2—also showed reduced allele sharing among discordant pairs. The comparison of concordant and discordant pairs yielded a p-value of 0.0006.

In designing studies to find genes involved in colorectal cancer, careful thought needs to be given to how polyps are to be handled. In the Wiesner et al. (2003) study, cancers and polyps were both treated as "affected," although a supplemental analysis indicated that counting individuals with smaller polyps as affected reduced the evidence for linkage. If the focus is on genes that affect the progression from polyps to cancer, then sampling of families based on sigmoidoscopy clinics might be desirable, and polyps would need to be treated as a covariate in the analysis. On the other hand, if the focus is on the initiating event, then the sampling should be population-based and individuals with polyps might be treated as cases, but then sigmoidoscopy should be offered to all at-risk individuals to overcome selection bias based on FH. Better yet, approaches to the analysis that treat polyps and cancer as bivariate phenotypes could be used.

It is increasingly being recognized, however, that linkage studies are only capable of identifying genes with relatively large effects on penetrance; hence, genome-wide association studies are beginning to be contemplated. In a widely quoted article, Risch and Merikangas (1996) suggested this approach and showed that the sample sizes needed using the TDT approach, restricted to cases ascertained as affected sib pairs, were much smaller than those for a corresponding linkage study. However, because LD is likely to be extremely variable across the genome and highly localized, a much greater density of markers is likely to be needed for such studies than is currently technically feasible; perhaps something of the order of a million polymorphisms might need to be tested. While the advent of modern DNA chip technologies may make this possible in the near future, it currently does not seem promising to begin with a genome-wide association scan unguided by prior hypotheses about possible candidate genes. Nevertheless, it is currently feasible to consider a scan of a large number of polymorphisms in many candidate genes simultaneously. Current efforts to understand the haplotype block structure of the human genome (Daly et al., 2000; Gabriel et al., 2002; Jeffreys et al., 2001; Patil et al., 2001) and to exploit this structure to identify a small subset of haplotype-tagging SNPs (Clayton, 2002; Zhang et al., 2002b; Stram et al., 2003a) will greatly simplify such efforts.

However, the data analysis challenges posed by such large-scale undertakings will remain formidable, as discussed below.

Implications for clinical management

As noted earlier, the standard treatment of FAP is complete removal of the colon to prevent colorectal cancer. The situation is different for HNPCC, for which there is no recognized precursor lesion. Although these patients do not develop the massive number of polyps that FAP patients do, they still develop some polyps. It has been suggested that MMR mutations do not initiate the polyps, but instead make them more likely to progress to carcinoma or accelerate their evolution (Lynch et al., 1996). Evidence for this comes from the much lower ratio of polyps to cancer in prospective screening studies of HNPCC families compared to the general population and, more important, from the high frequency of advanced cancers that develop within 2–5 years of a negative colonoscopy in individuals from HNPCC families (Vasen et al., 1995). On this basis, Lynch et al. (1996) recommended more frequent colonoscopy for individuals with MMR mutations, with the possibility of prophylactic subtotal colectomy. Muller et al. (2000) discussed some more speculative molecular approaches to prevention in MMR carriers by trying to prevent somatic mutations, increase selection against clonal development, or increasing genetic instability to the point of apoptosis. More immediately applicable, chemoprevention trials of beta carotene and vitamins C and E have shown no protective effect (Greenberg et al., 1994), but a trial of calcium found a significant protective effect on the risk of developing any polyps and on the number of polyps (J. Baron et al., unpublished data). Other trials of aspirin and folate are currently underway.

The Future

Genome-wide scans for association and interactions

With the advent of new chip-based technologies for high-volume genotyping and gene expression assays, it will soon be technically feasible to consider forms of exploratory analysis that were inconceivable only recently. The first of these is the possibility of a genome-wide scan for association mentioned above. A DNA chip with perhaps hundreds of thousands of SNP polymorphisms might soon become available that would make case-control comparisons of thousands of subjects feasible. Standard techniques for single SNP analysis, as described in Chapter 9, could be used, with some allowance for multiple comparisons. The traditional Bonferroni correction for, say, a million comparisons would thus require an individual association to have attained a significance level of 5×10^{-8}. While this might seem hopelessly conservative, it is not impossible: to attain a 5% significance level in a standard chi-square test for association on 1 degree of freedom requires a chi square of 3.84, whereas a Bonferroni correction requires a chi square of 28.37; thus, the sample size would only have to be about 7.4 times larger than the sample without that correction. This procedure does, however, ignore the correlation in test statistics between markers that are in LD and hence is somewhat conservative (Abney et al., 2002). A variety of alternative techniques have been proposed, such as ranking the n statistics and assessing the significance of the kth statistic against $k\alpha/n$. Lazzeroni (2001), Efron (2003), Sabatti et al. (2003), and Storey and Tibshirani (2003) provide reviews and comparisons of the alternative procedures. Wacholder et al. (2003) have advocated reporting gene association studies using a Bayesian calculation of the "False Positive Reporting Probability" rather than conventional significance tests. This calculation entails consideration of the prior probability for each hypothesis as well as their significance and power. They emphasize that the prior probability for a randomly selected SNP might be on the order of 10^{-5}, but offer some general guidelines for how to incorporate prior knowledge about their functional significance or previous linkage or association studies. Tabor et al. (2002) provide an excellent discussion of how to choose candidate polymorphisms and appropriate priors for various types of polymorphisms. Two general approaches to genome-wide association studies have been distinguished (Cargill and Daley, 2000; Botstein and Risch, 2003): a *genomics* approach, based on a dense panel of anonymous SNP markers, exploiting the pattern of LD in the hopes of localizing a signal that could indicate a causal variant in the region; and a *functional* approach, focusing on non-synonymous SNPs in coding regions, splice-site junctions, or presumed promoter regions of candidate genes. The latter strategy that is likely to require an order of magnitude fewer markers, but risks missing some associations. See also Reich and Lander (2001) and Pritchard and Cox (2002) for a population genetics perspective on priors for candidate polymorphism associations and their implications for the "Common Disease Common Variant" hypothesis; in particular, the latter point out that polymorphisms identified near a linkage peak will tend to have a different distribution of susceptibility alleles than putative functional loci. Rather than restrict such association scans to simple marker-by-marker tests, it is likely that better power could be obtained by looking for peaks in a region using multiple markers simultaneously or using haplotype-based methods, as discussed in Chapter 10.

Even setting aside the problem of multiple comparisons in genome-wide association scans, the history of candidate gene association studies has been checkered at best (Cardon and Bell, 2001; Colhoun et al., 2003; Dahlman et al., 2002; Hirschhorn et al., 2002; Ionnidis et al., 2001; Terwilliger and Weiss, 1998). There are numerous reasons for this beyond the problem of multiple comparisons, including methodological problems (Colhoun et al., 2003; London et al., 1994; Page et al., 2003), publication bias (Begg and Berlin, 1988), population stratification (Thomas and Witte, 2002), and heterogeneity in the strength of the association due to unrecognized modifying factors, either genetic or environmental. The widespread impression of rampant failure to replicate prompted *Nature Genetics* (Anonymous, 1999, p. 2) to issue some guidelines about publication of candidate gene associations:

> [T]hey should have large sample sizes, small P values, report associations that make biological sense and alleles that affect the gene product in a physiologically meaningful way. In addition, they should contain an initial study as well as an independent replication, the association should be observed both in family-based and population-based studies, and the odds ratio and/or attributable risk should be high.

These are generally sensible recommendations. Indeed, it is only by adherence to generally accepted principles of rigorous population-based epidemiologic study design, including avoidance of underpowered studies and careful attention to the relevant modifying factors (e.g., race, environmental and host risk factors, other genes), that consistent findings can be expected. Hirschhorn and Altschuler (2002) and Lohmueller et al. (2003) provide further discussion of the implications of replication for the "Common Disease Common Variant" hypothesis.

Problems of multiple comparisons are further accentuated if many $G \times G$ and $G \times E$ interactions are also considered. Arguably, progress in characterizing complex diseases may require that such effects be considered, often with only limited prior knowledge to restrict the range of the search. A variety of *data mining* techniques have been proposed for this purpose, such as artificial neural networks and cluster analysis methods (Moore, 2001; Moore and Hahn, 2001; Moore et al., 2002; Ritchie et al., 2001; Hoh and Ott, 2003). Allen (2001) and Boyer et al. (2001) offer more skeptical views on the potential for data mining, while Jansen (2003) discusses the importance of considering multiple genes in combination.

Gene expression assays

Similar issues arise in the analysis of data from new gene expression array technologies, such as cDNA *microarrays* (Schena et al., 1995) and oligonucleotide *DNA chips* (Lipshutz et al., 1999). These technologies typically assess the expression of thousands of genes, either their absolute level of expression or the ratio of expression levels in two samples (e.g., tumor and control) assessed by comparative hybridization. The typical data analysis thus entails examining a two-dimensional array of a large number of samples by a large number of genes in an attempt to discern patterns. A variety of techniques have been proposed, including hierarchical cluster analysis (Eisen et al., 1998), multidimensional scaling (Khan et al., 1998), deterministic annealing (Alon et al., 1999), self-organizing maps (Golub et al., 1999; Tamayo et al., 1999), gene shaving (Hastie et al., 2000), tree harvesting (Hastie et al., 2001), and, more recently, model-based cluster analysis (Yeung et al., 2001) and plaid models (Lazzeroni and Owen, 2002). Michaels et al. (1998), Sherlock (2001), and the collection of articles in a special issue of *Genetic Epidemiology* on microarrays (Schaid, 2002b) contain general reviews. Such techniques might entail, for example, two-way clustering, in which the rows and columns of the array are rearranged in such a way as to reflect a hierarchical clustering of samples in which similar genes are expressed and a clustering of genes that are similarly expressed across samples, each clustering being represented in terms of a dendogram.

For example, Alon et al. (1999) used Affymetrix oligonucleotide arrays to study the expression of 6500 genes in 40 samples of colorectal tumors and 22 samples of normal colorectal mucosa. Using two-way clustering, they found coherent patterns in which, for example, ribosomal proteins tended to cluster together and cancer and normal cells could be distinguished based on their overall patterns, even though no individual genes differed greatly. In another experiment using the serial analysis of gene expression (SAGE) technique (Velculescu et al., 1995), Buckhaults et al. (2001) examined over 290,000 transcripts from normal, polyps, and colorectal cancer samples. Only 957 genes were differentially expressed, and of these, only 49 were expressed more than 20-fold in adenomas, 40 in cancers, and 9 in both. Six of these (*TGFBI, LYS, RDP, MIC-1, REGA,* and *DEHL*) were expressed on the cell surface, and their abnormal expression was subsequently confirmed by PCR analysis. Riggins and Morin (2002) provide a general review of gene expression techniques.

Proteomics offers the prospect of direct assessment of the proteins actually produced on a genome-wide basis, using mass spectrometry on two-dimensional gel electrophoresis, as opposed to the expression of RNA, but the field is in its infancy. Jungblut et al. (1999), Sellers and Yates (2003) provided general reviews of this field. As one example, Stierum et al. (2001) described a project to develop a colon epithelial cell line-based screening assay for nutrients with presumed anticolorectal carcinogenic properties by selecting genes that are involved in colorectal carcinogenesis, identifying cell lines that differentially express these genes, and determining the effects of nutrients thought to have anticarcinogenic effects. Once this is validated, the hope is that these panels will be useful for screening other nutrients for anticarcinogenic effects. McKerrow et al. (2000) described an application of proteomics methods to detecting the four major classes of proteases in 15 biopsy specimens of colorectal tumors, normal mucosa, and liver metastases. Petricoin et al. (2002) described an application of proteomic patterns in serum to distinguish ovarian cancer from other conditions, using a training set of 50 ovarian cancer cases and 50 unaffected women to construct an index that completely discriminated the two groups. They then showed that in an independent masked sample, the index could correctly identify all 50 cases and 63 of 66 noncases. If validated, this approach offers great potential for early detection. Statistical analysis techniques for these kinds of data are in their infancy, the first data mining conference on proteomics having occurred only in the fall of 2002. The mathematical challenge is in estimating the concentration of a potentially large number of proteins from a tracing of peaks as a function of molecular weight, each measured with some uncertainty and possibly overlapping.

So far, very little thought has been given to incorporation of gene expression and proteomics approaches in a wholistic approach to genetic epidemiology, in part because of the cost, but as this approach becomes more feasible, the potential is considerable. Much of the early work seems to have been an attempt to identify patterns that distinguish various disease groups, but of much greater interest is using them to investigate mechanistic pathways—the environmental or developmental signals that lead to gene expression, the effect of genotype (at the same locus as well as at modifier loci) on expression patterns, and its ultimate influence on disease risk (including, where appropriate, precursor lesions). Schadt et al. (2003) describe an approach to linkage analysis of expression levels to identify genetic loci controlling expression levels and integrate this information into linkage analysis of a phenotypic trait. See Jansen and Nap (2001) and Cheung and Spielman (2002) for further discussion of the potential for gene expression analysis in segregating populations to identify genetic loci whose sequence variation affects only their own expression (*cis*-acting factors) or that of many other genes (*trans*-acting factors). This merger of expression and genomic analysis has come to be called *genetical genomics* (Jansen and Nap, 2001). Jansen (2003) discusses ways in which variation at many loci can be exploited to disentangle complex gene networks. Kraft et al. (2003) describe a family-based expression-association test (FEXAT) to study correlations among expression levels and traits within sibships. Sellers and Yates (2003) discuss potential applications of proteomics in elucidating the genetic epidemiology of ovarian cancer and breast mammographic densities (a strong risk factor for breast cancer). In the latter example, they suggest a comparison of proteomic profiles from dense and nondense tissues from the same woman, thereby eliminating differences in serum proteins that might be found between women at the extremes of the distribution of average mammographic densities. Careful consideration of study design, including the choice of tissue to sample in cases and controls and the possibility of longitudinal observations on unaffected individuals, will be needed.

DNA methylation and loss of imprinting

Up to this point, we have focused on the effects of mutations in the DNA sequence on disease risk, but equally important are modifications of the genome that are heritable by cell progeny that do not affect the primary sequence but do affect the *expression* of genes, a field known as *epigenetics* (Cuthill, 1994; Laird, 1997; Prehn, 1994; Rubin, 1992). These include such mechanisms as histone modification, which affects chromatin structure, and the complement of transcription factors, but perhaps the best understood is DNA methylation. DNA methylation is an enzymatic addition of a methyl group to cytosine residues at the C-5 position and occurs at CpG sequences (meaning a C nucleotide followed by a G nucleotide). Although isolated CpG's are usually methylated, the human genome contains regions rich in CpG's, known as *CpG islands,* which typically are unmethylated. Promoter regions of genes often contain a CpG island and are normally unmethylated, except for imprinted or X-inactivated genes. Methylation of these genes in cancer or perhaps with aging can lead to their irreversible silencing. How abnormal methylation may depend on environmental or developmental stimuli is largely unknown but of great interest.

In the Knudson two-event model of carcinogenesis described above, two mutations (inherited or acquired) in a tumor-suppressor gene were thought to be required to produce a cancer. It is now appreciated that one of these events could be abnormal hypermethylation of the promoter region of a normal copy of the gene (Jones and Laird, 1999). Methylation patterns are generally conserved during mitosis but are largely eliminated very early in development, at around the blastocyst stage. Very soon thereafter, there is a wave of de novo methylation that re-establishes the original pattern by some mechanism that is not yet understood. Methylation profiles vary between genes (and regions of genes), between individuals, between tissues, between cells within a tissue, and over time (possibly reflecting exposure to environmental agents [Jirtle et al., 2000]). Thus, the profile of methylation is extremely rich in information. Laird (2003) estimates that there are 50 million CpG sites, and the total number of distinct profiles observed in cancer cells is far greater than the number of genetic changes; Laird calls this "a diagnostic dream and an analytical nightmare!" Statistical methods for the analysis of such data are in their infancy (see Siegmund and Laird, 2002, for a general review).

Using very simple manual clustering, Toyota et al. (1999) studied the methylation level of 30 CpG islands and classified them into what they called *Group A,* which are methylated in colon cancer but also in normal cells at an increasing rate with age, and *Group C,* where methylation was found only in a subset of *CpG island methylator phenotype (CIMP)* colorectal cancers. The first application of formal agglomerative clustering methods like those used in expression array analysis to methylation data were reported by Adorjan et al. (2002) and Virmani et al. (2002).

In colorectal polyps, two distinct profiles of methylation are observed: on the one hand, the overall methylation content is reduced (*hypomethylation*); on the other, CpG islands tend to be hypermethylated. A frequent change in colorectal cancers is hypermethylation of the estrogen receptor (*ER*) gene (Issa et al., 1994), generally leading to reduced expression or silencing of gene expression, even in early-stage tumors. *P16* and other genes have also been reported to show hypermethylation in cancer, with varying degrees of tumor specificity (Jones and Baylin, 2002). It has been suggested that folate deficiency produces this global hypomethylation, which in turn is compensated for by de novo methylation of CpG islands, suggesting potential prevention by folate supplementation.

Whereas most analyses have tended to focus on a small number of CpG islands separately, there is growing evidence that CpG island hypermethylation is a genome-wide phenomenon. Costello et al. (2000) examined 1184 CpG islands in 98 tumor samples and identified methylation profiles that were shared within tumor types. The mechanism for genome-wide hypermethylation is poorly understood. One possibility is loss of control of some trans-acting factors that regulate DNA methylation. Another possibility is accumulation of random methylation errors, with multiple stem cells passing through *bottlenecks* that result in a complete turnover of the progenitor cells over a lifetime (Yatabe et al., 2001). It has been suggested that cells with an MMR defect have an increased capacity to silence viral promoters by DNA methylation (Lengauer et al., 1997). However, Pao et al. (2000) found that although MMR+ and MMR− cells clearly differed in their extent of viral promoter expression, the difference could not be explained by DNA methylation. Thus, they question the existence of mutually exclusive DNA methylation and DNA repair (MMR) phenotypes. In a population-based study of 15 MSI+ and 47 MSI− tumors, Xiong et al. (2001) found a significantly increased level of methylation in four out of the five CpG islands examined in tumor tissue compared with adjacent normal mucosa, but found no significant difference in methylation levels by MSI status for any of the CpG islands other than *hMLH1*.

One of the potentially most important implications of DNA methylation is that it is potentially reversible by agents such as 5-aza-cytidine, although results are currently limited to cell culture and animal experiments, and the procedure could have both beneficial and adverse consequences (Barletta et al., 1997; Laird et al., 1995). Clinical trials of this agent are now ongoing (Aparicio et al., 2003; Daskalakis et al., 2002; Momparler et al., 2000). In any event, the potential clinical utility of methylation for early detection, prognosis, or response to treatment remains a very exciting area (Laird, 2003).

In Mendelian inheritance, both maternal and paternal copies of each gene are expressed equally, so penetrance is a function only of the number of copies of a mutant allele. *Imprinting* refers to the expression of only one copy of a gene (Crouse, 1960). A familiar example is the difference between a mule (a cross between a maternal horse and a paternal donkey) and a hinny (the reverse cross). DNA methylation is thought to be a fundamental mechanism underlying imprinting (Li et al., 1993).

Recently, it has been recognized that loss of imprinting (LOI) is another possible mechanism by which the copy of a gene that is normally silenced can become expressed abnormally. The initial work was done on Wilms' tumor and the insulin-like growth factor-II (*IGF2*) gene (Rainier et al., 1993). This gene was examined because of evidence of LOH at 11p15, where it is located. In individuals who are heterozygous at this locus, it is possible to determine which copy of the gene is preferentially expressed, and in normal individuals it turns out to be the paternal copy. However, in 70% of Wilms' tumors, both copies are expressed.

In colorectal cancer, Cui et al. (1998) found that 44% of cases had LOI in their tumor tissue as well as in their normal mucosa compared with only 12% of unaffected controls, suggesting that this was an early event in the carcinogenesis process. Furthermore, 4 of 27 patients examined showed evidence of LOI in peripheral blood, raising the possibility that a simple screening test could be developed. Among the cases, there was also a dramatic difference in the prevalence of LOI by MSI status (91% in MSI+ vs. 12% in MSI−). In a subsequent report, Cui et al. (2003a) found *OR*s for LOI of 5.15 in unaffected individuals with an FH of colorectal cancer, 3.26 for adenoma cases, and 21.7 for colorectal cancer cases. The elevated *OR* in unaffected individuals with a positive FH suggests the possibility of using LOI as a prediagnostic screening test, but this could reflect an underlying constitutional susceptibility to *both* LOI and cancer and does not necessarily indicate that an elevation of LOI is indicative of an incipient disease process or even an increased risk of cancer, given the underlying genetic risk. Feinberg et al. (1999, 2002) provide further discussions of the mechanisms of LOI in cancer.

Table 12.1 Stereotypical Differences Between the Fields of Genetic and Molecular Epidemiology

Aspect	Genetic Epidemiology	Molecular Epidemiology
Principal aim	Gene discovery	Gene characterization
Sampling scheme	High-risk families	Population-based
Study design	Family-based studies	Case-control studies
Parent discipline	Statistical genetics	Molecular biology
Treatment of environment	Primitive or nonexistent	Focus on $G \times E$ interactions
Genes considered	Single, rare, major genes	Multiple common polymorphisms

Conclusions

This chapter has tried to show how progress in understanding the mechanisms of disease—using colorectal cancer as an archetypal example of a complex disease—requires a multidisciplinary interaction between such fields as genetics, epidemiology, molecular biology, and statistics. I have also tried to show how the actual practice of genetic epidemiology often differs from the simple linear progression of studies laid out in the earlier chapters of this book.

Two subdisciplines, have emerged—*genetic epidemiology* and *molecular epidemiology*—which some see as essentially synonymous and others as quite different (Khoury and Dorman, 1998). The perceived differences between the two fields are illustrated in Table 12.1. While some of the differences are exaggerated and some are real, progress requires collaboration between these subdisciplines. Indeed, as Khoury and Dorman point out "However, there is one issue that we both agree on: the critical role of population-based studies in translating findings of the Human Genome Project into applications for medicine and public health." In writing this chapter, I was particularly struck by how quickly what started out to be a review of the application of the study design and statistical principles presented earlier in this book to the study of the etiology of colorectal cancer turned into an exploration of numerous molecular biology aspects that seemed to play a central role in elucidating this story. Thus, if this chapter has a single message, it is the close interplay between molecular and classical genetic epidemiology methods.

Glossary

Additive: A model for dominance in which the heterozygote is at an intermediate risk between the two homozygotes (synonymous with Dose-dependent).

Additive genetic variance: The component of variance of a phenotype that is attributable to the additive effect of both alleles at all relevant loci.

Admixed population: A population consisting of a mixture of two or more subpopulations, typically with differing allele frequencies, that have been inter-marrying for several generations.

Admixture (A-test): A likelihood ratio test comparing the joint MLE of α (the proportion of families linked) and θ (the recombination fraction) to the restricted MLE at $\alpha = 1$ (i.e., assuming that all families are linked).

Adoption design: A class of study designs aimed at estimating genetic and environmental contributions to a phenotype by comparing adopted individuals with their natural and adoptive parents or siblings.

Affected relative pair method: A class of linkage analysis methods based on comparing the distribution of identity by descent (q.v.) or identity by state (q.v.) of a marker between pairs of affected relatives with the distribution for that relative type.

Affected sib pair method: A special case of the affected relative pair method using only pairs of affected siblings and identity by descent (q.v.).

Allele: One of two or more states in which either copy of a gene can exist.

Amino acids: The building blocks of proteins.

Ancestral inference: A class of statistical methods aimed at inferring the ancestral relationships between a set of individuals or genetic sequences; can be used for gene mapping.

Ancestral recombination graph: A representation of the ancestry of a set of DNA sequences back to a most recent common ancestor (q.v.), allowing for recombination events within the segment.

367

Aneuploid: Cells with excess or missing individual chromosomes.

Ascertainment: The process of identifying a family for inclusion in a genetic analysis.

Ascertainment correction: Including terms in a likelihood function or other methods of statistical modeling to allow for the way in which the studied families were ascertained in order to remove bias in the estimates of population parameters (penetrance and allele frequencies); used particularly in segregation analysis.

Ascertainment probability: The probability that a random case in the population will be selected as a proband.

Association: A tendency for a particular genotype to occur more commonly in cases of a disease (or be correlated with a continuous phenotype) than expected by chance.

Association study: A study designed to test or characterize (q.v.) the association between a phenotype and a specific candidate gene or to try to localize an unknown gene using linkage disequilibrium (q.v.).

Assortive mating: A tendency for individuals with similar genotypes to mate.

Asymptotic relative efficiency (ARE): The ratio of the large-sample variances for estimators from alternative study designs and/or methods of analysis; equivalently, the ratio of sample sizes that would be required to attain the same degree of statistical precision.

Autosome: One of 22 of chromosomes that occur in pairs in the human genome (as distinct from the 2 sex chromosomes).

Base pair (bp): The unit of physical distance along a chromosome, measured in nucleotides.

Broad sense heritability: The total proportion of variance of a phenotype due to genotype, σ_G^2/σ^2, including additive, dominance, and epistatic components.

Candidate gene: A gene whose location and biologic function are already known, which may be plausibly related to the phenotype under study.

Carrier: An individual who has one copy (or more) of a disease susceptibility allele.

Case-cohort design: A study design in which a random sample of all subjects at entry to the cohort is used as a control group for the cases that occur in the total cohort.

Case-control design: A design used to detect association by comparing the genotypes (and other risk factors) of cases with those of unaffected controls.

Case-only design: A design for studying $G \times E$ or $G \times G$ interactions using only cases, under the assumption that the interacting factors are independently distributed in the source population; also known as a *case-case* design.

Case-parent trio design: A design for studying gene associations using the genotypes of affected cases and their parents; also known as *case-parent* triads.

Censored data: Data for which the values of some variables are known only to exceed some value; in survival analysis, a phenotype in which, for affected individuals, the age of disease onset is known, but for unaffected individuals, only the last age known to be disease free is known.

centiMorgan (cM): The unit of recombination, equaling 1/100th of a Morgan, or a 1% probability of a crossover.

Centromere: The point at which the chromatids are joined.

Characterization: The process of estimating the penetrance of a gene, variation in its population allele frequencies for all mutations, and interactions with other genes, environment, age, or other factors, once it has been cloned.

Chromatid: One of two strands of DNA that separate during meiosis to form a gamete.

Chromosome: One of 46 double strands of DNA that form the human genome.

Clone: A DNA fragment that has been amplified and purified by growth in bacterial cells.

Cloning: In gene discovery, the process of obtaining a DNA fragment that carries a gene.

Coalescent: A mathematical representation of the evolution of alleles in a population, leading backward in time to a most recent common ancestor (q.v.).

Coding region: A sequence of DNA that codes for a protein sequence.

Codominant: A model for dominance in which each of the three genotypes has a distinct effect on the phenotype.

Codon: A sequence of three bases specifying one amino acid.

Coefficient of inbreeding: The probability that the child of a consanguineous union will be autozygous for a particular allele (not necessarily a disease-causing one) descended through both parents from the common ancestors [the probability of having two alleles identical by descent (q.v.)].

Coefficient of relationship: The expected number of alleles shared identical by descent (q.v.) between two individuals $= 2^{-R}$ where R is the degree of relationship (q.v.).

Cohort study: An epidemiologic study design based on follow-up (possibly retrospectively) of a group of individuals whose risk factor characteristics are defined at the start of observation. In genetic epidemiology, a cohort study can be used to study familial aggregation or association with candidate genes; members of the cohort can be unrelated or can be enrolled as families for this purpose (a familial cohort study).

Complete ascertainment: A process of ascertainment in which all families in a defined population with at least one case are included.

Complex disease: A disorder that appears to have a genetic component but with no simple Mendelian pattern of single-gene inheritance; multiple genes, polygenes, environmental factors, age effects, and their interactions may be involved.

Concordance rate: The proportion of twin pairs with an affected member in which both members are affected (see Pairwise and Probandwise concordance rate).

Confounding: A spurious association caused by one or more uncontrolled variables that are related to both the risk factor and the disease under study.

Consanguinity: When two parents have one or more ancestors in common (results in inbred offspring).

Cosegregation: A tendency for alleles at two linked loci to be transmitted from parent to offspring together.

Covariate: A measured variable related to the risk of disease in a multivariate model for penetrance.

Crossover: The exchange of material between two homologous chromatids during meiosis; crossovers are not directly observable, but an odd number appears as a recombination (q.v.) event.

Cytogenetic rearrangement: Deletion, insertion, or inversion of a piece of a chromosome, or the exchange of pieces of two separate chromosomes. Rearrangements that disrupt a gene may result in disease.

Cytogenetics: The study of whole chromosomes as seen in individual cells.

Degree of relationship: An integer representing the closeness of the genetic relationship equaling $-\log_2(\varphi)$ where φ is the coefficient of relationship (q.v.): full sibs, parents, and offspring are first-degree relatives; half-sibs, grandparents, aunts, uncles, nieces, and nephews are second-degree relatives; first-cousins are third-degree relatives; and so on.

Diploid: Fertilized eggs and most body cells containing two copies of the genome.

Direct counting: A method of linkage analysis based on the observed number of recombinants in a set of informative meioses (q.v.).

Disease susceptibility allele: The allele at a disease locus that confers increased risk.

Dizygotic (DZ) twins: Twins that share only half of their genes, resulting from the independent fertilization of two ova by separate sperm; DZ twins are genetically related to the same extent as sibs but may have stronger sharing of environmental influences, particularly in utero; fraternal twins.

DNA: Deoxyribonucleic acid, which makes up genes and chromosomes, composed of a double-stranded string of nucleotides.

Dominance: The joint effect of the two copies of a gene in influencing the phenotype probability (see Additive, Codominant, Dominant, Recessive).

Dominance genetic variance: The component of the variance of a phenotype that is attributable specifically to the differential effect of two copies of the same allele (relative to that predicted from the sum of their separate allelic effects) across all relevant genes.

Dominant: A model for dominance in which individuals with a single copy of a disease susceptibility allele have the same risk of disease as those with two copies.

Dose-dependent: A model for dominance in which the heterozygote is at intermediate risk between the two homozygotes (synonymous with Additive).

Double helix: The physical structure of DNA, in which two complementary pairs of nucleotide bases are chemically bound and twisted around each other.

Double heterozygote: An individual who is heterozygous at two loci, such as a disease and a marker locus.

Effect modification: Modification of the magnitude of some measure of association between a risk factor and disease by a third variable; also known as interaction (q.v.).

Elston-Stewart algorithm: A method for computing the likelihood of a pedigree by recursively computing the probability of all possible pairs of genotypes of each mating, conditional on the phenotypes of all their descendants. See peeling.

Environmentality: The proportion of variance of an underlying liability to disease that is due to shared unmeasured environmental factors.

Epidemiology: The study of the distribution and causes of disease in populations.

Epigenetics: Any of several phenomena involving modifications of the genome not involving the primary DNA sequence that are heritable by the progeny of a cell and affect gene expression; includes DNA methylation.

Epistasis: An interactive effect between two or more genes, such as suppression or alteration of the expression of one gene by another locus.

Epistatic genetic variance: The component of variance of a phenotype that is attributable to the interactive effect of two or more genes.

Exclusion mapping: A genome-wide search technique that proceeds by eliminating regions for which there is convincing evidence against the existence of any gene with an effect larger than some specified minimal amount.

Exons: The remaining sequences of DNA that remain in the mature mRNA after the introns are removed by RNA splicing.

Expectation-maximization (E-M) algorithm: An iterative modelfitting procedure that maximizes a likelihood function by alternately computing the expectation of sufficient statistics under the current model parameters and then updating the parameters by maximizing the likelihood given these expectations.

Familial: Cases of disease with a positive family history.

Familial aggregation: A tendency for a disease to occur in multiple family members more often than would be expected by chance, or a positive correlation in a continuous phenotype within families, whether due to genetic (hence, hereditary) or shared environmental factors.

Familial relative risk (FRR): The ratio of the familial risk to the risk in the general population or to the risk given no affected family members.

Familial risk: The probability that an individual will be affected by a disease, given that he or she has an affected family member.

Family-based association test (FBAT): A class of association tests that use genetic data on family members (e.g., sibships and/or parents) to compute the distribution of a suitable test statistic under the null hypothesis, conditional on the phenotypes.

Fine mapping: The process of localizing a disease gene below the level of resolution of linkage analysis.

Fisher information: The expectation of the negative of the matrix of second derivatives of the loglikelihood; the inverse of the information evaluated at the parameter estimates gives the covariance matrix of the estimates.

Flanking markers: Two marker loci located on opposite sides of a disease susceptibility locus.

Founder: A member of a pedigree whose parents do not appear in the pedigree; sometimes restricted to the top generation.

Founder effect: Gene frequencies among offspring of a small sample of the original gene pool that are not representative of the general population.

Frailty model: A model for dependent survival data based on the assumption that individuals' survival times are independent conditional on an unobserved risk factor (frailty) shared by all members of the family.

Frameshift: A DNA variant resulting from insertion or deletion of one or two (but not three) nucleotides in a coding region that completely changes the amino acid sequence downstream of the mutation.

Fully penetrant: A gene for which the probability of being affected is 1 for individuals carrying the susceptible genotype (one or two copies of the mutant allele, depending on its dominance).

Gamete: A germ cell (sperm or ovum) that carries only one of each pair of the parent's genes.

Gene: The fundamental unit of genetic information that is transcribed to form a single protein.

Gene expression: The process by which the transcript and translation (q.v.) of genes into proteins is controlled by various environmental or developmental influences on a cell.

Gene identity: The number of alleles shared identical by descent (q.v.) by a pair of individuals.

Gene pool: The total collection of alleles present in a population.

Generalized Estimating Equations (GEE): A statistical method for fitting models based on solving an equation that equates the average of certain moments of the marginal distribution of the observed data and their predicted values under the model.

Genetic code: The relationship between the 64 possible triplets of nucleotides in DNA and the 20 amino acids they encode.

Genetic drift: Cumulative changes in gene frequency due to random variation in allele transmissions between generations in finite populations (rather than systematic changes due to selective forces).

Genetic epidemiology: The study of the joint action of genes and environmental factors in causing disease in human populations and their patterns of inheritance in families.

Genetic heterogeneity: Variation in the recombination rate between families with respect to a marker of interest (beyond what would be expected by chance), including the possibility that only a subset of families are carrying the mutation linked to the marker.

Genetic mapping: A class of methods for discovering the location of genes related to a phenotype using recombination.

Genetic modeling: Postulation of an explicit model for the unobserved (latent) variables—major genes and/or polygenes—and fitting of the model using maximum likelihood by summing or integrating over all possible values of the unobserved quantities.

Genetic relationship: The relationship between members of a pedigree defined by the possible transmissions of genes from a common ancestor.

Genetic relative risk (GRR): The ratio of the risk of a disease in individuals with different genotypes.

Genetic variance: The component of variance of a phenotype that can be attributed to all genetic influences; includes additive, dominance, and epistatic variance components (q.v.).

Genome scan: The process of searching for a disease gene using widely spaced markers scattered throughout the entire genome; also known as a *genome scan*.

Genotype: The (possibly unobserved) state of an individual's gene at one or more loci relating to the phenotype of interest.

Germ cell mutation: A mutation in a gamete that can be transmitted to offspring and their descendants.

Gibbs sampling: An iterative method for fitting models based on random sampling of each unobservable quantity (parameters and/or latent variables) in turn from their full conditional distribution given the observed data and the current values of the other quantities; a particular form of the Markov chain Monte Carlo (q.v.) method.

Haploid: Cells containing one copy of the genome, such as sperm or unfertilized egg cells.

Haplotype: A combination of alleles at multiple linked loci that are transmitted together.

Haplotype block structure: The organization of extended sequences into blocks with high linkage disequilibrium and limited numbers of haplotypes, separated by regions of low linkage disequilibrium.

Haplotype sharing statistic: Any statistic based on a comparison of the distribution of lengths of shared haplotype segments surrounding a possible location across all possible pairs of case haplotypes against an expected distribution obtained by a randomization procedure.

Hardy-Weinberg equilibrium: A tendency for the population allele frequencies to remain invariant across generations, with genotype probabilities that are a particular function of the population allele frequency.

Hazard function: The instantaneous risk of disease in individuals currently not affected as a function of age and possibly other factors; used to specify penetrance for censored age-at-onset traits.

Hazard ratio: The ratio of two hazard functions at the same age, say for carriers and noncarriers; see also Relative risk.

Hereditary: A tendency for disease susceptibility to be transmitted from parents to offspring through a genetic mechanism; a case that is likely to have been caused by an inherited gene.

Heritability: The proportion of variance of an underlying liability to disease that is due to shared genetic factors.

Heterozygote: An individual who carries two different alleles for a particular gene.

Hidden Markov models: A class of statistical methods based on an unobserved set of latent variables that are assumed to have the Markov property that each variable is independent of the others, conditional on its immediate neighbors. Used in the Lander-Green algorithm (q.v.) to compute identical by descent (q.v.) probabilities on pedigrees by proceeding locus by locus, using only the probabilities saved for the previous locus.

Homologous: Referring to two chromosomes that are paired or to two loci within paired chromosomes that code for the same gene.

Homozygote: An individual who carries two identical copies of an allele for a particular gene.

Hybridization: The process by which single-stranded DNA or RNA will recognize and bind to complementary DNA or RNA sequences.

Identical by descent (IBD): Alleles shared by two relatives that were transmitted from the same ancestor.

Identical by state (IBS): Any alleles shared by two relatives, regardless of their ancestral origin.

Imprinting: A temporary modification of a DNA sequence (e.g, methylation), which leads to different expression by the unimprinted and imprinted alleles. Imprinting is stable during mitosis but is removed before or during meiosis (but could be reapplied or reversed).

Inbreeding: See Consanguinity.

Incidence: The rate at which previously unaffected individuals in a population develop new disease over time (see Prevalence).

Independent assortment: A tendency for genotypes of spouses to be uncorrelated; one of two fundamental Mendelian principles.

Indirectly standardized rate ratio (SRR): A ratio of standardized incidence rates (q.v.) comparing groups with different baseline characteristics (e.g., genotypes).

Information: See Fisher information.

Informative meiosis: Transmission of two or more loci from a parent who is doubly heterozygous (q.v.) with phase (q.v.) known, so that the transmitted haplotype can be scored definitively as either a recombinant (q.v.) or a nonrecombinant.

Interaction: Any pattern of deviation between the joint effect of two or more factors (such as genes, environment, or age) on a trait and what would be predicted from a model for their separate effects.

Interference: The phenomenon that the occurrence of a recombination at one location alters the probability of other recombinations occurring in its neighborhood.

Introns: Long noncoding sequences interrupting the coding region of most genes.

Karyogram: Photographic display of chromosomes from largest to smallest, followed by the sex chromosomes.

Karyotype: A precise description of the chromosomes (including the overall count, identification of any extra or lost chromosomes, identification of regions of a chromosome that may have been deleted or inverted or moved to another chromosome, etc.).

Kin cohort design: A design for characterizing candidate gene associations by comparing the incidence of the disease in relatives of carriers to that in relatives of noncarriers; allows estimation of penetrance.

Kinship coefficient: The probability that a randomly selected allele from each member of a pair of individuals is identical by descent (q.v.) (one-half of the coefficient of relationship) (q.v.).

Lander-Green algorithm: An approach to multipoint linkage analysis using hidden Markov models (q.v.), allowing the calculation of identical by descent (q.v.) probabilities at any location along a chromosome given the complete marker information in the region available for pedigrees of moderate size.

Liability: An unobservable susceptibility to disease, composed of the sum of environmental and genetic contributions.

Likelihood: The probability of the observed data given a postulated form of model, viewed as a function of its parameters; in the genetic context, the probability of the phenotypes in a pedigree or set of pedigrees.

Likelihood ratio test: The ratio of the logarithm of the likelihood evaluated at the maximum likelihood estimates of the parameter to that evaluated at their null value; twice the natural logarithm of the likelihood ratio has a chi-square distribution; the log of the likelihood ratio to the base 10 is known as the lod score (q.v.).

Linkage: A tendency for genes that are located nearby on the same chromosome to cosegregate (q.v.); a form of analysis aimed at detecting linkage.

Linkage analysis: The process of determining the approximate chromosomal location of a gene by looking for evidence of cosegregation (q.v.) with other genes whose locations are already known [i.e., marker (q.v.) genes].

Linkage disequilibrium (LD): A tendency for certain pairs of alleles at two linked loci to be associated with each other in the population more than would be expected by chance.

Linkage disequilibrium mapping: Any of a number of techniques used to localize a trait gene by the disequilibrium between the trait locus and marker loci.

Locus: The location on a chromosome of a particular gene (pl. *loci*).

Lod score: The logarithm of the likelihood ratio to the base 10; also called lods.

Loss of heterozygosity (LOH): The unbalanced mitotic recombination (usually in cancer cells) as a mechanism for loss of DNA from one chromosome. If the region lost contains a tumor-suppressor gene and the retained allele is inactive (through mutation), the recombination results in loss of the only functioning allele of the tumor-suppressor gene.

Major gene: A single gene that has a large influence on the phenotype probability.

Map: An assumed assignment of locations to a set of markers, including both their order and distances between them.

Map function: An assumed mathematical relationship between physical distance along a chromosome [measured in base pairs (q.v.)] and the corresponding recombination rate [measured in centiMorgans (q.v.)].

Marker: A polymorphic gene whose physical location is known; used in linkage analysis.

Markov chain Monte Carlo (MCMC): Any of a number of iterative methods for fitting models based on random sampling of unobservable quantities (parameters and/or latent variables) conditional on the observed data and the current values of the other quantities; Gibbs sampling (q.v.) is a particular example.

Marry-in: A member of a pedigree whose parents do not appear in the pedigree and who is not a member of the topmost generation.

Mating type: The joint genotype of both parents in a nuclear family.

Maximum likelihood: The principle of statistical inference that favors the parameter estimate that maximizes the likelihood, together with the mathematical theory that provides confidence limits and significance tests based on the likelihood function.

Maximum likelihood estimate (MLE): The parameter value that maximizes the likelihood function for a particular dataset.

Meiosis: The process of cell division leading to the creation of gametes containing one of each pair of the parental genes.

Mendelian: Following an inheritance pattern predicted by Mendel's laws.

Mendel's laws: (1) Law of segregation (q.v.) of alleles; (2) law of independent assortment (q.v.).

Microsatellite: Repeated regions throughout the genome containing a very simple repetitive motif (e.g., CA repeat).

Mitosis: The process of cell division leading to replication of the full complement of chromosomes that is identical to the original set.

Mixed model: A penetrance model involving one or more major genes as well as polygenes; also known as a multifactorial model.

Mod score (mods): The maximum of the likelihood ratio for linkage over all possible values of the segregation parameters at the disease locus; can be shown to be equivalent to the retrospective likelihood of the marker data given the phenotypes.

Molecular epidemiology: The branch of epidemiology concerned with the use of molecular markers for exposure, genes, or disease processes.

Monozygotic (MZ) twins: Twins with identical genes, resulting from the separation of an oocyte after fertilization; identical twins.

Morgan: A measure of map distance corresponding to the expected number of crossovers equaling 1.

Most recent common ancestor (MRCA): The most recent ancestor of a set of individuals or DNA sequences from whom (which) all their genes at a particular locus (or region) are derived.

Multifactorial: A phenotype that is influenced by both genetic and environmental factors; mixed model.

Multilocus: Penetrance models involving more than one distinct genetic locus for a trait.

Multiple ascertainment: Identification of families through probands where the ascertainment probability is substantially larger than 0 and less than 1, so that some families are likely to be identified through multiple probands but not every case is a proband.

Multiplex: A family with two or more cases of the disease of interest; an ascertainment scheme that requires two or more cases for a family to be included in the study.

Multipoint linkage: A form of linkage analysis involving two or more marker loci, aimed at identifying flanking markers.

Mutation: Any change in the sequence of a DNA molecule produced in mitosis or meiosis. A mutation may result in disease if it occurs in the small fraction of the genome that contains coding sequences, or it may be a totally harmless polymorphism. Mutation forms the basis for the difference between alleles. Some mutations are beneficial and may be the substrate for positive natural selection. The term *mutation* is sometimes limited to those polymorphisms that have a serious effect on the function of the gene (e.g., cause premature truncation of the protein product); there are usually rare and deleterious.

Narrow sense heritability: The proportion of variance of a phenotype due specifically to additive genetic effects (the sum of individual allelic effects).

Nested case-control design: A study design in which, for each case in a cohort, one or more controls are selected at random from the set of subject that were at risk at that time.

Newton–Raphson method: An iterative method of maximizing a likelihood function by moving from a current parameter value in the direction of increasing likelihood by an amount depending on the first and second derivatives.

Nitrogenous base: The four nitrogenous bases found in DNA are adenine, cytosine, thymine, and guanine. Thus, there are four different types of nucleotides that can be used to build a DNA molecule.

Nonparametric: A class of statistical tests that do not require assumptions about the probability distributions of the observed random variables, often using ranks and permutation tests; for example, in linkage analysis, affected relative pairs methods.

Nuclear family: A portion of a pedigree (q.v.) containing a single pair of parents and their immediate offspring [a single sibship (q.v.)].

Nucleic acid: A polymer (chain) of nucleotides. The two types of nucleic acid are DNA and RNA.

Nucleotide: A nitrogenous base linked to a sugar (ribose or deoxyribose) and a phosphate. Nucleotides are the building blocks for nucleic acids (DNA and RNA).

Odds ratio (OR): The ratio of the odds of disease between two groups, where the odds is the probability of being affected divided by the probability of not being affected; see Relative risk.

Oligogenic: A trait that is determined by two or more major genes (and possibly other factors).

Once removed: Separated by one generation as a pedigree would be drawn. *First cousins once removed* describe the relationship between an individual and the child of his or her first cousin. This is an intermediate relationship between first and second cousins in the numbers of genes shared.

Ousiotype: A hypothetical discrete factor postulated to be transmitted within families that could provide an alternative to a Mendelian major gene to account for an observed familial aggregation.

Pairwise concordance rate: An estimator of the proportion of twinships in the population who are concordant when twinships have been identified by complete ascertainment.

Path analysis: A form of statistical analysis aimed at fitting the correlations between phenotypes of different types of relatives to a model of genetic and environmental influences.

Pedigree: A collection of genetically related individuals, such as a collection of interrelated nuclear families.

Peeling: The process of computing the probabilities of genotypes for a mating given the phenotypes of their descendants used in the Elston-Stewart algorithm (q.v.).

Penetrance: The probability of a phenotype given the genotype (this could be a function, including modifying effects of age or other factors).

Phase: For doubly heterozygous individuals, the pairing of alleles at the two loci (i.e., $dm \mid DM$ vs. $dM \mid Dm$). A person is phase-known when study of his or her parents has shown that there is only one possible arrangement of his or her alleles into specific haplotypes at the loci of interest. A person is phase-unknown when study has been unable to establish the arrangement of his or her alleles into haplotypes.

Phenocopy: An affected individual with the normal genotype.

Phenotype: The observable trait or disease status that may be influenced by a genotype.

Polygene: The net effect of a large number of genes, each of which contributes only a small effect.

Polymerase chain reaction (PCR): A laboratory technique that allows a small sample of DNA to be replicated millions of times to allow genotyping by other methods.

Polymorphism: A tendency for gene to exist in more than one form or the specific alleles thereof. The term *polymorphism* is often distinguished from *mutation* by requiring it to be relatively common (e.g., greater than 1%).

Polymorphism information content (PIC): The probability that an individual is heterozygous and that the spouse and children have genotypes that allow the determination of the source of each allele; a measure of the informativeness of an allele for linkage analysis.

Polyploid: Cells containing one or more extra sets of chromosomes.

Population allele frequencies: The probability distribution in the general population of each allele for a gene.

Population genetics: The study of the distribution and evolution of genes in populations.

Positional cloning: Identification of a gene by location through linkage analysis.

Prevalence: The proportion of individuals in a designated population who have a particular disease or condition (see Incidence).

Proband: The individual who caused a family to be identified and included in a genetic analysis, usually an affected individual.

Probandwise concordance rate: An estimator of the risk of disease to an individual with an affected cotwin.

Promoter: A cluster of cis-acting regulatory sequences, usually situated just upstream (at the 5′ end) of the coding region, that regulate the initiation of gene transcription.

Proportional hazards model: A model for the hazard function that assumes that the hazard ratio is constant over time for any pair of covariate values (e.g., genotypes).

Prospective study: A design study in which subjects are enrolled and exposures are measured in the present. The cohort is then followed into the future for ascertainment of their health outcome development.

Qualitative trait: A phenotype that takes only a discrete set of possible values, such as present or absent.

Quantitative trait: A phenotype that can take any value (within some range), such as height.

Quantitative trait locus (QTL): A genetic locus that influences the distribution of a quantitative trait.

Randomization test: A class of statistical significance tests based on a comparison of some test statistic for the observed data with a distribution of that statistic across data sets obtained by randomly permuting or resampling the observed data in some way. A statistical test for familiality might be performed by randomly permuting family memberships, keeping family structures intact.

Recessive: A model for dominance in which individuals with only one copy of the susceptibility allele have the same risk as those with none.

Recombinant: A specific recombination event observed in a transmission.

Recombination: The phenomenon in which genes from two different homologous chromosomes are joined during the process of meiosis, reflecting an odd number of crossover events.

Regressive model: A multivariate model in which one includes as covariates for each individual the phenotypes of all individuals in the family who appear before him or her in the dataset.

Relative risk (RR): The ratio of some measure of disease frequency between two groups, such as carriers and noncarriers of a particular allele (genetic RR) or relatives of cases and relatives of controls (familial RR).

Restriction fragment length polymorphism (RFLP): A type of polymorphism that causes variation in the length of a restriction fragment. It can result from insertions or deletions between two restriction sites, from deletion of a restriction site, or from creation of a new restriction site. This type of polymorphism is often used as a marker locus.

Retrospective study: Any study design based on past records up to the present (could be the cohort or case-control type).

RNA: A type of single-stranded nucleic acid that serves as an intermediary between the genomic information (DNA) and its phenotypic expression (protein).

Score test: A significance test derived from the likelihood function by comparing the score (the first derivative of the loglikelihood) evaluated at the null hypothesis to the Fisher information (q.v.).

Segregation: The phenomenon in which an individual inherits half of his or her genes from each parent; one of the two fundamental Mendelian principles.

Segregation analysis: Statistical analyses aimed at testing hypotheses about the existence of major genes, polygenes, and environmental influences in pedigree data on phenotypes, and at estimating penetrance and allele frequency parameters in such models, without reference to measured genetic markers.

Segregation ratio: The probability that an offspring of a particular mating type (q.v.) of interest is affected.

Sense strand: The nontemplate DNA strand.

Sequential sampling of pedigrees: The process of assembling large pedigrees by extending smaller pedigrees in directions thought to be potentially informative without using prior knowledge of the actual phenotypes in the new branches.

Sex chromosome: One of two chromosomes that are not homologous and carry sex-determining genes.

Sex-linked: A trait determined by genes on one of the sex chromosomes (specifically, X-linked if the gene is located on the X chromosome).

Sib pair analysis: A form of linkage analysis based on comparison of the sharing of markers identical by descent (q.v.) by sib pairs in relation to their sharing of phenotypes; affected pair methods use only sib pairs with both members affected and compare their allele sharing with a distribution expected by chance; for continuous traits, the squared difference in phenotypes is regressed on the number of shared alleles.

Sibship: An entire collection of the offspring of a single pair of parents.

Simplex: A family with only a single case of the disease of interest; an ascertainment scheme for which a single case is sufficient to bring the family into the study.

Single ascertainment: A process of ascertainment in which families are ascertained with probability proportional to the number of affected members.

Single nucleotide polymorphism (SNP): A DNA sequence variation consisting of a change in a single base pair.

Sister chromatid exchange (SCE): Recombination between sister chromatids during mitosis.

Somatic cells: Any cell in the body other than germ cells.

Somatic mutation: A mutation to a somatic cell that is not transmitted to offspring.

Sporadic: An isolated case in a family with no other members affected; it is distinguished from a phenocopy (q.v.), which is a case who does not have the susceptible genotype.

Standardized incidence rate (SIR): A ratio between the observed and the expected number of events in a cohort based on the rates from some reference population.

Tetrachoric correlation: The correlation in the hypothetical bivariate normal correlation of liabilities underlying the observable distribution of affection status of pairs of individuals under a threshold model.

Threshold ascertainment: An ascertainment model that assumes that probands are representative of all members of the population with phenotypes greater than some minimum value (the threshold). Used for continuous traits.

Trans: On different members of a pair of homologous chromosomes.

Transcription: The first step in the conversion of genomic information (DNA) to protein: the process of copying genetic information from DNA to RNA.

Transition probability: The probability of an offspring's genotype, given his or her parents' genotypes.

Transitions: The substitution of one purine for another ($A \leftrightarrow G$) or one pyrimidine for another ($C \leftrightarrow T$).

Translation: The second step in the conversion of genomic information (DNA) to protein: the process of copying genetic information from messenger RNA (mRNA) to protein.

Transmission/disequilibrium test (TDT): A test for association based on comparing the alleles transmitted to a proband to the parental alleles not transmitted using matched case-control methods.

Transmission probability: The probability that a given allele will be transmitted from parent to offspring.

Transversions: Replacement of a purine by a pyrimidine or vice versa.

Twin study: A design for determining genetic and environmental influences on a trait by comparing the similarity or concordance of monozygotic (q.v.) and dizygotic (q.v.) twins.

Two-point linkage: A form of linkage analysis involving the use of a single marker locus at a time.

Variable number of terminal repeats (VNTR): A type of polymorphism that results from differences in the number of repeats in a repeated DNA sequence (e.g., CACACACA . . .). This type of polymorphism is often used as a marker locus.

Variance components: Decomposition of the variance of a phenotype into components that are attributable to genes [additive, dominance, epistatic (q.v.)], shared environment, or random individual influences.

Wald test: A significance test derived from the likelihood function, based on a comparison of the maximum likelihood estimate to its asymptotic standard error.

Wild type: The normal allele, not associated with an increased risk of the phenotype.

X inactivation: Random selection of one of the two X chromosomes in females that is not expressed.

X-linked: On the X chromosome, with a distinctive pattern of inheritance.

References

Aaltonen LA, Peltomaki P, Leach FS, et al. Clues to the pathogenesis of familial colorectal cancer. *Science* 1993; 260:812–816.

Aaltonen LA, Salovaara R, Kristo P, et al. Incidence of hereditary nonpolyposis colorectal cancer and the feasibility of molecular screening for the disease. *New England Journal of Medicine* 1998; 338:1481–1487.

Aarnio M, Sankila R, Pukkala E, et al. Cancer risk in mutation carriers of DNA-mismatch-repair genes. *International Journal of Cancer* 1999; 81:214–218.

Abecasis GR, Cardon LR, Cookson WO. A general test of association for quantitative traits in nuclear families. *American Journal of Human Genetics* 2000; 66:279–292.

Abecasis G, Noguchi E, Heinzmann A, et al. Extent and distribution of linkage disequilibrium in three genomic regions. *American Journal of Human Genetics* 2001; 68:191–197.

Abney M, Ober C, McPeek MS. Quantitative-trait homozygosity and association mapping and empirical genomewide significance in large, complex pedigrees: fasting serum-insulin level in the Hutterites. *American Journal of Human Genetics* 2002; 70:920–934.

Adorjan P, Distler J, Lipscher E, et al. Tumour class prediction and discovery by microarray-based DNA methylation analysis. *Nucleic Acids Research* 2002; 30:e21.

Ahsan H, Neugut AI, Garbowski GC, et al. Family history of colorectal adenomatous polyps and increased risk for colorectal cancer. *Annals of Internal Medicine* 1998; 128:900–905.

Akaike H. Information theory and an extension of the maximum likelihood principle. In: Petrov BN and Csaki F (eds.), *Second International Symposium on Information Theory*. Budapest, Akademia Kiado, 1973: 267–281.

Akey J, Jin L, Xiong M. Haplotypes vs. single marker linkage disequilibrium tests: what do we gain? *European Journal of Human Genetics* 2001; 9:291–300.

Allen AS, Rathouz PJ, Satten GA. Informative missingness in genetic association studies: case-parent designs. *American Journal of Human Genetics* 2003; 72:671–680.

Allen JF. In silico veritas. Data-mining and automated discovery: the truth is in there. *EMBO Reports* 2001; 2:542–544.

Allison DB. Transmission-disequilibrium tests for quantitative traits. *American Journal of Human Genetics* 1997; 60:676–690.

Allison DB, Heo M, Kaplan N, et al. Sibling-based tests of linkage and association for quantitative traits. *American Journal of Human Genetics* 1999; 64:1754–1763.

Almasy L, Blangero J. Multipoint quantitative-trait linkage analysis in general pedigrees. *American Journal of Human Genetics* 1998; 62:1198–1211.

Alon U, Barkai N, Notterman DA, et al. Broad patterns of gene expression revealed by clustering analysis of tumor and normal colon tissues probed by oligonucleotide arrays. *Proceedings of the National Academy of Sciences* 1999; 96:6745–6750.

Altshuler D, Kruglyak L, Lander ES. Genetic polymorphism and disease [letter]. *New England Journal of Medicine* 1998; 338:1626.

Amos C. Robust variance-components approach for assessing genetic linkage in pedigrees. *American Journal of Human Genetics* 1994; 54:535–543.

Anderson D. Genetic study of breast cancer: identification of a high risk group. *Cancer* 1974; 34:1090–1097.

Andrieu N, Clavel F, Auquier A, et al. Association between breast cancer and family malignancies. *European Journal of Cancer* 1991; 27:244–248.

Andrieu N, Clavel F, Auquier A, et al. Variations in the risk of breast cancer associated with a family history of breast cancer according to age at onset and reproductive factors. *Journal of Clinical Epidemiology* 1993; 46:973–980.

Andrieu N, Demenais F. Interactions between genetic and reproductive factors in breast cancer risk in a French family sample. *American Journal of Human Genetics* 1997; 61:678–690.

Andrieu N, Goldstein A, Langholz B, et al. Counter-matching in gene-environment interaction studies: efficiency and feasibility. *American Journal of Epidemiology* 2001; 153:265–274.

Anglian-Breast-Cancer-Study-Group. Prevalence and penetrance of *BRCA1* and *BRCA2* mutations in a population-based series of breast cancer cases. *British Journal of Cancer* 2000; 83:1301–1308.

Annest JL, Sing CF, Biron P, et al. Familial aggregation of blood pressure and weight in adoptive families. I. Comparisons of blood pressure and weight statistics among families with adopted, natural, or both natural and adopted children. *American Journal of Epidemiology* 1979a; 110:479–491.

Annest JL, Sing CF, Biron P, et al. Familial aggregation of blood pressure and weight in adoptive families. II. Estimation of the relative contributions of genetic and common environmental factors to blood pressure correlations between family members. *American Journal of Epidemiology* 1979b; 110:492–503.

Annest JL, Sing CF, Biron P, et al. Familial aggregation of blood pressure and weight in adoptive families. III. Analysis of the role of shared genes and shared household environment in explaining family resemblance for height, weight and selected weight/height indices. *American Journal of Epidemiology* 1983; 117:492–506.

Anonymous. Freely associating. *Nature Genetics* 1999; 22:1–2.

Anonymous. Genes, drugs and race. *Nature Genetics* 2001; 29:239–240.

Anton-Culver H, Kurosaki T, Taylor T, et al. Validation of family history of breast cancer and identification of the *BRCA1* and other syndromes using a population-based cancer registry. *Genetic Epidemiology* 1996; 13:193–205.

Antoniou AC, Gayther S, Stratton J, et al. Risk models for familial ovarian and breast cancer. *Genetic Epidemiology* 2000; 18:173–190.

Antoniou AC, Pharoah P, McMullan G, et al. Evidence for further breast cancer susceptibility genes in addition to *BRCA1* and *BRCA2* in a population-based study. *Genetic Epidemiology* 2001; 21:1–18.

Antoniou AC, Pharoah PD, McMullan G, et al. A comprehensive model for familial breast cancer incorporating *BRCA1, BRCA2* and other genes. *British Journal of Cancer* 2002; 86:76–83.

Antoniou A, Pharoah PD, Narod S, et al. Average risks of breast and ovarian cancer associated with *BRCA1* or *BRCA2* mutations detected in case series unselected for family history: A combined analysis of 22 studies. *American Journal of Human Genetics* 2003; 72:1117–1130.

Aparicio A, Eads CA, Leong LA, et al. Phase I trial of continuous infusion 5-aza-2′-deoxycytidine. *Cancer Chemotherapy and Pharmacololgy* 2003; 51:231–239.

Apicella C, Andrews L, Hodgson S, et al. Log odds of carrying an ancestral mutation in *BRCA1* or *BRCA2* for a defined personal and family history in an Ashkenazi Jewish woman (LAMBDA). *Breast Cancer Research* 2003; 5: R206–R216.

Ardlie KG, Kruglyak L, Steiestad M. Patterns of linkage disequilibrium in the human genome. *Nature Reviews Genetics* 2002; 3:299–309.

Armitage P. *Statistical Methods in Medical Research.* Oxford: Blackwell Scientific, 1971.

Armitage P, Doll R. The age distribution of cancer and a multistage theory of carcinogenesis. *British Journal of Cancer* 1954; 8:1–12.

Armstrong BK, McMichael AJ. Cancer in migrants. *Medical Journal of Australia* 1984; 140:3–4.

Armstrong G, Woodings T, Stenhouse N, et al. Mortality from cancer in migrants to Australia—1962 to 1971. Perth, WA, Australia: NH&MRC Research Unit in Epidemiology and Preventive Medicine, Raind Medical Statistics Unit, Department of Medicine, University of Western Australia, 1983.

Arnheim N, Calabrese P, Nordborg M. Hot and cold spots of recombination in the human genome: the reason we should find them and how this can be achieved. *American Journal of Human Genetics* 2003; 73:5–16.

Aste H, Saccomanno S, Bonelli L, et al. Adenomatous polyps and familial incidence of colorectal cancer. *European Journal of Cancer and Clinical Oncology* 1984; 20:1401–1403.

Atwood LD, Heard-Costa NL. Limits of fine-mapping a quantitative trait. *Genetic Epidemiology* 2003; 24:99–106.

Bacanu S–A, Devlin B, Roeder K. The power of genomic control. *American Journal of Human Genetics* 2000; 66:1933–1944.

Bacanu S–A, Devlin B, Roeder K. Association studies for quantitative traits in structured populations. *Genetic Epidemiology* 2002; 22:78–93.

Bader JS. The relative power of SNPs and haplotype as genetic markers for association tests [comment]. *Pharmacogenomics* 2001; 2:11–24.

Bahlo M, Griffiths RC. Inference from gene trees in a subdivided population. *Theoretical Population Biology* 2000; 57:79–95.

Bahlo M, Griffiths RC. Coalescence time for two genes from a subdivided population. *Journal of Mathematical Biology* 2001; 43:397–410.

Bailey-Wilson JE, Elston RC, Schuelke GS, et al. Segregation analysis of hereditary nonpolyposis colorectal cancer. *Genetic Epidemiology* 1986; 3:27–38.

Balding DJ, Bishop M, Cannings C. *Handbook of Statistical Genetics.* Chichester, UK: Wiley, 2001.

Bale SJ, Chakravarti A, Strong LC. Aggregation of colon cancer in family data. *Genetic Epidemiology* 1984; 1:53–61.

Bamshad MJ, Wooding S, Watkins WS et al. Human population genetic structure and inference of group membership. *American Journal of Human Genetics* 2003; 72:578–589.

Bao MZ, Wang JX, Dorman JS, et al. HLA-DQ beta non-ASP-57 allele and incidence of diabetes in China and the USA. *Lancet* 1989; 2:497–498.

Barletta JM, Rainier S, Feinberg AP. Reversal of loss of imprinting in tumor cells by 5-aza-2′-deoxycytidine. *Cancer Research* 1997; 57:48–50.

Begg CB. On the use of familial aggregation in population-based case probands for calculating penetrance. *Journal of the National Cancer Institute* 2002; 94:1221–1226.

Begg CB, Berlin JA. Publication bias: a problem in interpreting medical data. *Journal of the Royal Statistical Society, Series A* 1988; 151:419–463.

Bell G, Horita S, Karam JH. A polymorphic locus near the human insulin gene is associated with insulin-dependent diabetes mellitus. *Diabetes* 1984; 33:176–183.

Bernstein J, Haile R, Thompson WD, et al. Challenges in designing a study evaluating the role of gene-environment interactions in the etiology of breast cancer: the WECARE study. Under review.

Berry D, Parmigiani G, Sanchez J, et al. Probability of carrying a mutation of breast-ovarian cancer gene *BRCA1* based on family history. *Journal of the National Cancer Institute* 1997; 89:227–238.

Bickeboller H, Clerget-Darpoux F. Statistical properties of the allelic and genotypic transmission/disequilibrium test for multiallelic markers. *Genetic Epidemiology* 1995; 12:865–870.

Bink MC, Janss LL, Quaas RL. Markov chain Monte Carlo for mapping a quantitative trait locus in outbred populations. *Genetic Research* 2000; 75:231–241.

Blackwelder WC, Elston RC. A comparison of sib-pair linkage tests for disease susceptibility loci. *Genetic Epidemiology* 1985; 2:85–97.

Bleeker-Wagemakers LM, Gal A, Kumar-Singh R, et al. Evidence for nonallelic genetic heterogeneity in autosomal recessive retinitis pigmentosa. *Genomics* 1992; 14:811–812.

Blum K, Noble EP, Sheridan PJ, et al. Allelic association of human dopamine D2 receptor gene in alcoholism. *Journal of the American Medical Association* 1990; 263:2055–2060.

Bodmer WF, Bailey CJ, Bodmer J, et al. Localization of the gene for familial adenomatous polyposis on chromosome 5. *Nature* 1987; 328:614–616.

Boehnke M. Allele frequency estimation from data on relatives. *American Journal of Human Genetics* 1991; 48:22–25.

Boehnke M. Limits of resolution of genetic linkage studies: implications for the positional cloning of human disease genes. *American Journal of Human Genetics* 1994; 55:379–390.

Boehnke M, Arnheim N, Li H, et al. Fine-structure genetic mapping of human chromosomes using the polymerase chain reaction on single sperm: experimental design considerations. *American Journal of Human Genetics* 1989; 45:21–32.

Boehnke M, Young MR, Moll PP. Comparison of sequential and fixed-structure sampling of pedigrees in complex segregation analysis of a quantitative trait. *American Journal of Human Genetics* 1988; 43:336–343.

Boland CR. Hereditary nonpolyposis colorectal cancer (HNPCC). In: Vogelstein B and Kinzler KW (eds.), *The Genetic Basis of Human Cancer*. New York, McGraw-Hill, 2002: 307–321.

Bonney G. Regressive models for familial and other binary traits. *Biometrics* 1986; 42:611–625.

Boon M, Nolte IM, Bruinenberg M, et al. Mapping of a susceptibility gene for multiple sclerosis to the 51 kb interval between G511525 and D6S1666 using a new method of haplotype sharing analysis. *Neurogenetics* 2001; 3:221–230.

Borecki IB. The impact of marker allele frequency misspecification in variance components quantitative trait locus analysis using sibship data. *Genetic Epidemiology* 1999; 17(Suppl 1):S73–S77.

Botstein D, Risch N. Discovering genotypes underlying human phenotypes: past successes for Mendelian disease, future approaches for complex diseases. *Nature Genetics Supplement* 2003; 33:228–237.

Bourgain C, Genin E, Holopainen P, et al. Use of closely related affected individuals for the genetic study of complex diseases in founder populations. *American Journal of Human Genetics* 2001a; 68:154–159.

Bourgain C, Genin E, Margaritte-Jeannin P, et al. Maximum identity length contrast: a powerful method for susceptibility gene detection in isolated populations. *Genetic Epidemiology* 2001b; 21:S560–S564.

Bourgain C, Genin E, Quesneville H, et al. Search for multifactorial disease susceptibility genes in founder populations. *Annals of Human Genetics* 2000; 64:255–265.

Bourgain C, Hoffjan S, Nicolae R, et al. Novel case-control test in a founder population identifies p-selection as an atopy-susceptibility locus. *American Journal of Human Genetics* 2003; 73:612–626.

Boyer TG, Chen PL, Lee WH. Genome mining for human cancer genes: wherefore art thou? *Trends in Molecular Medicine* 2001; 7:187–189.

Brennan P. Gene-environment interaction and aetiology of cancer: what does it mean and how can we measure it? *Carcinogenesis* 2002; 23:381–387.

Breslow NE, Cain K. Logistic regression for two-stage case-control data. *Biometrika* 1988; 75:11–20.

Breslow NE, Day NE. *Statistical Methods in Cancer Research: I. The Analysis of Case-Control Studies*. Lyon: IARC Scientific Publications, 1980.

Breslow NE, Day NE. *Statistical Methods in Cancer Research. II. The Design and Analysis of Cohort Studies*. Lyon: IARC Scientific Publications, 1987.

Briscoe D, Stephens J, O'Brien J. Linkage disequilibrium in admixed populations: applications in gene mapping. *Journal of Heredity* 1994; 85:59–63.

Brown D, Gorin M, Weeks D. Efficient strategies for genomic searching using the affected-pedigree-member method of linkage analysis. *American Journal of Human Genetics* 1994; 54:544–552.

Bryant H, Brasher P. Risks and probabilities of breast cancer: short-term versus lifetime probabilities. *Canadian Medical Association Journal* 1994; 150:211–216.

Buckhaults P, Rago C, St Croix B, et al. Secreted and cell surface genes expressed in benign and malignant colorectal tumors. *Cancer Research* 2001; 61: 6996–7001.

Burchard EG, Ziv E, Coyle N, et al. The importance of race and ethnic background in biomedical research and clinical practice. *New England Journal of Medicine* 2003; 348:1170–1175.

Burns TL, Moll PP, Schork MA. Comparisons of different sampling designs for the determination of genetic transmission mechanisms in quantitative traits. *American Journal of Human Genetics* 1984; 36:1060–1074.

Burt RW, Bishop DT, Cannon LA, et al. Dominant inheritance of adenomatous colonic polyps and colorectal cancer. *New England Journal of Medicine* 1985; 312:1540–1544.

Burton PR, Palmer LJ, Jacobs K, et al. Ascertainment adjustment: where does it take us? *American Journal of Human Genetics* 2000; 67:1505–1514.

Cahill DP, Lengauer C, Yu J, et al. Mutations of mitotic checkpoint genes in human cancers. *Nature* 1998; 392:300–303.

Cain K, Breslow N. Logistic regression analysis and efficient design for two-stage studies. *American Journal of Epidemiology* 1988; 128:1198–1206.

Cannings C, Thompson E. Ascertainment in the sequential sampling of pedigrees. *Clinical Genetics* 1977; 12:208–212.

Cannings C, Thompson EA, Skolnick MH. Probability functions on complex pedigrees. *Advances in Applied Probability* 1978; 10:26–91.

Cannon-Albright LA, Skolnick MH, Bishop DT, et al. Common inheritance of susceptibility to colonic adenomatous polyps and associated colorectal cancers. *New England Journal of Medicine* 1988; 319:533–537.

Cardon LR, Abecasis GR. Using haplotype blocks to map human complex trait loci. *Trends in Genetics* 2003; 19:135–140.

Cardon LR, Bell JI. Association study designs for complex diseases. *Nature Reviews Genetics* 2001; 2:91–99.

Cargill M, Altshuler D, Ireland J, et al. Characterization of single-nucleotide polymorphisms in coding regions of human genes. *Nature Genetics* 1999; 22:231–238.

Cargill M, Daley GQ. Mining for SNPs: putting the common variants—common disease hypothesis to the test. *Pharmacogenomics* 2000; 1:27–37.

Carstensen B, Soll-Johanning H, Villadsen E, et al. Familial aggregation of colorectal cancer in the general population. *International Journal of Cancer* 1996; 68:428–435.

Cavalli-Sforza LL, Menozzi P, Piazza A. *The History and Geography of Human Genes.* Princeton, NJ: Princeton University Press, 1994.

Chakraborty R, Weiss K, Majumder P, et al. A method to detect excess risk of disease in structured data: cancer in relatives of retinoblastoma patients. *Genetic Epidemiology* 1984; 1:229–244.

Chen J, Giovannucci E, Kelsey K, et al. A methylenetetrahydrofolate reductase polymorphism and the risk of colorectal cancer. *Cancer Research* 1996; 56:4862–4864.

Cheung VG, Spielman RS. The genetics of variation in gene expression. *Nature Genetics Supplement* 2002; 32:522–525.

Chiano M, Clayton D. Fine genetic mapping using haplotype analysis and the missing data problem. *Annals of Human Genetics* 1998; 62:55–60.

Childs B, Scriver CR. Age at onset and causes of disease. *Perspectives in Biology and Medicine* 1986; 29:437–460.

Clark AG, Weiss KM, Nickerson DA, et al. Haplotype structure and population genetic inferences from nucleotide-sequence variation in human lipoprotein lipase. *American Journal of Human Genetics* 1998; 63:595–612.

Clarke C. ABO blood groups and secretor character in duodenal ulcer. *British Medical Journal* 1956; 2:725–731.

Claus EB, Risch N, Thompson W. Age at onset as an indicator of familial risk of breast cancer. *American Journal of Epidemiology* 1990; 131:961–972.

Claus EB, Risch N, Thompson WD. Genetic analysis of breast cancer in the Cancer and Steroid Hormone study. *American Journal of Human Genetics* 1991; 48:232–242.

Claus EB, Schildkraut J, Iversen ES, Jr, et al. Effect of *BRCA1* and *BRCA2* on the association between breast cancer risk and family history. *Journal of the National Cancer Institute* 1998; 90:1824–1829.

Clayton DG. A Monte Carlo method for Bayesian inference in frailty models. *Biometrics* 1991; 47:467–485.

Clayton DG. A generalization of the transmission/disequilibrium test for uncertain-haplotype transmission. *American Journal of Human Genetics* 1999; 65:1170–1177.

Clayton DG. Choosing a set of haplotype tagging SNPs from a larger set of diallelic loci. Unpublished manuscript cited in Johnson et al. (2001) available from http://www.nature.com/ng/journal/v29/n2/extref/ng1001-233-S10.html.

Clayton DG, Jones H. Transmission/disequilibrium tests for extended marker haplotypes. *American Journal of Human Genetics* 1999; 65:1161–1169.

Clayton D, McKeigue PM. Epidemiological methods for studying genes and environmental factors in complex diseases. *Lancet* 2001; 358:1356–1360.

Clerget-Darpoux F, Bonaiti-Pellie C, Hochez J. Effects of misspecifying genetic parameters in lod score analysis. *Biometrics* 1986; 42:393–399.

Cleves MA, Olson JM, Jacobs KB. Exact transmission-disequilibrium tests with multiallelic markers. *Genetic Epidemiology* 1997; 14:337–347.

Cohen J. *Statistical Power Analysis for the Behavioral Sciences.* New York: New York Academy of Sciences Press, 1988.

Colhoun HM, McKeigue PM, Davey Smith G. Problems of reporting genetic associations with complex outcomes. *Lancet* 2003; 361:865–872.

Collaborative-Group-on-Hormonal-Factors-in-Breast-Cancer. Breast cancer and hormonal contraceptives: collaborative reanalysis of individual data on 53 297 women with breast cancer and 100 239 women without breast cancer from 54 epidemiological studies. *Lancet* 1996; 347:1713–1727.

Collins A, Lonjou C, Morton N. Genetic epidemiology of single-nucleotide polymorphisms. *Proceedings of the National Academy of Sciences of the United States of America* 1999; 96:15173–15177.

Collins-Schramm HE, Phillips CM, Operario DJ, et al. Ethnic-difference markers for use in mapping by admixture linkage disequilibrium. *American Journal of Human Genetics* 2002; 70:737–750.

Conti DV, Cortessis V, Molitor J, et al. Bayesian modeling of complex metabolic pathways. *Human Heredity* 2003: in press.

Conti DV, Witte JS. Hierarchical modeling of linkage disequilibrum: genetic structure and spatial relations. *American Journal of Human Genetics* 2003; 72: 351–363.

Cooper RS. Race, genes, and health—new wine in old bottles? *International Journal of Epidemiology* 2003; 32:23–25.

Cooper RS, Kaufman JS, Ward R. Race and genomics. *New England Journal of Medicine* 2003; 348:1166–1170.

Cordell H. Epistasis: what it means, what it doesn't mean, and statistical methods to detect it in humans. *Human Molecular Genetics* 2002; 11:2463–2468.

Cordell H, Elston R. Fieller's theorem and linkage disequilibrium mapping. *Genetic Epidemiology* 1999; 17:237–252.

Cortessis V, Thomas DC. Toxicokinetic genetics: an approach to gene-environment and gene-gene interactions in complex metabolic pathways. In: Bird P, Boffetta P, Buffler P, et al. (eds.), *Mechanistic Considerations in the Molecular Epidemiology of Cancer*. Lyon: IARC Scientific Publications, 2003: in press.

Costello JF, Fruhwald MC, Smiraglia DJ, et al. Aberrant CpG-island methylation has non-random and tumour-type-specific patterns. *Nature Genetics* 2000; 24:132–138.

Cotton RGH, Scriver CR. Proof of "disease causing" mutation. *Human Mutation* 1998; 12:1–3.

Couzin J. Genomics. New mapping project splits the community. *Science* 2002; 296:1391–1393.

Cozen W, Gill PS, Ingles SA, et al. IL-6 levels and genotype are associated with risk of young adult Hodgkin's lymphoma. *Blood* 2003, in press.

Cox D. Regression models and life tables (with discussion). *Journal of the Royal Statistical Society, Series B* 1972; 34:187–220.

Cramer DW, Hutchison GB, Welch WR, et al. Determinants of ovarian cancer risk. I. Reproductive experiences and family history. *Journal of the National Cancer Institute* 1983; 71:711–716.

Cross HS, Bajna E, Bises G, et al. Vitamin D receptor and cytokeratin expression may be progression indicators in human colon cancer. *Anticancer Research* 1996; 16:2333–2337.

Crouse H. The controlling element in sex chromosome behavior in Sciara. *Genetics* 1960; 45:1429.

Cui H, Cruz-Correa M, Giardiello FM, et al. Loss of *IGF2* imprinting: a potential marker of colorectal cancer risk. *Science* 2003a; 299:1753–1755.

Cui H, Horon IL, Ohlsson R, et al. Loss of imprinting in normal tissue of colorectal cancer patients with microsatellite instability. *Nature Medicine* 1998; 4:1276–1280.

Cui JS, Antoniou AC, Dite GS, et al. After *BRCA1* and *BRCA2*—what next? Multifactorial segregation analyses of three-generation, population-based Australian families affected by female breast cancer. *American Journal of Human Genetics* 2001; 68:420–431.

Cui JS, Hopper JL. Why are the majority of hereditary cases of early-onset breast cancer sporadic? A simulation study. *Cancer Epidemiology, Biomarkers, and Prevention* 2000; 9:805–812.

Cui JS, Spurdle AB, Southey MC, et al. Regressive logistic and proportional hazards disease models for within-family analyses of measured genotypes, with application to a *CYP17* polymorphism and breast cancer. *Genetic Epidemiology* 2003b; 24:161–172.

Curtis D. Genetic dissection of complex traits [letter]. *Nature Genetics* 1996; 12:356–357.

Curtis D. Use of siblings as controls in case-control association studies. *Annals of Human Genetics* 1997; 61:319–333.

Curtis D, Sham PC. A note on the application of the transmission disequilibrium test when a parent is missing. *American Journal of Human Genetics* 1995; 56:811–812.

Cuthill S. Cellular epigenetics and the origin of cancer. *Bioessays* 1994; 16:393–394.

Dahlman I, Eaves IA, Kosoy R, et al. Parameters for reliable results in genetic association studies in common disease. *Nature Genetics* 2002; 30:149–150.

Daly MB, Offit K, Li F, et al. Participation in the cooperative family registry for breast cancer studies: issues of informed consent. *Journal of the National Cancer Institute* 2000; 92:452–456.

Daly MB, Rioux JD, Schaffner SF, et al. High-resolution haplotype structure in the human genome. *Nature Genetics* 2001; 29:229–232.

Darwish H, DeLuca HF. Vitamin D–regulated gene expression. *Critical Reviews in Eukaryotic Gene Expression* 1993; 3:89–116.

Daskalakis M, Nguyen TT, Nguyen C, et al. Demethylation of a hypermethylated *P15/INK4B* gene in patients with myelodysplastic syndrome by 5-aza-2'-deoxycytidine (decitabine) treatment. *Blood* 2002; 100:2957–2964.

Dawid AP. Causal inference without counterfactuals (with discussion). *Journal of the American Statistical Association* 2000; 95:407–448.

Dawson DV, Elston RC. A bivariate problem in human genetics: ascertainment of families through a correlated trait. *American Journal of Medical Genetics* 1984; 18:435–448.

de Jong MM, Nolte IM, te Meerman GJ, et al. Low penetrance genes and their involvement in colorectal cancer susceptibility. *Cancer Epidemiology, Biomarkers and Prevention* 2002; 11:1332–1352.

Dean M, Stephens J, Winkler C, et al. Polymorphic admixture typing in human ethnic populations. *American Journal of Human Genetics* 1994; 55:788–808.

Devlin B, Risch N. A comparison of linkage disequilibrium measures for fine-scale mapping. *Genomics* 1995; 29:311–337.

Devlin B, Roeder K. Genomic control for association studies. *Biometrics* 1999; 55:997–1004.

Devlin B, Roeder K, Bacanu S-A. Unbiased methods for population-based association studies. *Genetic Epidemiology* 2001; 21:273–284.

Devlin B, Roeder K, Wasserman L. Genomic control for association studies: a semiparametric test to detect excess-haplotype sharing. *Biostatistics* 2000; 1:369–387.

Dietmaier W, Wallinger S, Bocker T, et al. Diagnostic microsatellite instability: definition and correlation with mismatch repair protein expression. *Cancer Research* 1997; 57:4749–4756.

Dite GS, Jenkins MA, Southey MC, et al. Familial risks, early-onset breast cancer, and *BRCA1* and *BRCA2* germline mutations. *Journal of the National Cancer Institute* 2003; 95:448–457.

Douglas JA, Boehnke M, Gallanders E, et al. Experimentally-derived haplotypes substantially increase the efficiency of linkage disequilibrium studies. *Nature Genetics* 2001; 28:361–364.

Drigalenko E. How sib pairs reveal linkage. *American Journal of Human Genetics* 1998; 63:1242–1245.

Dunlop MG, Farrington SM, Carothers AD, et al. Cancer risk associated with germline DNA mismatch repair gene mutations. *Human Molecular Genetics* 1997; 6:105–110.

Dunning A, Durocher F, Healey C, et al. The extent of linkage disequilibrium in four populations with distinct demographic histories. *American Journal of Human Genetics* 2000; 67:1544–1554.

Dupuis J, Van Eerdewegh P. Multipoint linkage analysis of the pseudoautosomal regions, using affected sibling pairs. *American Journal of Human Genetics* 2000; 67:462–475.

Easton D. Cancer risks in A-T heterozygotes. *International Journal of Radiation Biology* 1994; 66:S177–S182.

Easton D. Breast cancer—not just whether but when? *Nature Genetics* 2000; 26:390–391.

Easton D, Bishop D, Ford D, et al. Genetic linkage analysis in familial breast and ovarian cancer: results from 214 families. *American Journal of Human Genetics* 1993; 52:678–701.

Easton D, Ford D, Bishop D. Breast and ovarian cancer incidence in *BRCA1*-mutation carriers. *American Journal of Human Genetics* 1995; 56:265–271.

Edwards AWF. The measure of association in a 2 × 2 table. *Journal of the Royal Statistical Society, Series A* 1963; 126:109–114.

Edwards JH. Exclusion mapping. *Journal of Medical Genetics* 1987; 24:539–543.

Efron B. Large-scale simultaneous hypothesis testing: the choice of a null hypothesis. *Journal of the American Statistical Association* 2003; 98: in press.

Efron G, Tibshirani RJ. *An Introduction to the Bootstrap.* New York: Chapman and Hall, 1994.

Eisen MB, Spellman PT, Brown PO, et al. Cluster analysis and display of genome-wide expression patterns. *Proceedings of the National Academy of Sciences of the United States of America* 1998; 95:14863–14868.

Elston RC. 'Twixt cup and lip: how intractable is the ascertainment problem? *American Journal of Human Genetics* 1995; 56:15–17.

Elston RC, Buxbaum S, Jacobs KB, et al. Haseman and Elston revisited. *Genetic Epidemiology* 2000; 19:1–17.

Elston RC, Guo X, Williams LV. Two-stage global search designs for linkage analysis using pairs of affected relatives. *Genetic Epidemiology* 1996; 13:535–558.

Elston RC, Stewart J. A general model for the genetic analysis of pedigrees. *Human Heredity* 1971; 21:523–542.

Epstein MP, Satten GA. Inference on haplotype effects in case-control studies using unphased genotype data. *American Journal of Human Genetics* 2003, in press.

Ewens WJ. *Mathematical Population Genetics.* Berlin: Springer-Verlag, 1979.

Ewens WJ, Spielman RS. The transmission/disequilibrium test: history, subdivision, and admixture. *American Journal of Human Genetics* 1995; 57:455–464.

Excoffier L, Slatkin M. Maximum-likelihood estimation of molecular haplotype frequencies in a diploid population. *Molecular Biology and Evolution* 1995; 12:921–927.

Falconer DS. The inheritance of liability to certain diseases estimated from the incidence among relatives. *Annals of Human Genetics* 1967; 29:51–76.

Falconer DS, MacKay TFC. *Introduction to Quantitative Genetics (4th ed.).* New York: Addison-Wesley, 1994.

Falk CT, Rubinstein P. Haplotype relative risks: an easy reliable way to construct a proper control sample for risk calculations. *Annals of Human Genetics* 1987; 51:227–233.

Faraway JJ. Distribution of the admixture test for the detection of linkage under heterogeneity. *Genetic Epidemiology* 1993; 10:75–83.

Faraway JJ. Testing for linkage under heterogeneity: A test versus C test. *American Journal of Human Genetics* 1994; 54:563–564; discussion 564–567.

Farrington SM, Lin-Goerke J, Ling J, et al. Systematic analysis of *hMSH2* and *hMLH1* in young colon cancer patients and controls. *American Journal of Human Genetics* 1998; 63:749–759.

Fearon ER. Molecular genetics of colorectal cancer. *Annals of the New York Academy of Sciences* 1995; 768:101–110.

Fearon ER, Hamilton SR, Vogelstein B. Clonal analysis of human colorectal tumors. *Science* 1987; 238:193–197.

Fearon ER, Vogelstein B. A genetic model for colorectal tumorigenesis. *Cell* 1990; 61:759–767.

Fears T, Brown C. Logistic regression methods for retrospective case-control studies using complex sampling procedures. *Biometrics* 1986; 42:955–960.

Feigelson H, Henderson B. Estrogens and breast cancer: an epidemiologic perspective. In: Manni A (ed.), *Contemporary Endocrinology: Endocrinology of Breast Cancer*. Totowa, NJ: Humana Press, 1998: 55–67.

Feigelson H, McKean-Cowdin R, Coetzee G, et al. Building a multigenic model of breast cancer susceptibility: *CYP17* and *HSD17B1* are two important candidates. *Cancer Research* 2001; 61:785–789.

Feinberg AP. Imprinting of a genomic domain of 11p15 and loss of imprinting in cancer: an introduction. *Cancer Research* 1999; 59:1743s–1746s.

Feinberg AP. Genomic imprinting and cancer. In: Vogelstein B and Kinzler KW (eds.), *The Genetic Basis of Human Cancer* (2nd ed.). New York, McGraw-Hill, 2002: 43–55.

Fischer C, Beckmann L, Marjoram P, et al. Haplotype sharing analysis with SNPs in candidate genes: the *GAW12* example. *Genetic Epidemiology* 2003; 24:68–73.

Fishel R, Lescoe MK, Rao MR, et al. The human mutator gene homolog *MSH2* and its association with hereditary nonpolyposis colon cancer. *Cell* 1993; 75:1027–1038.

Ford D, Easton D, Bishop D, et al. Risks of cancer in *BRCA1*-mutation carriers. *Lancet* 1994; 343:692–695.

Ford D, Easton D, Stratton M, et al. Genetic heterogeneity and penetrance analysis of the *BRCA1* and *BRCA2* genes in breast cancer families. *American Journal of Human Genetics* 1998; 62:676–689.

Forsti A, Jin Q, Sundqvist L, et al. Use of monozygotic twins in search for breast cancer susceptibility loci. *Twin Research* 2001; 4:251–259.

Foster DP, George EI. The risk inflation criterion for multiple regression. *Annals of Statistics* 1994; 22:1947–1975.

Freimer N, Sandkuijl L, Blower S. Incorrect specification of marker allele frequencies: effects on linkage analysis. *American Journal of Human Genetics* 1993; 52:1102–1110.

Frisse L, Hudson RR, Bartoszewicz A, et al. Gene conversion and different population histories may explain the contrast between polymorphism and linkage disequilibrium levels. *American Journal of Human Genetics* 2001; 69:831–843.

Fuchs CS, Giovannucci EL, Colditz GA, et al. A prospective study of family history and the risk of colorectal cancer. *New England Journal of Medicine* 1994; 331:1669–1674.

Fulker DW, Cherny SS, Sham PC, et al. Combined linkage and association sib-pair analysis for quantitative traits. *American Journal of Human Genetics* 1999; 64:259–267.

Gabriel SB, Schaffner SF, Nguyen H, et al. The structure of haplotype blocks in the human genome. *Science* 2002; 296:2225–2229.

Gail M, Pee D, Benichou J, et al. Designing studies to estimate the penetrance of an identified autosomal dominant mutation: cohort, case-control, and genotype-proband designs. *Genetic Epidemiology* 1999a; 16:15–39.

Gail M, Pee D, Carroll R. Kin-cohort designs for gene characterization. *Monographs of the National Cancer Institute* 1999b; 26:55–60.

Garcia-Closas M, Lubin JH. Power and sample size calculations in case-control studies of gene–environment interactions: comments on different approaches. *American Journal of Epidemiology* 1999; 149:689–692.

Gatti RA, Tward A, Concannon P. Cancer risk in ATM heterozygotes: a model of phenotypic and mechanistic differences between missense and truncating mutations. *Molecular Genetics and Metabolism* 1999; 68:419–423.

Gauderman WJ. Candidate gene association analysis for a quantitative trait, using parent–offspring trios. *Genetic Epidemiology* 2003, in press.

Gauderman WJ. Sample size calculations for association studies of gene–gene interaction. *American Journal of Epidemiology* 2002b; 155:478–484.

Gauderman WJ. Sample size requirements for matched case-control studies of gene–environment interaction. *Statistics in Medicine* 2002c; 21:35–50.

Gauderman WJ. A method for simulating familial disease data with variable age at onset and genetic and environmental effects. *Statistics and Computation* 1995; 5:237–243.

Gauderman WJ, Faucett CL. Detection of gene–environment interactions in joint segregation and linkage analysis. *American Journal of Human Genetics* 1997; 61:1189–1199.

Gauderman WJ, Faucett CL, Morrison JL, et al. Joint segregation and linkage analysis of a quantitative trait compared to separate analyses. *Genetic Epidemiology* 1997a; 14:993–998.

Gauderman WJ, Macgregor S, Briollais L, et al. Longitudinal data analysis in pedigree studies. *Genetic Epidemiology* 2003, in press.

Gauderman WJ, Millstein J. The case-only design to detect G × E interaction for a survival trait [Abstract IGES-55]. *Genetic Epidemiology* 2002; 23:282.

Gauderman WJ, Morrison JL, Carpenter CL, et al. Analysis of gene–smoking interaction in lung cancer. *Genetic Epidemiology* 1997b; 14:199–214.

Gauderman WJ, Thomas DC. Censored survival models for genetic epidemiology: a Gibbs sampling approach. *Genetic Epidemiology* 1994; 11:171–188.

Gauderman WJ, Witte JS, Thomas DC. Family-based association studies. *Monographs of the National Cancer Institute* 1999; 26:31–37.

Gayther S, Mangion J, Russell P, et al. Variation of risks of breast and ovarian cancer associated with different germline mutations of the *BRCA2* gene. *Nature Genetics* 1997; 15:103–105.

Gelernter J, Goldman D, Risch N. The *A1* allele at the D2 dopamine receptor gene and alcoholism. A reappraisal. *Journal of the American Medical Association* 1993; 269:1673–1677.

Gelman A, Bois F, Jiang J. Physiological pharmacokinetic analysis using population modeling and informative prior distributions. *Journal of the American Statistical Association* 1996; 91:1400–1412.

Geman S, Geman D. Stochastic relaxation, Gibbs distribution, and the Bayesian restoration of images. *IEEE Transactions on Pattern Analysis and Machine Intelligence* 1984; 6:721–741.

George EI, Foster DP. Calibration and empirical Bayes variable selection. *Biometrika* 2000; 87:731–747.

Geyer C, Thompson E. Annealing Markov chain Monte Carlo with applications to ancestral inference. *Journal of the American Statistical Association* 1995; 90:909–920.

Gilks W, Richardson S, Spiegelhalter D (eds.). *Markov Chain Monte Carlo in practice*. London: Chapman and Hall, 1996.

Go RC, Elston RC, Kaplan EB. Efficiency and robustness of pedigree segregation analysis. *American Journal of Human Genetics* 1978; 30:28–37.

Goldstein DB. Islands of linkage disequilibrium. *Nature Genetics* 2001; 29:109–111.

Golub TR, Slonim DK, Tamayo P, et al. Molecular classification of cancer: class discovery and class prediction by gene expression monitoring. *Science* 1999; 286:531–537.

Gong G, Whittemore AS. Optimal designs for estimating penetrance of rare mutations of a disease susceptibility gene. *Genetic Epidemiology* 2003; 24:173–180.

Gordis L. *Epidemiology*. Philadelpha: W.B. Saunders, 1996.

Grabrick DM, Hartmann LC, Cerhan JR, et al. Risk of breast cancer with oral contraceptive use in women with a family history of breast cancer. *Journal of the American Medical Association* 2000; 284:1791–1798.

Graham J, Thompson E. Disequilibrium likelihoods for fine-scale mapping of a rare allele. *American Journal of Human Genetics* 1998; 63:1517–1530.

Green P. Reversible jump Markov chain Monte Carlo computation and Bayesian model determination. *Journal of the Royal Statistical Society, Series B* 1995; 82:711–732.

Greenberg D. Inferring mode of inheritance by comparison of lod scores. *American Journal of Human Genetics* 1989; 35:480–486.

Greenberg ER, Baron JA, Tosteson TD, et al. A clinical trial of antioxidant vitamins to prevent colorectal adenoma. Polyp Prevention Study Group [see comments]. *New England Journal of Medicine* 1994; 331:141–147.

Greenland S. Randomization, statistics, and causal inference. *Epidemiology* 1990; 1:421–429.

Greenland S, Thomas D. On the need for the rare disease assumption in case-control studies. *American Journal of Epidemiology* 1982; 116:547–553.

Griffiths AJF, Miller JH, Suzuki DT, et al. *An Introduction to Genetic Analysis* (7th Ed.). New York: WH Freeman & Co., 2000.

Griffiths R, Marjoram P. Ancestral inference from samples of DNA sequences with recombination. *Journal of Computational Biology* 1996; 3:479–502.

Griffiths R, Marjoram P. An ancestral recombination graph. In: Donnelly P and Tavaré S (eds.), *Progress in Population Genetics and Human Evolution/IMA Volumes in Mathematics and Its Applications*. Berlin: Springer-Verlag, 1997: 257–270.

Griffiths R, Tavaré S. Ancestral inference in population genetics. *Statistical Science* 1994a; 9:307–319.

Griffiths R, Tavaré S. Simulating probability distributions in the coalescent. *Theoretical Population Biology* 1994b; 46:131–159.

Griffiths R, Tavaré S. Computational methods for the coalescent. In: Donnelly P and Tavaré S (eds.), *Population Genetics and Human Evolution*. Berlin: Springer-Verlag, 1997; 87:165–182.

Groden J, Thliveris A, Samowitz W, et al. Identification and characterization of the familial adenomatous polyposis coli gene. *Cell* 1991; 66:589–600.

Guo X, Elston R. Two-stage global search designs for linkage analysis II: including discordant relative pairs in the study. *Genetic Epidemiology* 2000; 18:111–127.

Haenszel W. Cancer mortality among the foreign born in the United States. *Journal of the National Cancer Institute* 1961; 26:37–132.

Haenszel W, Kurihara M. Studies of Japanese migrants. I. Mortality from cancer and other diseases among Japanese in the United States. *Journal of the National Cancer Institute* 1968; 40:43–68.

Haiman CA, Stram DO, Pike MC, et al. A comprehensive haplotype analysis of *CYP19* and breast cancer risk. The Multiethnic Cohort. *Human Molecular Genetics* 2003; 12:2679–2692.

Haines JL, Pericak-Vance MA (eds.). *Approaches to Gene Mapping in Complex Human Diseases*. New York: Wiley-Liss, 1998.

Haldane JBS. The combination of linkage values and the calculation of distances between the loci of linked factors. *Journal of Genetics* 1919; 8:299–309.

Hall JM, Friedman L, Guenther C, et al. Closing in on a breast cancer gene on chromosome 17q. *American Journal of Human Genetics* 1992; 50:1235–1242.

Hall JM, Lee MK, Newman B, et al. Linkage of early-onset familial breast cancer to chromosome 17q21. *Science* 1990; 250:1684–1689.

Hamilton AS, Mack TM. Use of twins as mutual proxy respondents in a case-control study of breast cancer: effect of item nonresponse and misclassification. *American Journal of Epidemiology* 2000; 152:1093–1103.

Hamilton AS, Mack TM. Puberty and genetic susceptibility to breast cancer in a case-control study in twins. *New England Journal of Medicine* 2003; 348:2313–2322.

Hanson RL, Kobes S, Lindsay RS, et al. Assessment of parent-of-origin effects in linkage analysis of quantitative traits. *American Journal of Human Genetics* 2001; 68:951–962.

Hartl DL. *A Primer of Population Genetics*. Sunderland, MA: Sinauer, 2000.

Hartl DL, Clark AG. *Principles of Population Genetics* (3rd ed.). Sunderland, MA: Sinauer Associates, 1997.

Hartge P. Genes, hormones, and pathways to breast cancer. *New England Journal of Medicine* 2003; 348:2352–2354.

Haseman J, Elston R. The investigation of linkage between a quantitative trait and a marker locus. *Behavioral Genetics* 1972; 2:3–19.

Hasstedt SJ. A mixed-model likelihood approximation on large pedigrees. *Computers and Biomedical Research* 1982; 15:295–307.

Hasstedt SJ. A variance components/major locus likelihood approximation on quantitative data. *Genetic Epidemiology* 1991; 8:113–125.

Hastbacka J, De La Chapelle A, Kaitila I, et al. Linkage disequilibrium mapping in isolated founder populations: diastrophic dysplasia in Finland. *Nature Genetics* 1992; 2:204–211.

Hastie T, Tibshirani R, Botstein D, et al. Supervised harvesting of expression trees. *Genome Biology* 2001; 2:RESEARCH0003.

Hastie T, Tibshirani R, Eisen MB, et al. "Gene shaving" as a method for identifying distinct sets of genes with similar expression patterns. *Genome Biology* 2000; 1:RESEARCH0003.

Hauser ER, Boehnke M, Guo SW, et al. Affected-sib-pair interval mapping and exclusion for complex genetic traits: sampling considerations. *Genetic Epidemiology* 1996; 13:117–137.

Heath SC. Markov chain Monte Carlo segregation and linkage analysis for oligogenic models. *American Journal of Human Genetics* 1997; 61:748–760.

Hedrick P. Gametic disequilibrium measures: proceed with caution. *Genetics* 1987; 117:331–341.

Henderson BE, Pike MC, Bernstein L, et al. Breast cancer. In: Schottenfeld D and Fraumeni JFJ (eds.), *Cancer Epidemiology and Prevention* (2nd ed.). Oxford: Oxford University Press, 1996: 1022–1039.

Herbots H. The structured coalescent. In: Donnelly P and Tavare S (eds.), *Progress in Population Genetics and Human Evolution*. New York: Springer, 1997: 231–255.

Herrera L, Kakati S, Gibas L, et al. Gardner syndrome in a man with an interstitial deletion of 5q. *American Journal of Medical Genetics* 1986; 25:473–476.

Hey J, Machado CA. The study of structured populations—new hope for a difficult and divided science. *Nature Reviews Genetics* 2003; 4:535–543.

Higgins J. Effects of child rearing by schizophrenic mothers: a follow-up. *Journal of Psychiatric Research* 1976; 13:1–9.

Hill AB. The environment and disease: association or causation? *Journal of the Royal Society of Medicine* 1965; 58:295–300.

Hill MJ, Morson BC, Bussey HJ. Aetiology of adenoma–carcinoma sequence in large bowel. *Lancet* 1978; 1:245–247.

Hill W. Estimation of linkage disequilibrium in randomly mating populations. *Heredity* 1974; 33:229–239.

Hill W, Weir B. Maximum-likelihood estimation of gene location by linkage disequilibrium. *American Journal of Human Genetics* 1994; 54:705–714.

Hirschhorn JN, Altschuler D. Once and again—issues surrounding replication in genetic association studies. *Journal of Clinical Endocrinology Metabolism* 2002; 87:4438–4441.

Hirschhorn JN, Lohmueller K, Byrne E, et al. A comprehensive review of genetic association studies. *Genetics in Medicine* 2002; 4:45–61.

Hodge SE. The information contained in multiple sibling pairs. *Genetic Epidemiology* 1984; 1:109–122.

Hodge SE, Elston RC. Lods, wrods, and mods: the interpretation of lod scores calculated under different models. *Genetic Epidemiology* 1994; 11:329–342.

Hodge SE, Greenberg DA. Sensitivity of lod scores to changes in diagnostic status. *American Journal of Human Genetics* 1992; 50:1053–1066.

Hodge SE, Anderson CE, Neiswanger K, et al. The search for heterogeneity in insulin-dependent diabetes mellitus (IDDM): linkage studies, two-locus models, and genetic heterogeneity. *American Journal of Human Genetics* 1983; 35:1139–1155.

Hodge SE, Vieland VJ. The essence of single ascertainment. *Genetics* 1996; 144:1215–1223.

Hoggart CJ, Parra EJ, Shriver MD et al. Control of confounding of genetic associations in stratified populations. *American Journal of Human Genetics* 2003; 72:1492–1504.

Hoh J, Ott J. Mathematical multi-locus approaches to localizing complex human trait genes. *Nature Reviews Genetics* 2003; 4:701–709.

Holm NV. Studies of cancer etiology in the Danish twin population. I. Breast cancer. *Progress in Clinical and Biological Research* 1981; 69:211–216.

Holm NV, Hauge M, Harvald B. Etiologic factors of breast cancer elucidated by a study of unselected twins. *Journal of the National Cancer Institute* 1980; 65:285–298.

Holmans P, Craddock N. Efficient strategies for genome scanning using maximum-likelihood affected-sib-pair analysis. *American Journal of Human Genetics* 1997; 60:657–666.

Hopper JL. Genetic epidemiology of female breast cancer. *Seminars in Cancer Biology* 2001; 11:367–374.

Hopper JL. Commentary: case-control-family designs: a paradigm for future epidemiology research. *International Journal of Epidemiology* 2003; 32:48–50.

Hopper JL, Chenevix-Trench G, Jolley DJ, et al. Design and analysis issues in a population-based, case-control-family study and the Co-operative Family Registry for Breast Cancer Studies (CFRBCS). *Journal of the National Cancer Institute Monographs* 1999a; 26:95–100.

Hopper JL, Southey MC, Dite GS, et al. Population-based estimate of the average age-specific cumulative risk of breast cancer for a defined set of protein-truncating mucations in *BRCA1* and *BRCA2*. *Cancer Epidemiology, Biomarkers and Prevention* 1999b; 8:741–747.

Horvath S, Laird NM. A discordant-sibship test for disequilibrium and linkage: no need for parental data. *American Journal of Human Genetics* 1998; 63:1886–1897.

Horvath S, Laird NM, Knapp M. The transmission/disequilibrium test and parental-genotype reconstruction for X-chromosomal markers. *American Journal of Human Genetics* 2000; 66:1161–1167.

Horvath S, Xu X, Laird NM. The family based association test method: strategies for studying general genotype–phenotype associations. *European Journal of Human Genetics* 2001; 9:301–306.

Horvitz D, Thompson D. A generalization of sampling without replacement from a finite population. *Journal of the American Statistical Association* 1952; 47:663–685.

Hougaard P, Thomas D. Frailty. In: Elston RC, Palmer L, and Olson JH (eds.), *Encyclopedia of Genetics.* Oxford: Oxford University Press, 2002: 277–283.

Houlston RS, Collins A, Kee F, et al. Segregation analysis of colorectal cancer in Northern Ireland. *Human Heredity* 1995; 45:41–48.

Houwen R, Baharloo S, Blankenship K, et al. Genome screening by searching for shared segments: mapping a gene for benign recurrent intrahepatic cholestasis. *Nature Genetics* 1994; 8:380–386.

Hrubek Z, Floderus-Myrhed B, de Faire U, et al. Familial factors in mortality with control of epidemiological covariables: Swedish twins born 1886–1925. *Acta Geneticae Medicae et Gemellologiae* 1984; 33:403–412.

Huang Q, Fu Y-X, Boerwinkle E. Comparison of strategies for selecting single nucleotide polymorphisms for case/control association studies. *Human Genetics* 2003; 113:253–257.

Hubert R, MacDonald M, Gusella J, et al. High resolution localization of recombination hot spots using sperm typing. *Nature Genetics* 1994; 7:420–424.

Hubinette A, Lichtenstein P, Ekbom A, et al. Birth characteristics and breast cancer risk: a study among like-sexed twins. *International Journal of Cancer* 2001; 91:248–251.

Huelsenbeck JP, Ronquist F, Nielsen R, et al. Bayesian inference of phylogeny and its impact on evolutionary biology. *Science* 2001; 294:2310–2314.

Humphries P, Kenna P, Farrar GJ. On the molecular genetics of retinitis pigmentosa. *Science* 1992; 256:804–808.

Ingraham LJ, Kety SS. Adoption studies of schizophrenia. *American Journal of Medical Genetics* 2000; 97:18–22.

Ionnidis JPA, Ntzani EE, Trikalinos TA, et al. Replication validity of genetic association studies. *Nature Genetics* 2001; 29:306–309.

Ionov Y, Peinado MA, Malkhosyan S, et al. Ubiquitous somatic mutations in simple repeated sequences reveal a new mechanism for colonic carcinogenesis. *Nature* 1993; 363:558–561.

Issa JP, Ottaviano YL, Celano P, et al. Methylation of the oestrogen receptor CpG island links ageing and neoplasia in human colon. *Nature Genetics* 1994; 7:536–540.

Jansen RC. Studying complex biological systems using multifactorial perturbation. *Nature Reviews Genetics* 2003; 4:145–151.

Jansen RC, Nap J-P. Genetical genomics: the added value from segregation. *Trends in Genetics* 2001; 17:388–391.

Jass JR. Diagnosis of hereditary non-polyposis colorectal cancer. *Histopathology* 1998; 32:491–497.

Jeffreys AJ, LKauppi L, Neumann R. Intensely punctate meiotic recombination in the class II region of the major histocompatibility complex. *Nature Genetics* 2001; 29:217–222.

Jenkins MA, Baglietto L, Dite GS, et al. After *hMSH2* and *hMLH1*—what next? Analysis of three-generational, population-based, early-onset colorectal cancer families. *International Journal of Cancer* 2002; 102:166–171.

Jirtle RL, Sander M, Barrett JC. Genomic imprinting and environmental disease susceptibility. *Environmental Health Perspectives* 2000; 108:271–278.

Johnson GC, Esposito L, Barratt BJ, et al. Haplotype tagging for the identification of common disease genes. *Nature Genetics* 2001; 29:233–237.

Jones PA, Baylin SB. The fundamental role of epigenetic events in cancer. *Nature Reviews Genetics* 2002; 3:415–428.

Jones PA, Laird PW. Cancer epigenetics comes of age. *Nature Genetics* 1999; 21:163–167.

Judson R, Stephens JC, Windemuth A. The predictive power of haplotypes in clinical response. *Pharmacogenomics* 2000; 1:15–26.

Jungblut PR, Zimny-Arndt U, Zeindl-Eberhart E, et al. Proteomics in human disease: cancer, heart and infectious diseases. *Electrophoresis* 1999; 20:2100–2110.

Kaijser M, Lichtenstein P, Granath F, et al. In utero exposures and breast cancer: a study of opposite-sexed twins. *Journal of the National Cancer Institute* 2001; 93:60–62.

Kainu T, Juo SH, Desper R, et al. Somatic deletions in hereditary breast cancers implicate 13q21 as a putative novel breast cancer susceptibility locus. *Proceedings of the National Academy of Sciences of the United States of America* 2000; 97:9603–9608.

Kaplan E, Elston R. A subroutine package for maximum likelihood estimation (MAXLIK). Chapel Hill: University of North Carolina, 1972.

Kaplan NL, Hill W, Weir B. Likelihood methods for locating disease genes in nonequilibrium populations. *American Journal of Human Genetics* 1995; 56:18–32.

Kaplan NL, Hudson R, Langley C. The "hitchhiking effect" revisited. *Genetics* 1989; 123:887–899.

Kaplan NL, Martin ER, Weir BS. Power studies for the transmission/disequilibrium tests with multiple alleles. *American Journal of Human Genetics* 1997; 60:691–702.

Kaplan NL, Weir BS. Expected behavior of conditional linkage disequilibrium. *American Journal of Human Genetics* 1992; 51:333–343.

Karter AJ. Commentary: Race, genetics, and disease—in search of a middle ground. *International Journal of Epidemiology* 2003; 32:26–28.

Kass R, Raftery A. Bayes factors. *Journal of the American Statistical Association* 1995; 90:773–795.

Kaufman JS, Cooper RS. Commentary: considerations for use of racial/ethnic classification in etiologic research. *American Journal of Epidemiology* 2001; 154:291–298.

Kelly J, Wade M. Molecular evolution near a two-locus balanced polymorphism. *Journal of Theoretical Biology* 2000; 204:83–101.

Kerber RA, Amos CI, Finkelstein D, et al. Design issues in a multi-center study of linkage for susceptibility loci in cancer. Under review.

Kerem B, Rommens J, Buchanan J, et al. Identification of the cystic fibrosis gene: genetic analysis. *Science* 1989; 245:1073–1080.

Khan J, Simon R, Bittner M, et al. Gene expression profiling of alveolar rhabdomyosarcoma with cDNA microarrays. *Cancer Research* 1998; 58:5009–5013.

Khoury MJ, Beaty TH. Applications of the case-control method in genetic epidemiology. *Epidemiologic Reviews* 1994; 16:134–150.

Khoury MJ, Beaty TH, Cohen B. *Fundamentals of Genetic Epidemiology*. Oxford: Oxford University Press, 1993.

Khoury MJ, Beaty TH, Liang KY. Can familial aggregation of disease be explained by familial aggregation of environmental risk factors? *American Journal of Epidemiology* 1988; 127:674–683.

Khoury MJ, Dorman JS. The Human Genome Epidemiology Network. *American Journal of Epidemiology* 1998; 148:1–3.

Khoury MJ, Flanders WD. On the measurement of susceptibility to genetic factors. *Genetic Epidemiology—Supplement* 1989; 6:699–711.

Khoury MJ, James LM. Population and familial relative risks of disease associated with environmental factors in the presence of gene–environment interaction. *American Journal of Epidemiology* 1993; 137:1241–1250.

Khoury MJ, Yang Q. The future of genetic studies of complex human diseases: an epidemiologic perspective. *Epidemiology* 1998; 9:350–354.

Kim L-L, Fijal BA, Witte JS. Hierarchical modeling of the relation between sequence variants and a quantitative trait: addressing multiple comparison and population stratification issues. *Genetic Epidemiology* 2001; 21:S668–S673.

King M-C, Marks JH, and Mandell JB. Breast and ovarian cancer risks due to inherited mutations in *BRCA1* and *BRCA2*. *Science* 2003; 302:643–646.

Kingman JFC. On the genealogy of large populations. *Journal of Applied Probability* 1982; 19A:27–43.

Kinzler KW, Vogelstein B. Colorectal tumors. In: Vogelstein B and Kinzler KW (eds.), *The Genetic Basis of Human Cancer* (2nd ed.). New York: McGraw-Hill, 2002a: 583–610.

Kinzler KW, Vogelstein B. Familial cancer syndromes: the role of caretakers and gatekeepers. In: Vogelstein B and Kinzler KW (eds.), *The Genetic Basis of Human Cancer* (2nd ed.). New York: McGraw-Hill, 2002b: 209–210.

Kirk KM, Cardon LR. The impact of genotyping error on haplotype reconstruction and frequency estimation. *European Journal of Human Genetics* 2002; 10:616–622.

Kittles RA, Weiss KM. Race, ancestry, and genes: Implications for defining disease risk. *Annual Review of Genomics and Human Genetics* 2003; 4:33–67.

Klienbaum DG, Kupper LL, Morgentern H. *Epidemiologic Research: Principles and Quantitative Methods.* Belmont, CA: Lifetime Learning, 1982.

Knapp M. The transmission/disequilibrium test and parental-genotype reconstruction: the reconstruction-combined transmission/disequilibrium test. *American Journal of Human Genetics* 1999; 64:861–870.

Knowler WC, Williams RC, Pettitt DJ, et al. Gm3,5,13,14 and type 2 diabetes mellitus: an association in American Indians with genetic admixture. *American Journal of Human Genetics* 1988; 43:520–526.

Knudson A. Mutation and cancer: statistical study of retinoblastoma. *Cancer Investigations* 1971; 1:187–193.

Koch R. Die aetiology der tuberculose (1882). Reprinted in Clark D (ed.), *Source book of medical history.* New York: Dover Publications, 1942.

Kong A, Cox NJ. Allele-sharing models: LOD scores and accurate linkage tests. *American Journal of Human Genetics* 1997; 61:1179–1188.

Kong A, Gudbjartsson DF, Sainz J, et al. A high-resolution recombination map of the human genome. *Nature Genetics* 2001; 31:241–247.

Korczak JF, Pugh EW, Premkumar S, et al. Effects of marker information on sib-pair linkage analysis of a rare disease. *Genetic Epidemiology—Supplement* 1995; 12:625–630.

Kosambi D. The estimation of map distances from recombination values. *Annals of Eugenics* 1944; 12:172–175.

Kraft P. A robust score test for linkage disequilibrium in general pedigrees. *Genetic Epidemiology* 2001; 21(Suppl 1):S447–S452.

Kraft P, Schadt EE, Aten J, et al. A family-based test for correlation between gene expression and trait values. *American Journal of Human Genetics* 2003; 72:1323–1330.

Kraft P, Thomas DC. Bias and efficiency in family-matched gene-characterization studies: conditional, prospective, retrospective, and joint likelihoods. *American Journal of Human Genetics* 2000; 66:1119–1131.

Kraft P, Thomas DC. Case-sibling gene-association studies for diseases with variable age at onset. *Statistics in Medicine,* 2003, in press.

Kraft P, Wilson M. Family-based association tests incorporating parental genotypes [letter]. *American Journal of Human Genetics* 2002; 71:1239–1240.

Kruglyak L. Prospects for whole-genome linkage disequilibrium mapping. *Nature Genetics* 1999; 22:139–144.

Kruglyak L, Daly MJ, Lander ES. Rapid multipoint linkage analysis of recessive traits in nuclear families, including homozygosity mapping. *American Journal of Human Genetics* 1995; 56:519–527.

Kruglyak L, Daly MJ, Reeve-Daly MP, et al. Parametric and nonparametric linkage analysis: a unified multipoint approach. *American Journal of Human Genetics* 1996; 58:1347–1363.

Kruglyak L, Lander ES. Complete multipoint sib-pair analysis of qualitative and quantitative traits. *American Journal of Human Genetics* 1995; 57:439–454.

Kuhner M, Felsenstein J. Sampling among haplotype resolutions in a coalescent-based genealogy sampler. *Genetic Epidemiology* 2000; 19:S15–S21.

Kuhner M, Yamato J, Felsenstein J. Estimating effective population size and mutation rate from sequence data using Metropolis-Hastings sampling. *Genetics* 1995; 140:1421–1430.

Laird NM, Horvath S, Xu X. Implementing a unified approach to family-based tests of association. *Genetic Epidemiology* 2000; 19(Suppl 1):S36–S42.

Laird PW. Oncogenic mechanisms mediated by DNA methylation. *Molecular Medicine Today* 1997; 3:223–229.

Laird PW. The power and promise of DNA methylation markers. *Nature Reviews Cancer* 2003; 3:253–266.

Laird PW, Jackson-Grusby L, Fazeli A, et al. Suppression of intestinal neoplasia by DNA hypomethylation. *Cell* 1995; 81:197–205.

Lake SL, Blacker D, Laird NM. Family-based tests of association in the presence of linkage. *American Journal of Human Genetics* 2000; 67:1515–1525.

Laken SJ, Petersen GM, Gruber SB, et al. Familial colorectal cancer in Ashkenazim due to a hypermutable tract in APC. *Nature Genetics* 1997; 17:79–83.

Lalouel JM, Morton NE. Complex segregation analysis with pointers. *Human Heredity* 1981; 31:312–321.

Lander ES, Green P. Construction of multilocus genetic linkage maps in humans. *Proceedings of the National Academy of Sciences of the United States of America* 1987; 84:2363–2367.

Lander ES, Kruglyak L. Genetic dissection of complex traits: guidelines for interpreting and reporting linkage results. *Nature Genetics* 1995; 11:241–247.

Lander ES, Linton LM, Birren B, et al. Initial sequencing and analysis of the human genome. *Nature* 2001; 409:860–921.

Lander ES, Schork NJ. Genetic dissection of complex traits. *Science* 1994; 265:2037–2048.

Langholz B, Borgan O. Counter-matching: a stratified nested case-control sampling method. *Biometrika* 1995; 82:69–79.

Langholz B, Rothman N, Wacholder S, et al. Cohort studies for characterizing measured genes. *Monographs of the National Cancer Institute* 1999a; 26:39–42.

Langholz B, Thomas DC. Nested case-control and case-cohort sampling: a critical comparison. *American Journal of Epidemiology* 1990; 131:169–176.

Langholz B, Zyogas A, Thomas D, et al. Ascertainment bias in rate ratio estimation from case-sibling control studies of variable age-at-onset disease. *Biometrics* 1999b; 55:1129–1136.

LaPorte RE, Tajima N, Akerblom HK, et al. Geographic differences in the risk of insulin-dependent diabetes mellitus: the importance of registries. *Diabetes Care* 1985; 8:101–107.

Last J. *A Dictionary of Epidemiology*. Oxford: Oxford University Press, 1993.

Lathrop M, Lalouel J, Jullier C, et al. Strategies for multilocus linkage analysis in humans. *Proceedings of the National Academy of Sciences of the United States of America* 1984; 81:3443–3446.

Lathrop G, Lalouel J, White R. Calculation of human linkage maps: likelihood calculations for multilocus linkage analysis. *Genetic Epidemiology* 1986; 3:39–52.

Laurent-Puig P, Beroud C, Soussi T. APC gene: database of germline and somatic mutations in human tumors and cell lines. *Nucleic Acids Research* 1998; 26:269–270.

Lazzeroni LC. Linkage disequilibrium and gene mapping: an empirical least squares approach. *American Journal of Human Genetics* 1998; 62:159–170.

Lazzeroni LC. A chronology of fine-scale gene mapping by linkage disequilibrium. *Statistical Methods in Medical Research* 2001; 10:57–76.

Lazzeroni LC, Arnheim N, Schmitt K, et al. Multipoint mapping calculations for sperm-typing data. *American Journal of Human Genetics* 1994; 55:431–436.

Lazzeroni LC, Lange K. A conditional inference framework for extending the transmission/disequilibrium test. *Human Heredity* 1998; 48:67–81.

Lazzeroni LC, Owen A. Plaid models for gene expression data. *Statistica Sinica* 2002; 12:61–86.

Leach FS, Nicolaides NC, Papadopoulos N, et al. Mutations of a *mutS* homolog in hereditary nonpolyposis colorectal cancer. *Cell* 1993; 75:1215–1225.

Lee H, Stram DO. Segregation analysis of continuous phenotypes by using higher sample moments. *American Journal of Human Genetics* 1996; 58:213–224.

Lee H, Stram DO, Thomas D. A generalized estimating equations approach to fitting major gene models in segregation analysis of continuous phenotypes. *Genetic Epidemiology* 1993; 10:61–74.

Lee J, Thomas D. Performance of Markov chain Monte Carlo approaches for mapping genes in oligogenic models with an unknown number of loci. *American Journal of Human Genetics* 2000; 67:1232–1250.

Lehesjoki AE, Koskiniemi M, Norio R, et al. Localization of the *EPM1* gene for progressive myoclonus epilepsy on chromosome 21: linkage disequilibrium allows high resolution mapping. *Human Molecular Genetics* 1993; 2:1229–1234.

Lengauer C, Kinzler KW, Vogelstein B. Genetic instability in colorectal cancers. *Nature* 1997; 386:623–627.

Leppert M, Dobbs M, Scambler P, et al. The gene for familial polyposis coli maps to the long arm of chromosome 5. *Science* 1987; 238:1411–1413.

Levi F, Randimbison L, La Vecchia C. Incidence of colorectal cancer following adenomatous polyps of the large intestine. *International Journal of Cancer* 1993; 55:415–418.

Levin ML. The occurrence of lung cancer in man. *Acta Unio Internationalis Contra Cancrum* 1953; 19:531–541.

Lewin B. *Genes*. Oxford: Oxford University Press, 1997.

Lewontin R. The interaction of selection and linkage. I. General considerations: heterotic models. *Genetics* 1964; 49:49–67.

Lewontin R. On measures of gametic diesquilibrium. *Genetics* 1988; 120:849–852.

Li E, Beard C, Jaenisch R. Role for DNA methylation in genomic imprinting. *Nature* 1993; 366:362–365.

Li FP, Fraumeni JF Jr, Mulvihill JJ, et al. A cancer family syndrome in twenty-four kindreds. *Cancer Research* 1988; 48:5358–5362.

Li H, Fan J. A general test of association for complex diseases with variable age of onset. *Genetic Epidemiology* 2000; 19:S43–S49.

Li H, Hsu L. Effects of age at onset on the power of the affected sib pair and transmission/disequilibrium tests. *Annals of Human Genetics* 2000; 64:239–254.

Li H, Yang P, Schwartz A. Analysis of age of onset data from case-control family studies. *Biometrics* 1998; 54:1030–1039.

Li J, Wang D, Dong J, et al. The power of transmission disequilibrium tests for quantitative traits. *Genetic Epidemiology* 2001; 21(Suppl 1):S632–S637.

Liang KY, Beaty T, Cohen B. Application of odds ratio regression models for assessing familial aggregation from case-control studies. *American Journal of Epidemiology* 1986; 124:678–683.

Liang KY, Zeger SL. Longitudinal data analysis using generalized linear models. *Biometrika* 1986; 73:13–22.

Liang KY, Zeger S, Qaqish B. Multivariate regression analysis for categorical data. *Journal of the Royal Statistical Society, Series B* 1992; 54:3–40.

Lichtenstein P, Holm NV, Verkasalo PK, et al. Environmental and heritable factors in the causation of cancer—analyses of cohorts of twins from Sweden, Denmark, and Finland. *New England Journal of Medicine* 2000; 343:78–85.

Lilienfeld A, Levin M, Kessler I. *Cancer in the United States*. Cambridge, MA: Harvard University Press, 1972.

Lin KM, Shashidharan M, Thorson AG, et al. Cumulative incidence of colorectal and extracolonic cancers in *MLH1* and *MSH2* mutation carriers of hereditary nonpolyposis colorectal cancer. *Journal of Gastrointestinal Surgery* 1998; 2:67-71.

Lin S. A scheme for constructing an irreducible Markov chain for pedigree data. *Biometrics* 1995; 51:318–322.

Lin S, Cutler DJ, Zwick ME, et al. Haplotype inference in random population samples. *American Journal of Human Genetics* 2002; 71:1129–1137.

Lin S, Thompson E, Wijsman E. Achieving irreducibility of the Markov chain Monte Carlo method applied to pedigree data. *IMA Journal of Mathematical Applications in Medicine and Biology* 1993; 10:1–17.

Lin S, Thompson E, Wijsman E. Finding non-communicating sets of Markov chain Monte Carlo estimates on pedigrees. *American Journal of Human Genetics* 1994; 54:695–704.

Lin SS, Kelsey JL. Use of race and ethnicity in epidemiologic research: concepts, methodological issues, and suggestions for research. *Epidemiologic Reviews* 2000; 22:187–202.

Lindblom A, Tannergard P, Werelius B, et al. Genetic mapping of a second locus predisposing to hereditary non-polyposis colon cancer. *Nature Genetics* 1993; 5:279–282.

Lipshutz RJ, Fodor SP, Gingeras TR, et al. High density synthetic oligonucleotide arrays. *Nature Genetics* 1999; 21:20–24.

Little R, Rubin D. *Statistical Analysis with Missing Data*. New York: Wiley, 1989.

Liu B, Farrington SM, Petersen GM, et al. Genetic instability occurs in the majority of young patients with colorectal cancer. *Nature Medicine* 1995; 1:348–352.

Liu B, Parsons R, Papadopoulos N, et al. Analysis of mismatch repair genes in hereditary non-polyposis colorectal cancer patients. *Nature Medicine* 1996; 2:169–174.

Liu JS, Sabatti C, Teng J, et al. Bayesian analysis of haplotypes for linkage disequilibrium mapping. *Genome Research* 2001; 11:1716–1724.

Liu Y, Tritchler D, Bull SB. A unified framework for transmission-disequilibrium test analysis of discrete and continuous traits. *Genetic Epidemiology* 2002; 22:26–40.

Loeb LA. Microsatellite instability: marker of a mutator phenotype in cancer. *Cancer Research* 1994; 54:5059–5063.

Lohmueller KE, Pearce CL, Pike M, et al. Meta-analysis of genetic association studies supports a contribution of common variants to susceptibility to common disease. *Nature Genetics* 2003; 33:177–182.

London S, Daly A, Thomas D, et al. Methodological issues in the interpretation of studies of the CYP 2D6 genotype in relation to lung cancer risk. *Pharmacogenetics* 1994; 4:107–108.

Long AD, Langley CH. The power of association studies to detect the contribution of candidate genetic loci to variation in complex traits. *Genome Research* 1999; 9:720–731.

Lopez A, Xamena N, Marcos R, et al. Germ cells microsatellite instability. The effect of different mutagens in a mismatch repair mutant of *Drosophila (spel1)*. *Mutation Research* 2002; 514:87–94.

Los H, Postmus PE, Boomsma DI. Asthma genetics and intermediate phenotypes: a review from twin studies. *Twin Research* 2001; 4:81–93.

Lovett E. Family studies in cancer of the colon and rectum. *British Journal of Surgery* 1976; 63:13–18.

Lubin JH, Gail MH. Biased selection of controls for case-control analysis of cohort studies. *Biometrics* 1984; 40:63–75.

Lunetta KL, Faraone SV, Biederman J, et al. Family-based tests of association and linkage that use unaffected sibs, covariates, and interactions. *American Journal of Human Genetics* 2000; 66:605–614.

Lynch HT, Guirgis H, Swartz M, et al. Genetics and colon cancer. *Archives of Surgery* 1973; 106:669–675.

Lynch HT, Kimberling WJ, Biscone KA, et al. Familial heterogeneity of colon cancer risk. *Cancer* 1986; 57:2089–2096.

Lynch HT, Krush AJ. Cancer family "G" revisited: 1895–1970. *Cancer* 1971; 27:1505–1511.

Lynch HT, Shaw MW, Magnuson CW, et al. Hereditary factors in cancer. Study of two large midwestern kindreds. *Archives of Internal Medicine* 1966; 117:206–212.

Lynch HT, Smyrk T, Lynch JF. Overview of natural history, pathology, molecular genetics and management of HNPCC (Lynch syndrome). *International Journal of Cancer* 1996; 69:38–43.

Lyttle TW. Cheaters sometimes prosper: distortion of mendelian segregation by meiotic drive. *Trends in Genetics* 1993; 9:205–210.

Ma J, Stampfer MJ, Giovannucci E, et al. Methylenetetrahydrofolate reductase polymorphism, dietary interactions, and risk of colorectal cancer. *Cancer Research* 1997; 57:1098–1102.

MacDonald M, Lin C, Srinidhi L, et al. Complex patterns of linkage disequilibrium in the Huntington's disease region. *American Journal of Human Genetics* 1991; 49:723–734.

MacDonald M, Novelletto A, Lin C, et al. The Huntington's disease candidate region exhibits many different haplotypes. *Nature Genetics* 1992; 1:99–103.

Mack TM, Deapen D, Hamilton AS. Representativeness of a roster of volunteer North American twins with chronic disease. *Twin Research* 2000; 3:33–42.

Mack W, Langholz B, Thomas D. Survival models for familial aggregation of cancer. *Environmental Health Perspectives* 1990; 87:27–35.

MacLean CJ, Morton NE, Lew R. Analysis of family resemblance. IV. Operational characteristics of segregation analysis. *American Journal of Human Genetics* 1975; 27:365–384.

Macklin M. Inheritance of cancer of the stomach and large intestine. *Journal of the National Cancer Institute* 1960; 24:551–571.

MacMahon B, Pugh TF. *Epidemiology: Principles and Methods*. Boston: Little, Brown, 1970.

Malécot G. *Les Mathématiques de l'Hérédité*. Paris: Masson, 1948.

Maldonado G, Greenland S. Estimating causal effects (with discussion). *International Journal of Epidemiology* 2002; 31:422–438.

Mallows CL. Some comments on C_p. *Technometrics* 1973; 15:661–676.

Mandal DM. Effects of misspecification of allele frequencies on the type I error rate of model-free linkage analysis. *Human Heredity* 2000; 50:126–132.

Mannila H, Koivisto M, Perola M, et al. Minimum description length block finder, a method to identify haplotype blocks and to compare the strength of block boundaries. *American Journal of Human Genetics* 2003; 73:86–94.

Manuila A. Blood groups and disease—hard facts and delusions. *Journal of the American Medical Association* 1958; 167:2047–2053.

Martin ER, Bass MP, Kaplan NL. Correcting for a potential bias in the pedigree disequilibrium test. *American Journal of Human Genetics* 2001; 68:1065–1067.

Martin ER, Kaplan NL, Weir B. Tests for linkage and association in nuclear families. *American Journal of Human Genetics* 1997; 61:439–448.

Martin ER, Monks S, Warren L, et al. A test for linkage and association in general pedigrees: the pedigree disequilibrium test. *American Journal of Human Genetics* 2000; 67:146–154.

McGuffin P, Huckle P. Simulation of Mendelism revisited: the recessive gene for attending medical school. *American Journal of Human Genetics* 1990; 46:994–999.

McKeigue P. Mapping genes underlying ethnic differences in disease risk by linkage disequilibrium in recently admixed populations. *American Journal of Human Genetics* 1997; 60:188–196.

McKerrow JH, Bhargava V, Hansell E, et al. A functional proteomics screen of proteases in colorectal carcinoma. *Molecular Medicine* 2000; 6:450–460.

McMichael AJ, Giles GG. Cancer in migrants to Australia: extending the descriptive epidemiological data. *Cancer Research* 1988; 48:751–756.

McPeek M, Strahs A. Assessment of linkage disequilibrium by the decay of haplotype sharing, with application to fine-scale genetic mapping. *American Journal of Human Genetics* 1999; 65:858–875.

Meng Z, Zaykin DV, Xu C-F, et al. Selection of genetic markers for association analysis, using linkage disequilibrium and haplotypes. *American Journal of Human Genetics* 2003; 73:115–130.

Merriman TR, Eaves IA, Twells RC, et al. Transmission of haplotypes of microsatellite markers rather than single marker alleles in the mapping of a putative type 1 diabetes susceptibility gene (*IDDM6*). *Human Molecular Genetics* 1998; 7:517–524.

Michaels GS, Carr DB, Askenazi M, et al. Cluster analysis and data visualization of large-scale gene expression data. *Pacific Symposium on Biocomputing* 1998; 42–53.

Miki Y, Swensen J, Shattuck-Eldens D, et al. A strong candidate for the breast and ovarian cancer susceptibility gene BRCA1. *Science* 1994; 266:66–71.

Miller RG. The jackknife—a review. *Biometrika* 1074; 61:1–15.

Miyaki M, Konishi M, Tanaka K, et al. Germline mutation of *MSH6* as the cause of hereditary nonpolyposis colorectal cancer. *Nature Genetics* 1997; 17:271–272.

Modan B, Hartge P, Hirsh-Yechezkel G, et al. Parity, oral contraceptives, and the risk of ovarian cancer among carriers and noncarriers of a *BRCA1* or *BRCA2* mutation. *New England Journal of Medicine* 2001; 345:235–240.

Mohlke K, Lange E, Valle T, et al. Linkage disequilibrium between microsatellite markers extends beyond 1 cM on chromosome 20 in Finns. *Genome Research* 2001; 11:1221–1226.

Mokliatchouk O, Blacker D, Rabinowitz D. Association tests for traits with variable age at onset. *Human Heredity* 2001; 51:46–53.

Molitor J, Marjoram P, Thomas DC. Application of Bayesian spatial statistical methods to the analysis of haplotype effects and gene mapping. *Genetic Epidemiology* 2003a; 25:95–105.

Molitor J, Marjoram P, Thomas DC. Fine-scale mapping of disease genes with multiple mutations via spatial clustering techniques. *American Journal of Human Genetics* 2003b; in press.

Moll PP, Berry TD, Weidman WH, et al. Detection of genetic heterogeneity among pedigrees through complex segregation analysis: an application to hypercholesterolemia. *American Journal of Human Genetics* 1984; 36:197–211.

Momparler RL, Eliopoulos N, Ayoub J. Evaluation of an inhibitor of DNA methylation, 5-aza-2'-deoxycytidine, for the treatment of lung cancer and the future role of gene therapy. *Advances in Experimental Medicine and Biology* 2000; 465:433–446.

Mongeau JG, Biron P, Sing CF. The influence of genetics and household environment upon the variability of normal blood pressure: the Montreal Adoption Survey. *Clinical and Experimental Hypertension—Part A, Theory and Practice* 1986; 8:653–660.

Moody DA. *Genetics of Man*. New York: Norton Publishing, 1975.

Moolgavkar SH, Knudson A. Mutation and cancer: a model for human carcinogenesis. *Journal of the National Cancer Institute* 1981; 66:1037–1052.

Moolgavkar SH, Luebeck EG. Multistage carcinogenesis: population-based model for colon cancer. *Journal of the National Cancer Institute* 1992; 84:610–618.

Moore JH. Improved power of sib-pair linkage analysis using measures of complex trait dynamics. *Human Heredity* 2001; 52:113–115.

Moore JH, Hahn L. Power of cellular automata for identifying gene–gene and gene–environment interactions [abstract]. *Genetic Epidemiology* 2001; 21:168.

Moore JW, Parker JS, Olsen NJ, et al. Symbolic discriminant analysis of microarray data in autoimmune disease. *Genetic Epidemiology* 2002; 23:57–69.

Morris A, Pedder A, Ayres K. Linkage disequilibrium assessment via log-linear modeling of SNP haplotype frequencies. *Genetic Epidemiology* 2003; 25:106–114.

Morris AP, Whittaker JC, Balding DJ. Bayesian fine-scale mapping of disease loci by hidden Markov models. *American Journal of Human Genetics* 2000; 67:155–169.

Morris AP, Whittaker JC, Balding DJ. Fine-scale mapping of disease loci via shattered coalescent modeling of genealogies. *American Journal of Human Genetics* 2002; 70:686–707.

Morris RW, Kaplan NL. On the advantage of haplotype analysis in the presence of multiple disease susceptibility alleles. *Genetic Epidemiology* 2002; 23:221–233.

Morton NE. Sequential tests for the detection of linkage. *American Journal of Human Genetics* 1955; 7:277–318.

Morton NE. The detection and estimation of linkage between the genes for elliptocytosis and the Rh blood type. *American Journal of Human Genetics* 1956; 8:80–96.

Morton NE. *Outline of Genetic Epidemiology*. Berlin: S. Karger, 1982.

Morton NE, Chung CS. *Genetic Epidemiology*. New York: Academic Press, 1978.

Morton NE, MacLean CJ. Analysis of family resemblance. 3. Complex segregation of quantitative traits. *American Journal of Human Genetics* 1974; 26:489–503.

Morton NE, Rao DC, Lalouel J-M. *Methods in Genetic Epidemiology*. Berlin: S. Karger, 1983.

Moslein G, Tester DJ, Lindor NM, et al. Microsatellite instability and mutation analysis of *hMSH2* and *hMLH1* in patients with sporadic, familial and hereditary colorectal cancer. *Human Molecular Genetics* 1996; 5:1245–1252.

Muller HH, Heinimann K, Dobbie Z. Genetics of hereditary colon cancer—a basis for prevention? *European Journal of Cancer* 2000; 36:1215–1223.

Nagase H, Nakamura Y. Mutations of the *APC* (adenomatous polyposis coli) gene. *Human Mutation* 1993; 2:425–434.

Nakama H, Zhang B, Fukazawa K, et al. Family history of colorectal adenomatous polyps as a risk factor for colorectal cancer. *European Journal of Cancer* 2000; 36:2111–2114.

Nakamura Y, Lathrop M, Leppert M, et al. Localization of the genetic defect in familial adenomatous polyposis within a small region of chromosome 5. *American Journal of Human Genetics* 1988; 43:638–644.

Narod SA. Modifiers of risk of hereditary breast and ovarian cancer. *Nature Reviews Cancer* 2002; 2:113–123.

Narod SA, Boyd J. Current understanding of the epidemiology and clinical implications of *BRCA1* and *BRCA2* mutations for ovarian cancer. *Current Opinion in Obstetrics and Gynecology* 2002; 14:19–26.

Narod SA, Dubé M-P, Klijn J, et al. Oral contraceptives and the risk of breast cancer in BRCA1 and BRCA2 mutation carriers. *Journal of the National Cancer Institute* 2002; 94:1773–1779.

Narod SA, Goldgar D, Cannon-Albright L, et al. Risk modifiers in carriers of *BRCA1* mutations. *International Journal of Cancer* 1995; 64:394–398.

Narod SA, Risch HA, Moslehi R, et al. Oral contraceptives and the risk of hereditary ovarian cancer. *New England Journal of Medicine* 1998; 339:424–428.

Narod SA, Sun P, Risch HA. Ovarian cancer, oral contraceptives, and *BRCA* mutations [letter]. *New England Journal of Medicine* 2001; 345:1706–1707.

Neale MC, Cardon LR. *Methodology for Genetic Studies of Twins and Families*. Berlin: Kluwer Academic, 1992.

Neel J. Editorial. *Genetic Epidemiology* 1984; 1:5–6.

Neel JV, Schull WJ. *Human Heredity*. Chicago: University of Chicago Press, 1954.

Nemesure B, He Q, Mendell N. Integration of linkage analyses and disease association studies. *Genetic Epidemiology* 1995; 12:653–658.

Neuhausen S, Swensen J, Miki Y, et al. A P1-based physical map of the region from D17S776 to D17S78 containing the breast cancer susceptibility gene *BRCA1*. *Human Molecular Genetics* 1994; 3:1919–1926.

Neuman R, Rice J. Note on linkage analysis when the mode of transmission is unknown. *Genetic Epidemiology* 1990; 7:349–358.

Nishisho I, Nakamura Y, Miyoshi Y, et al. Mutations of chromosome 5q21 genes in FAP and colorectal cancer patients. *Science* 1991; 253:665–669.

Niu T, Qin ZS, Xu X, et al. Bayesian haplotype inference for multiple linked single-nucleotide polymorphisms. *American Journal of Human Genetics* 2002; 70:157–169.

Nolte IM. The Haplotype Sharing Statistic: fine-mapping of disease gene loci by comparing patients and controls for the length of haplotype sharing. Ph.D. dissertation. Groningen: University of Groningen, 2002.

Novis BH, Naftali TE. Family history of colorectal adenomatous polyps and increased risk of colorectal cancer. *Gastrointestinal Endoscopy* 1999; 49:266–268.

Nowell PC. The clonal evolution of tumor cell populations. *Science* 1976; 194:23–28.

O'Connell J, Weeks D. The VITESSE algorithm for rapid exact multilocus linkage analysis via genotype set-recording and fuzzy inheritance. *Nature Genetics* 1995; 11:402–408.

Ophoff RA, Escamilla MA, Service SK, et al. Genomewide linkage disequilibrium mapping of severe bipolar disorder in a population isolate. *American Journal of Human Genetics* 2002; 71:565–574.

Ott J. Linkage analysis and family classification under heterogeneity. *Annals of Human Genetics* 1983; 47:311–320.

Ott J. Y-linkage and pseudoautosomal linkage. *American Journal of Human Genetics* 1986; 38:891–897.

Ott J. Statistical properties of the haplotype relative risk. *Genetic Epidemiology* 1989; 6:127–130.

Ott J. *Analysis of Human Genetic Linkage* (3rd ed.). Baltimore: Johns Hopkins University Press, 1999.

Ott J. Predicting the range of linkage disequilibrium. *Proceedings of the National Academy of Sciences of the United States of America* 2000; 97:2–3.

Ottman R. Epidemiologic approach to gene-environment interaction. *Genetic Epidemiology* 1990; 7:177–185.

Page GP, George V, Go R, et al. "Are we there yet?" Deciding when one has demonstrated specific genetic causation in complex diseases and complex traits. *American Journal of Human Genetics* 2003; 73:711–719.

Palmer LJ, Jacobs KB, Elston RC. Haseman and Elston revisited: the effects of ascertainment and residual familial correlations on power to detect linkage [letter]. *Genetic Epidemiology* 2000; 19:456–460.

Pao MM, Liang G, Tsai YC, et al. DNA methylator and mismatch repair phenotypes are not mutually exclusive in colorectal cancer cell lines. *Oncogene* 2000; 19:943–952.

Parascandola M, Weed DL. Causation in epidemiology. *Journal of Epidemiology and Community Health* 2001; 55:905–912.

Parkin DM, Whelan SL, Ferlay J, et al. *Cancer Incidence in Five Continents*, Vol. VII. Lyon: IARC Scientific Publications, No. 143, 1997.

Parmigiani G, Berry D, Aguilar O. Determining carrier probabilities for breast cancer susceptibility genes *BRCA1* and *BRCA2*. *American Journal of Human Genetics* 1998; 62:145–158.

Patil N, Berno AJ, Hinds DA, et al. Blocks of limited haplotype diversity revealed by high-resolution scanning of human chromosome 21. *Science* 2001; 294:1719–1723.

Pawlowitzki I-H, Edwards JH, Thompson EA (eds.). *Genetic Mapping of Disease Genes*. San Diego, CA: Academic Press, 1997.

Pearl J. *Causality: models, reasoning, and inference*. Cambridge: Cambridge University Press, 2000.

Peltomaki P, Aaltonen LA, Sistonen P, et al. Genetic mapping of a locus predisposing to human colorectal cancer. *Science* 1993; 260:810–812.

Peltonen L, Palotie A, Lange K. Use of population isolates for mapping complex traits. *Nature Reviews Genetics* 2000; 1:182–190.

Penrose L. Some practical considerations in testing for genetic linkage in sib data. *Ohio Journal of Science* 1939; 39:291–296.

Peterson G, Parmigiani G, Thomas D. Missense mutations in disease genes: a Bayesian approach to evaluate causality. *American Journal of Human Genetics* 1998; 62:1516–1524.

Peto J. Genetic predisposition to cancer. In: Cairns J, Lyon J, and Skolnick M (eds.), *Cancer Incidence in Defined Populations* (Banbury Report No 5). Cold Spring Harbor, NY: Cold Spring Harbor Laboratory, 1980: 203–213.

Peto J, Collins N, Barfoot R, et al. Prevalence of *BRCA1* and *BRCA2* gene mutations in patients with early-onset breast cancer. *Journal of the National Cancer Institute* 1999; 91:943–949.

Peto J, Mack T. High constant incidence in twins and other relatives of women with breast cancer. *Nature Genetics* 2000; 26:411–414.

Petricoin EF, Ardekani AM, Hitt BA, et al. Use of proteomic patterns in serum to identify ovarian cancer. *Lancet* 2002; 359:572–577.

Pharoah PD, Day NE, Duffy S, et al. Family history and the risk of breast cancer: a systematic review and meta-analysis. *International Journal of Cancer* 1997; 71:800–809.

Phillips MS, Lawrence R, Sachidanandam R, et al. Chromosome-wide distribution of haplotype blocks and the role of recombination hot spots. *Nature Genetics* 2003; 33:382–387.

Phimister EG. Medicine and the racial divide. *New England Journal of Medicine* 2003; 348:1081–1082.

Piegorsch W, Weinberg C, Taylor J. Non-hierarchical logistic models and case-only designs for assessing susceptibility in population-based case-control studies. *Statistics in Medicine* 1994; 13:153–162.

Pike M, Krailo M, Henderson B, et al. "Hormonal" risk factors, "breast tissue age" and the age-incidence of breast cancer. *Nature* 1983; 303:767–770.

Ploughman L, Boehnke M. Estimating the power of a proposed linkage study for a complex genetic trait. *American Journal of Human Genetics* 1989; 44:543–551.

Ponz de Leon M, Antonioli A, Ascari A, et al. Incidence and familial occurrence of colorectal cancer and polyps in a health-care district of northern Italy. *Cancer* 1987; 60:2848–2859.

Potter JD. Colorectal cancer: molecules and populations. *Journal of the National Cancer Institute* 1999; 91:916–932.

Potter JD, Slattery ML, Bostick RM, et al. Colon cancer: a review of the epidemiology. *Epidemiologic Reviews* 1993; 15:499–545.

Powell SM, Zilz N, Beazer-Barclay Y, et al. APC mutations occur early during colorectal tumorigenesis. *Nature* 1992; 359:235–237.

Powles T, Eeles R, Ashley S, et al. Interim analysis of the incidence of breast cancer in the Royal Marsden Hospital tamoxifen randomised chemoprevention trial. *Lancet* 1998; 352:98–101.

Prehn RT. Cancers beget mutations versus mutations beget cancers. *Cancer Research* 1994; 54:5296–5300.

Prentice RL. A case-cohort design for epidemiologic studies and disease prevention trials. *Biometrika* 1986; 73:1–11.

Prentice RL, Hsu L. Regression on hazard ratios and cross ratios in multivariate failure time analysis. *Biometrika* 1997; 84:349–363.

Prentice RL, Zhao LP. Estimating equations for parameters in means and covariances of multivariate discrete and continuous responses. *Biometrics* 1991; 47:825–839.

Prentice RL, Sheppard L. Dietary fat and cancer: consistency of the epidemiologic data, and disease prevention that may follow from a practical reduction in fat consumption. *Cancer Causes and Control* 1990; 1:81–97.

Press WH, Teukolsky SA, Vetterling WT, et al. *Numerical Recipies in C: The Art of Scientific Computing* (2nd ed.). Cambridge: Cambridge University Press, 1992.

Pritchard JK. Are rare variants responsible for susceptibility to complex diseases? *American Journal of Human Genetics* 2001; 69:124–137.

Pritchard JK, Cox NJ. The allelic architecture of human disease genes: common disease–common variant... or not? *Human Molecular Genetics* 2002; 11:2417–2423.

Pritchard JK, Donnelly P. Case-control studies of association in structured or admixed populations. *Theoretical Population Biology* 2001; 60:226–237.

Pritchard JK, Przeworski M. Linkage disequilibrium in humans: models and data. *American Journal of Human Genetics* 2001; 69:1–14.

Pritchard JK, Rosenberg NA. Use of unlinked genetic markers to detect population stratification in association studies. *American Journal of Human Genetics* 1999; 65:220–228.

Pritchard JK, Stephens M, Donnelly P. Inference of population structure using multilocus genotype data. *Genetics* 2000a; 155:945–959.

Pritchard JK, Stephens M, Rosenberg NA, et al. Association mapping in structured populations. *American Journal of Human Genetics* 2000b; 67:170–181.

Przeworski M, Wall J. Why is there so little intragenic linkage disequilibrium? *Genetical Research* 2001; 77:143–151.

Qian D, Thomas D. Genome scan of complex traits by haplotype sharing correlation. *Genetic Epidemiology* 2001; 21:S582–S587.

Rabinowitz D. A transmission disequilibrium test for quantitative trait loci. *Human Heredity* 1997; 47:342–350.

Rabinowitz D, Laird N. A unified approach to adjusting association tests for population admixture with arbitrary pedigree structure and arbitrary missing marker information. *Human Heredity* 2000; 50:211–223.

Rainier S, Johnson LA, Dobry CJ, et al. Relaxation of imprinted genes in human cancer. *Nature* 1993; 362:747–749.

Rannala B, Statkin M. Likelihood analysis of disequilibrium mapping and related problems. *American Journal of Human Genetics* 1998; 62:459–473.

Rao CR. *Linear Statistical Inference and Its Applications* (2nd ed.). New York: Wiley, 1973.

Rao D. Editorial comment. *Genetic Epidemiology* 1985; 1:3.

Reich DE, Cargill M, Bolk S, et al. Linkage disequilibrium in the human genome. *Nature* 2001; 411:199–204.

Reich DE, Goldstein DB. Detecting association in a case-control study while correcting for population stratification. *Genetic Epidemiology* 2001; 20:4–16.

Reich DE, Lander ES. On the allelic spectrum of human disease. *Trends in Genetics* 2001; 17:502–510.

Reich DE, Schaffner SF, Daly MJ, et al. Human genome sequence variation and the influence of gene history, mutation and recombination. *Nature Genetics* 2002; 5:5.

Renwick J. The mapping of human chromosomes. *Annual Review of Genetics* 1971; 5:81–120.

Riggins GJ, Morin PJ. Gene expression profiling in cancer. In: Vogelstein B and Kinzler KW (eds.), *The Genetic Basis of Human Cancer*. New York: McGraw-Hill, 2002: 131–141.

Rioux JD, Daly MJ, Silverberg MS, et al. Genetic variation in the 5q31 cytokine gene cluster confers susceptibility to Crohn disease. *Nature Genetics* 2001; 29:223–228.

Risch HA, McLaughlin JR, Cole DE, et al. Prevalence and penetrance of germline *BRCA1* and *BRCA2* mutations in a population series of 649 women with ovarian cancer. *American Journal of Human Genetics* 2001; 68:700–710.

Risch N. A new statistical test for linkage heterogeneity. *American Journal of Human Genetics* 1988; 42:353–364.

Risch N. Linkage strategies for genetically complex traits. II. The power of affected relative pairs. *American Journal of Human Genetics* 1990a; 46:229–241.

Risch N. Linkage strategies for genetically complex traits. I. Multilocus models. *American Journal of Human Genetics* 1990b; 46:222–228.

Risch N, Burchard E, Ziv E, et al. Categorization of humans in biomedical research: genes, race and disease. *Genome Biology* 2002; 3:1–12.

Risch N, Merikangas K. The future of genetic studies of complex human diseases. *Science* 1996; 273:1616–1617.

Risch N, Zhang H. Extreme discordant sib pairs for mapping quantitative trait loci in humans. *Science* 1995; 268:1584–1589.

Risch N, Zhang H. Mapping quantitative trait loci with extreme discordant sib pairs: sampling considerations. *American Journal of Human Genetics* 1996; 58:836–843.

Ritchie MD, Hahn LW, Roodi N, et al. Multifactor-dimensionality reduction reveals high-order interactions among estrogen-metabolism genes in sporadic breast cancer. *American Journal of Human Genetics* 2001; 69:138–147.

Rodriguez-Bigas MA, Boland CR, Hamilton SR, et al. A National Cancer Institute Workshop on Hereditary Nonpolyposis Colorectal Cancer Syndrome: meeting highlights and Bethesda guidelines. *Journal of the National Cancer Institute* 1997; 89:1758–1762.

Rosenberg NA, Pritchard JK, Weber JL, et al. Genetic structure of human populations. *Science* 2002; 298:2381–2385.

Rothman KJ. Causes. *American Journal of Epidemiology* 1976; 104:587–592.

Rothman KJ, Greenland S. *Modern Epidemiology*. Philadelphia: Lippencott-Raven, 1998.

Rothman N, Wacholder S, Caporaso NE, et al. The use of common polymorphisms to enhance the epidemiologic study of environmental carcinogens. *Biochemica et Biophysica Acta* 2001; 1471:C1–10.

Rozenblum E, Vahteristo P, Sandberg T, et al. A genomic map of a 6-Mb region at 13q21-q22 implicated in cancer development: identification and characterization of candidate genes. *Human Genetics* 2002; 110:111–121.

Rubin D. *Multiple Imputation for Nonresponse in Surveys*. New York: Wiley, 1987.

Rubin DB. Comment: Neyman (1923) and causal inference in experiments and observational studies. *Statistical Science* 1990; 5:472–480.

Rubin H. Cancer development: the rise of epigenetics. *European Journal of Cancer* 1992; 28:1–2.

Rubinstein P, Walker M, Carpenter C. Genetics of HLA disease association: the use of the haplotype relative risk (HRR) and the "Haplo-Delta" (DH) estimates in juvenile diabetes from three racial groups. *Human Immunology* 1981; 3:384.

Sabatti C, Service S, Freimer N. False discovery rate and correction for multiple comparisons in linkage disequilibrium genome screens. *Genetics* 2003; 164:829–833.

Sachidanandam R, Weissman D, Schmidt SC, et al. A map of human genome sequence variation containing 1.42 million single nucleotide polymorphisms. *Nature* 2001; 409:928–933.

Satagopan J, Yandell B, Newton M, et al. A Bayesian approach to detect quantitative trait loci using Markov chain Monte Carlo. *Genetics* 1996; 144:805–816.

Satten GA, Flanders WD, Yang Q. Accounting for unmeasured population substructure in case-control studies of genetic association using a novel latent-class model. *American Journal of Human Genetics* 2001; 68:466–477.

Sattin R, Rubin G, Webster L, et al. Family history and the risk of breast cancer. *Journal of the American Medical Association* 1985; 253:1908–1913.

Saunders CL, Begg CB. Kin-cohort evaluation of relative risks of genetic variants. *Genetic Epidemiology* 2003; 24:220–229.

Scapoli C, Ponz De Leon M, Sassatelli R, et al. Genetic epidemiology of hereditary non-polyposis colorectal cancer syndromes in Modena, Italy: results of a complex segregation analysis. *Annals of Human Genetics* 1994; 58:275–295.

Schadt EE, Monks SA, Drake TA, et al. Genetics of gene expression surveyed in maize, mouse and man. *Nature* 2003; 422:297–302.

Schaid DJ. Case-parents design for gene–environment interaction. *Genetic Epidemiology* 1999; 16:261–273.

Schaid DJ. Relative efficiency of ambiguous vs. directly measured haplotype frequencies. *Genetic Epidemiology* 2002a; 23:426–443.

Schaid DJ. Genetic epidemiology and microarrays. *Genetic Epidemiology* 2002b; 23:1–96.

Schaid DJ, Olson JM, Gauderman WJ, et al. Regression models for linkage: issues of traits, covariates, heterogeneity, and interaction. *Human Heredity* 2003; 55:86–96.

Schaid DJ, Rowland C. Use of parents, sibs and unrelated controls for detection of associations between genetic markers and disease. *American Journal of Human Genetics* 1998; 63:1492–1506.

Schaid DJ, Rowland CM, Tines DE, et al. Score tests for association between traits and haplotypes when linkage phase is ambiguous. *American Journal of Human Genetics* 2002; 70:425–434.

Schaid DJ, Sommer SS. Genotype relative risks: methods for design and analysis of candidate-gene association studies. *American Journal of Human Genetics* 1993; 53:1114–1126.

Schaid DJ, Sommer SS. Comparison of statistics for candidate-gene association studies. *American Journal of Human Genetics* 1994; 55:402–409.

Schena M, Shalon D, Davis RW, et al. Quantitative monitoring of gene expression patterns with a complementary DNA microarray. *Science* 1995; 270:467–470.

Schildkraut JM, Thompson WD. Relationship of epithelial ovarian cancer to other malignancies within families. *Genetic Epidemiology* 1988; 5:355–367.

Schork NJ, Fallin D, Thiel B, et al. The future of genetic case-control studies. In: Rao DC and Province M (eds.), *Genetic Dissection of Complex Traits*. San Diego, CA: Academic Press, 2001: 191–212.

Schork NJ, Thiel B, St Jean P. Linkage analysis, kinship, and the short-term evolution of chromosomes. *Journal of Experimental Zoology* 1999; 282:133–149.

Schwartz A, Boehnke M, Moll P. Family risk index as a measure of familial hetero-geneity of cancer risk. *American Journal of Epidemiology* 1988; 128:524–535.

Schwartz A, Kaufman R, Moll P. Heterogeneity of breast cancer risk in families of young breast cancer patients and controls. *American Journal of Epidemiology* 1991; 134:1325–1334.

Schwartz G. Estimating the dimension of a model. *Annals of Statistics* 1978; 6:461–464.

Schwartz RS. Racial profiling in medical research. *New England Journal of Medicine* 2001; 344:1392–1393.

Segal NL. New breast cancer research: mothers and twins. *Twin Research* 2000; 3:118–119, 122.

Self SG, Liang K-Y. Asymptotic properties of maximum likelihood estimators and likelihood ratio tests under nonstandard conditions. *Journal of the American Statistical Association* 1987; 82:605–610.

Self SG, Longton G, Kopecky KJ, et al. On estimating HLA/disease association with application to a study of aplastic anemia. *Biometrics* 1991; 47:53–61.

Selinger-Leneman H, Genin E, Norris JM, et al. Does accounting for gene-environment (G × E) interaction increase the power to detect the effect of a gene in a multifactorial disease? *Genetic Epidemiology* 2003; 24:200–207.

Sellers T, Bailey-Wilson J, Elston R, et al. Evidence for mendelian inheritance in the pathogenesis of lung cancer. *Journal of the National Cancer Institute* 1990; 82:1272–1279.

Sellers TA, Yates JR. Review of proteomics with applications to genetic epidemiology. *Genetic Epidemiology* 2003; 24:83–98.

Seltman H, Roeder K, Devlin B. Transmission/disequilibrium test meets measured haplotype analysis: family-based association analysis guided by evolution of haplotypes. *American Journal of Human Genetics* 2001; 68:1250–1263.

Sengul H, Weeks DE, Feingold E. A survey of affected-sibship statistics for nonparametric linkage analysis. *American Journal of Human Genetics* 2001; 69:179–190.

Serova OM, Mazoyer S, Puget N, et al. Mutations in *BRCA1* and *BRCA2* in breast cancer families: are there more breast cancer-susceptibility genes? *American Journal of Human Genetics* 1997; 60:486–495.

Service S. Linkage-disequilibrium mapping of disease genes by reconstruction of ancestral haplotypes in founder populations. *American Journal of Human Genetics* 1999; 64:1728–1738.

Sham PC. Sequential analysis and case-control candidate gene association studies: reply to Sobell et al. [letter; comment]. *American Journal of Medical Genetics* 1994; 54:154–157.

Sham PC, Curtis D. Monte Carlo tests for associations between disease and alleles at highly polymorphic loci. *Annals of Human Genetics* 1995; 59:97–105.

Sham PC, Purcell S, Cherny SS, et al. Powerful regression-based quantitative-trait linkage analysis of general pedigrees. *American Journal of Human Genetics* 2002; 71:238–253.

Shattuck-Eidens D, McClure M, Simard J, et al. A collaborative survey of 80 mutations in the *BRCA1* breast and ovarian cancer susceptibility gene. *Journal of the American Medical Association* 1995; 273:535–541.

Sheehan N. On the application of Markov chain Monte Carlo methods to genetic analyses on complex pedigrees. *International Statistical Reviews* 2000; 68:83–110.

Sheehan N, Thomas A. On the irreducibility of a Markov chain defined on a space of genotype configurations by a sampling scheme. *Biometrics* 1993; 49:163–175.

Sherlock G. Analysis of large-scale gene expression data. *Briefings in Bioinformatics* 2001; 2:350–362.

Shih MC, Whittemore AS. Tests for genetic association using family data. *Genetic Epidemiology* 2002; 22:128–145.

Siegmund KD, Gauderman WJ. Association tests in nuclear families. *Human Heredity* 2001; 52:66–76.

Siegmund KD, Gauderman WJ, Thomas DC. Gene characterization using high risk families: a sensitivity of the MOD score approach [Abstract 2251]. *American Journal of Human Genetics* 1999a; 65:A398.

Siegmund KD, Laird PW. Analysis of complex methylation data. *Methods* 2002; 27:170–178.

Siegmund KD, Langholz B, Kraft P, et al. Testing linkage disequilibrium in sibships. *American Journal of Human Genetics* 2000; 67:244–248.

Siegmund KD, Morrison J, Gauderman WJ. Who should be genotyped for estimating gene main effects in family-based disease registries? [Abstract]. *Genetic Epidemiology* 2001; 21:176.

Siegmund KD, Whittemore AS, Thomas DC. Multistage sampling for disease family registries. *Monographs of the National Cancer Institute* 1999b; 26:43–48.

Siemiatycki J, Thomas DC. Biological models and statistical interactions: an example from multistage carcinogenesis. *International Journal of Epidemiology* 1981; 10:383–387.

Sillanpää MJ, Corander J. Model choice in gene mapping: what and why. *Trends in Genetics* 2002; 18:301–307.

Sillanpää MJ, Kilpikari R, Ripatti S, et al. Bayesian association mapping for quantitative traits in a mixture of two populations. *Genetic Epidemiology* 2001; 21 (Suppl 1):S692–S699.

Sinsheimer JS, Palmer CG, Woodward JA. Detecting genotype combinations that increase risk for disease: maternal-fetal genotype incompatibility test. *Genetic Epidemiology* 2003; 24:1–13.

Skolnick M, Bishop D, Carmelli D, et al. A population-based assessment of familial cancer risk in Utah Mormon genealogies. In: Frances E, Arrighi P, and Rao N (eds.), *Genes, Chromosomes, and Neoplasia*. New York: Raven Press, 1981: 477–500.

Slattery M, Kerber R. A comprehensive evaluation of family history and breast cancer risk: the Utah Population Database. *Journal of the American Medical Association* 1993; 270:1563–1568.

Slattery M, Kerber R. Family history of cancer and colon cancer risk: the Utah Population Database. *Journal of the National Cancer Institute* 1994; 86:1618–1626.

Smith C. Some comments on the statistical methods used in linkage investigations. *American Journal of Human Genetics* 1959; 11:289–304.

Smith C. Heritability of liability and concordance in monozygous twins. *Annals of Human Genetics* 1970; 34:85–91.

Smith KJ, Johnson KA, Bryan TM, et al. The *APC* gene product in normal and tumor cells. *Proceedings of the National Academy of Sciences of the United States of America* 1993; 90:2846–2850.

Smith MW, Lautenberger JA, Shin HD, et al. Markers for mapping by admixture linkage disequilibrium in African-American and Hispanic populations. *American Journal of Human Genetics* 2001; 69:1080–1094.

Sobell JL, Heston LL, Sommer SS. Novel association approach for determining the genetic predisposition to schizophrenia: case-control resource and testing of a candidate gene. *American Journal of Medical Genetics* 1993; 48:28–35.

Sorensen TI, Nielsen GG, Andersen PK, et al. Genetic and environmental influences on premature death in adult adoptees. *New England Journal of Medicine* 1988; 318:727–732.

Spielman RS, Baur MP, Clerget-Darpoux F. Genetic analysis of IDDM: summary of GAW5-IDDM results. *Genetic Epidemiology* 1989; 6:43–58.

Spielman RS, Ewens WJ. The TDT and other family-based tests for linkage disequilibrium and association. *American Journal of Human Genetics* 1996; 59:983–989.

Spielman RS, McGinnis RE, Ewens WJ. Transmission test for linkage disequilibrium: the insulin gene region and insulin-dependent diabetes mellitus (IDDM). *American Journal of Human Genetics* 1993; 52:506–516.

Steinberg KK, Thacker SB, Smith SJ, et al. A meta-analysis of the effect of estrogen replacement therapy on the risk of breast cancer. *Journal of the American Medical Association* 1991; 265:1985–1990.

Stephens J, Briscoe D, O'Brien S. Mapping by admixture linkage disequilibrium in human populations: limits and guidelines. *American Journal of Human Genetics* 1994; 55:809–824.

Stephens J, Schneider J, Tanguay D, et al. Haplotype variation and linkage disequilibrium in 313 human genes. *Science* 2001a; 293:489–493.

Stephens M, Smith NJ, Donnelly P. A new statistical method for haplotype reconstruction from population data. *American Journal of Human Genetics* 2001b; 68:978–989.

Stierum R, Burgemeister R, van Helvoort A, et al. Functional food ingredients against colorectal cancer. An example project integrating functional genomics, nutrition and health. *Nutrition, Metabolism, and Cardiovascular Disease* 2001; 11:94–98.

Storey JD, Tibshirani R. Statistical significance for genomewide studies. *Proceedings of the National Academy of Science of the United States of America* 2003; 100:9440–9445.

Strachan P, Read AP. *Human Molecular Genetics* (2nd ed.). New York: Wiley-Liss, 1999.

Stram DO, Haiman CA, Hirschhorn JN, et al. Choosing haplotype-tagging SNPs based on unphased genotype data from a preliminary sample of unrelated subjects: the Multiethnic Cohort Study. *Human Heredity* 2003a; 55:27–36.

Stram DO, Pearce L, Bretsky P, et al. Modeling and E-M estimation of haplotype-specific relative risks from genotype data for a case-control study of unrelated individuals. *Human Heredity* 2003b; 55:179–190.

Strand M, Prolla TA, Liskay RM, et al. Destabilization of tracts of simple repetitive DNA in yeast by mutations affecting DNA mismatch repair. *Nature* 1993; 365:274–276.

Strauch K, Fimmers R, Kurz T, et al. Parametric and nonparametric multipoint linkage analysis with imprinting and two-locus-trait models: application to mite sensitization. *American Journal of Human Genetics* 2000; 66:1945–1957.

Struewing J, Hartge P, Wacholder S, et al. The risk of cancer associated with specific mutations of *BRCA1* and *BRCA2* among Ashkenazi Jews. *New England Journal of Medicine* 1997; 336:1401–1408.

Stumpf MP, Goldstein DB. Demography, recombination hotspot intensity, and the block structure of linkage disequilibrium. *Current Biology* 2003; 13:1–8.

Sun FZ, Flanders WD, Yang QH, et al. Transmission/disequilibrium tests for quantitative traits. *Annals of Human Genetics* 2000; 64:555–565.

Swift M. Ionizing radiation, breast cancer, and ataxia-telangiectasia. *Journal of the National Cancer Institute* 1994; 86:1571–1572.

Swift M, Chase C, Morrell D. Incidence of cancer in 161 families affected by ataxia-telangiectasia. *New England Journal of Medicine* 1991; 325:1831–1836.

Szatkiewicz JP, T.Cuenco K, Feingold E. Recent advances in human quantitative-trait-locus mapping: comparison of methods for discordant sibling pairs. *American Journal of Human Genetics* 2003; 73:874–885.

T.Cuenco K, Szatkiewicz JP, Feingold E. Recent advances in human quantitative-trait-locus mapping: comparison of methods for selected sibling pairs. *American Journal of Human Genetics* 2003; 73:863–873.

Tabor HK, Risch NJ, Myers RM. Candidate-gene approaches for studying complex genetic traits: practical considerations. *Nature Reviews Genetics* 2002; 3:391–397.

Taillon-Miller P, Bauer-Sardinna I, Saccone N, et al. Juxtaposed regions of extensive and minimal linkage disequilibrium in human X125 and Xq28. *Nature Genetics* 2000; 25:324–328.

Tamayo P, Slonim D, Mesirov J, et al. Interpreting patterns of gene expression with self-organizing maps: methods and application to hematopoietic differentiation. *Proceedings of the National Academy of Sciences of the United States of America* 1999; 96:2907–2912.

Tang H-K, Siegmund D. Mapping quantitative trait loci in oligogenic models. *Biostatistics* 2001; 2:147–162.

Te Meerman G, Van Der Meulen M. Genomic sharing surrounding alleles identical by descent effects of genetic drift and population growth. *Genetic Epidemiology* 1997; 14:1125–1130.

Terwilliger JD. A powerful likelihood method for the analysis of linkage disequilibrium between trait loci and one or more polymorphic marker loci. *American Journal of Human Genetics* 1995; 60:777–787.

Terwilliger JD, Ott J. A haplotype based haplotype relative risk approach to detecting allelic associations. *Human Heredity* 1992; 42:337–346.

Terwilliger JD, Ott J. *Handbook of Human Genetic Linkage*. Baltimore: Johns Hopkins University Press, 1994.

Terwilliger JD, Weiss KM. Linkage disequilibrium mapping of complex disease: fantasy or reality? *Current Opinion in Biotechnology* 1998; 9:578–594.

Thibodeau SN, Bren G, Schaid D. Microsatellite instability in cancer of the proximal colon. *Science* 1993; 260:816–819.

Thibodeau SN, French AJ, Cunningham JM, et al. Microsatellite instability in colorectal cancer: different mutator phenotypes and the principal involvement
of *hMLH1*. *Cancer Research* 1998; 58:1713–1718.

Thomas D. Genetic epidemiology with a capital "E." *Genetic Epidemiology* 2000a;
19:289–3000.

Thomas DB, Karagas MR. Migrant studies. In: Schottenfeld D and Fraumeni JFJ
(eds.), *Cancer Epidemiology and Prevention* (2nd ed.). Oxford: Oxford University Press, 1996: 236–254.

Thomas DC. Re: "Case-parents design for gene-environment interaction" by
Schaid. *Genetic Epidemiology* 2000b; 19:461–463.

Thomas DC, Cortessis V. A Gibbs sampling approach to linkage analysis. *Human
Heredity* 1992; 42:63–76.

Thomas DC, Gauderman WJ. Gibbs sampling methods in genetics. In: Gilks WR,
Richardson S, and Spiegelhalter DJ (eds.), *Markov Chain Monte Carlo in
Practice*. London: Chapman and Hall, 1996; 1:419–440.

Thomas DC, Langholz B, Mack W, et al. Bivariate survival models for analysis
of genetic and environmental effects in twins. *Genetic Epidemiology* 1990;
7:121–135.

Thomas DC, Morrison J, Clayton DS. Bayes estimates of haplotype effects. *Genetic
Epidemiology* 2001; 21:S712–S717.

Thomas DC, Qian D, Gauderman WJ, et al. A generalized estimating equations
approach to linkage analysis in sibships in relation to multiple markers and
exposure factors. *Genetic Epidemiology* 1999; 17:S737–S742.

Thomas DC, Stram DO, Conti D, et al. Bayesian spatial modeling of haplotype
associations. *Human Heredity* 2003, in press.

Thomas DC, Witte JS. Point: population stratification: a problem for case-control
studies of candidate gene associations? *Cancer Epidemiology, Biomarkers and
Prevention* 2002; 11:505–512.

Thompson D, Easton D, Breast Cancer Linkage Consortium. Variation in cancer
risks, by mutation position, in *BRCA2* mutation carriers. *American Journal of
Human Genetics* 2001; 68:410–419.

Thompson D, Easton DF, Goldgar DE. A full-likelihood method for the evaluation
of causality of sequence variants from family data. *American Journal of Human
Genetics* 2003; 73:652–655.

Thompson D, Stram DO, Goldgar D, et al. Haplotype tagging single nucleotide
polymorphisms and association studies. *Human Heredity* 2003, in press.

Thompson D, Szabo CI, Mangion J, et al. Evaluation of linkage of breast cancer
to the putative *BRCA3* locus on chromosome 13q21 in 128 multiple case
families from the Breast Cancer Linkage Consortium. *Proceedings of the
National Academy of Sciences of the United States of America* 2002;
99:827–831.

Thompson EA. *Pedigree Analysis in Human Genetics*. Baltimore: Johns Hopkins
University Press, 1986.

Thompson EA, Guo SW. Evaluation of likelihood ratios for complex genetic models. *IMA Journal of Mathematical Applications in Medicine and Biology* 1991;
8:149–169.

Thompson EA, Heath S. Estimation of conditional multilocus gene identity among
relatives. In: Seillier-Niuseuwutsch F (ed.), *Statistics in Molecular Biology and
Genetics*. New York: Institute of Mathematical Statistics, American Mathematical Society, 1999: 95–113.

Thomson G. A review of theoretical aspects of HLA and disease associations. *Theoretical Population Biology* 1981; 20:168–208.

Thorlacius S, Struewing JP, Hartge P, et al. Population-based study of risk of breast cancer in carriers of *BRCA2* mutation [see comments]. *Lancet* 1998; 352:1337–1339.

Tishkoff SA, Verrelli BC. Patterns of human genetic diversity: Implications for human evolutionary history and disease. *Annual Review of Genomics and Human Genetics* 2003; 4:293–340.

Toyota M, Ahuja N, Ohe-Toyota M, et al. CpG island methylator phenotype in colorectal cancer. *Proceedings of the National Academy of Sciences of the United States of America* 1999; 96:8681–8686.

Trucco M, Dorman JS. Immunogenetics of insulin-dependent diabetes mellitus in humans. *Critical Reviews in Immunology* 1989; 9:201–245.

Tsao J, Yatabe Y, Salovaara R, et al. Genetic reconstruction of individual colorectal tumor histories. *Proceedings of the National Academy of Sciences of the United States of America* 2000; 97:1236–1241.

Tu IP, Balise RR, Whittemore AS. Detection of disease genes by use of family data. II. Application to nuclear families. *American Journal of Human Genetics* 2000; 66:1341–1350.

Tzeng J-Y, Devlin B, Wasserman L, et al. On the identification of disease mutations by the analysis of haplotype similarity and goodness of fit. *American Journal of Human Genetics* 2003; 72:891–902.

Umbach DM, Weinberg CR. The use of case-parent triads to study joint effects of genotype and exposure. *American Journal of Human Genetics* 2000; 66:251–261.

Ursin G, Henderson B, Haile R, et al. Is oral contraceptive use more common in women with *BRCA1/BRCA2* mutations than in other women with breast cancer? *Cancer Research* 1997; 57:3678–3681.

Van Der Meulen M, Meerman G. Haplotype sharing analysis in affected individuals from nuclear families with at least one affected offspring. *Genetic Epidemiology* 1997; 14:915–919.

Vasen HF, Mecklin JP, Khan PM, et al. The International Collaborative Group on Hereditary Non-Polyposis Colorectal Cancer (ICG-HNPCC). *Diseases of the Colon and Rectum* 1991; 34:424–425.

Vasen HF, Nagengast FM, Khan PM. Interval cancers in hereditary non-polyposis colorectal cancer (Lynch syndrome). *Lancet* 1995; 345:1183–1184.

Vasen HF, Wijnen JT, Menko FH, et al. Cancer risk in families with hereditary non-polyposis colorectal cancer diagnosed by mutation analysis. *Gastroenterology* 1996; 110:1020–1027.

Veale AM. *Intestinal Polyposis*. Cambridge: Cambridge University Press, 1965.

Velculescu VE, Zhang L, Vogelstein B, et al. Serial analysis of gene expression. *Science* 1995; 270:484–487.

Verkasalo PK, Kaprio J, Pukkala E, et al. Breast cancer risk in monozygotic and dizygotic female twins: a 20-year population-based cohort study in Finland from 1976 to 1995. *Cancer Epidemiology, Biomarkers and Prevention* 1999; 8:271–274.

Veronesi U, Maisonneuve P, Costa A, et al. Prevention of breast cancer with tamoxifen: preliminary findings from the Italian randomised trial among hysterectomised women. Italian Tamoxifen Prevention Study. *Lancet* 1998; 352:93–97.

Vieland VJ, Hodge SE. Inherent intractability of the ascertainment problem for pedigree data: a general likelihood framework. *American Journal of Human Genetics* 1995; 56:33–43.

Vieland VJ, Hodge SE. The problem of ascertainment for linkage analysis. *American Journal of Human Genetics* 1996; 58:1072–1084.

Vieland VJ, Logue M. HLODs, trait models, and ascertainment: implications of admixture for parameter estimation and linkage detection. *Human Heredity* 2002; 53:23–35.

Virmani AK, Tsou JA, Siegmund KD, et al. Hierarchical clustering of lung cancer cell lines using DNA methylation markers. *Cancer Epidemiology, Biomarkers and Prevention* 2002; 11:291–297.

Vogel F, Motulsky AG. *Human Genetics: Problems and Approaches* (2nd ed.). Berlin: Springer-Verlag, 1986.

Vogelstein B, Fearon ER, Hamilton SR, et al. Genetic alterations during colorectal-tumor development. *New England Journal of Medicine* 1988; 319:525–532.

Waagepeterson R, Sorensen D. A tutorial on reversible jump MCMC with a view toward applications in QTL-mapping. *International Statistical Review* 2001; 69:49–62.

Wacholder S, Chanock S, Garcia-Closas M, et al. Assessing the probability of false positive reports in association studies. *Journal of the National Cancer Institute* 2003, in press.

Wacholder S, Hartge P, Struewing J, et al. The kin cohort study for estimating penetrance. *American Journal of Epidemiology* 1998; 148:623–630.

Wacholder S, Rothman N, Caporaso N. Population stratification in epidemiologic studies of common genetic variants and cancer: quantification of bias. *Journal of the National Cancer Institute* 2000; 92:1151–1158.

Wacholder S, Rothman N, Caporaso N. Counterpoint: bias from population stratification is not a major threat to the validity of conclusions from epidemiologic studies of common polymorphisms and cancer. *Cancer Epidemiology, Biomarkers and Prevention* 2002; 11:513–520.

Wakefield J. The Bayesian analysis of population pharmacokinetic models. *Journal of the American Statistical Association* 1996; 91:1400–1412.

Wall JD, Pritchard JK. Haplotype blocks and linkage disequilibrium in the human genome. *Nature Reviews Genetics* 2003a; 4:587–597.

Wall JD, Pritchard JK. Assessing the performance of the haplotype block model of linkage disequilibrium. *American Journal of Human Genetics* 2003b; 73:502–515.

Wang N, Akey JM, Zhang K, et al. Distribution of recombination crossovers and the origin of haplotype blocks: the interplay of population history, recombination, and mutation. *American Journal of Human Genetics* 2002; 71:1227–1234.

Warthin AS. Heredity with respect to carcinoma. *Archives of Internal Medicine* 1913; 12:546.

Watts JA, Morley M, Busdick JT, et al. Gene expression phenotype in heterozygous carriers of Ataxia telangiectasia. *American Journal of Human Genetics* 2002; 71:791–800.

Weale ME, Depondt C, Macdonald SJ, et al. Selection and evaluation of tagging SNPs in the neuronal-sodium-chanel gene *SCN1A:* implications for linkage-disequilibrium gene mapping. *American Journal of Human Genetics* 2003; 73:551–565.

Weber TK, Conlon W, Petrelli NJ, et al. Genomic DNA-based *hMSH2* and *hMLH1* mutation screening in 32 Eastern United States hereditary nonpolyposis colorectal cancer pedigrees. *Cancer Research* 1997; 57:3798–3803.

Weeks DE, Lange K. The affected-pedigree-member method of linkage analysis. *American Journal of Human Genetics* 1988; 42:315–326.

Weinberg CR. Methods for detection of parent-of-origin effects in genetic studies of case-parents triads. *American Journal of Human Genetics* 1999; 65:229–235.

Weinberg CR, Umbach DM. Choosing a retrospective design to assess joint genetic and environmental contributions to risk. *American Journal of Epidemiology* 2000; 152:197–203.

Weinberg CR, Wilcox AJ, Lie RT. A log-linear approach to case-parent-triad data: assessing effects of disease genes that act either directly or through maternal effects and that may be subject to parental imprinting. *American Journal of Human Genetics* 1998; 62:969–978.

Wender PH, Rosenthal D, Kety SS, et al. Crossfostering. A research strategy for clarifying the role of genetic and experiential factors in the etiology of schizophrenia. *Archives of General Psychiatry* 1974; 30:121–128.

White J. A two stage design for the study of the relationship between a rare exposure and a rare disease. *American Journal of Epidemiology* 1982; 1982:119–128.

Whiteman DC, Murphy MF, Verkasalo PK, et al. Breast cancer risk in male twins: joint analyses of four twin cohorts in Denmark, Finland, Sweden and the United States. *British Journal of Cancer* 2000; 83:1231–1233.

Whittaker JC, Denham MC, Morris AP. The problems of using the transmission/disequilibrium test to infer tight linkage. *American Journal of Human Genetics* 2000; 67:523–526.

Whittemore AS. Genome scanning for linkage: an overview. *American Journal of Human Genetics* 1996; 59:704–716.

Whittemore AS, Halpern J. A class of tests for linkage using affected pedigree members. *Biometrics* 1994; 50:118–127.

Whittemore AS, Halpern J. Multi-stage sampling in genetic epidemiology. *Statistics in Medicine* 1997; 16:153–167.

Whittemore AS, Tu IP. Detection of disease genes by use of family data. I. Likelihood-based theory. *American Journal of Human Genetics* 2000; 66:1328–1340.

Wiesner GL, Daley D, Lewis S, et al. A subset of familial colorectal neoplasia kindreds linked to chromosome 9q22.2-31.2. *Proceedings of the National Academy of Sciences of the United States of America* 2003; 17:17.

Wijnen JT, Vasen HF, Khan PM, et al. Clinical findings with implications for genetic testing in families with clustering of colorectal cancer. *New England Journal of Medicine* 1998; 339:511–518.

Wilcox AJ, Weinberg CR, Lie RT. Distinguishing the effects of maternal and offspring genes through studies of "case-parent triads." *American Journal of Epidemiology* 1998; 148:893–901.

Williams RC, Long JC, Hanson RL, et al. Individual estimates of European genetic admixture associated with lower body-mass index, plasma glucose, and prevalence of type 2 diabetes in Pima Indians. *American Journal of Human Genetics* 2000; 66:527–538.

Williamson J, Amos I. On the asymptotic behavior of the estimate of the recombination fraction under the null hypothesis of no linkage when the model is misspecified. *Genetic Epidemiology* 1990; 7:309–318.